ROCKVILLE PUBLIC LIBRARY

3 4035 13164 6776

W9-BKG-535

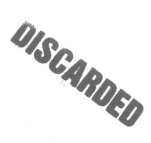

LIVING WITH RHEUMATOID ARTHRITIS

DISCARDED

A Johns Hopkins Press Health Book

ROCKVILLE PUBLIC LIBRARY
P. O. Box 1320 / 52 Union St.
Vernon, CT 06066

Living
with
Rheumatoid
Arthritis

3rd edition

TAMMI L. SHLOTZHAUER, M.D.

Johns Hopkins University Press
Baltimore

Note to the reader. This book is not meant to substitute for medical care of people with rheumatoid arthritis, and treatment should not be based solely on its contents. Instead, treatment must be developed in a dialogue between the individual and his or her physician. Our book has been written to help with that dialogue.

Drug dosage. The author and publisher have exerted every effort to ensure that the selection and dosage of drugs discussed in this text accord with current recommendations and practice at the time of publication. However, in view of ongoing research, changes in governmental regulations, and the constant flow of information relating to drug therapy and drug reactions, the reader is urged to check the package insert of each drug for any change in indications and dosage and for warnings and precautions. This is particularly important when the recommended agent is a new and/or infrequently used drug.

© 1993, 2003, 2014 Johns Hopkins University Press
All rights reserved. Published 2014
Printed in the United States of America on acid-free paper
9 8 7 6 5 4 3 2 1

Illustrations by Jacqueline Schaffer, except Figures 1 and 2. Figures 1 and 2 by Teresa Vaitkus.

Johns Hopkins University Press
2715 North Charles Street
Baltimore, Maryland 21218-4363
www.press.jhu.edu

Library of Congress Cataloging-in-Publication Data

Shlotzhauer, Tammi L.
    Living with rheumatoid arthritis / Tammi L. Shlotzhauer, M.D. — Third edition.
        pages cm
    Includes bibliographical references and index.
    ISBN 978-1-4214-1426-3 (hardcover : alk. paper) — ISBN 1-4214-1426-0
(hardcover : alk. paper) — ISBN 978-1-4214-1427-0 (pbk. : alk. paper) —
ISBN 1-4214-1427-9 (pbk. : alk. paper) — ISBN 978-1-4214-1428-7 (electronic) —
ISBN 1-4214-1428-7 (electronic) 1. Rheumatoid arthritis—Popular works. I. Title.
    RC933.S445 2014
    616.7'227—dc23
                                                                            2013043619

A catalog record for this book is available from the British Library.

Special discounts are available for bulk purchases of this book. For more information, please contact Special Sales at 410-516-6936 or specialsales@press.jhu.edu.

Johns Hopkins University Press uses environmentally friendly book materials, including recycled text paper that is composed of at least 30 percent post-consumer waste, whenever possible.

*The first edition was dedicated
with love and appreciation to our parents,
Richard and Carole Shlotzhauer,
Jean and Mickey McGuire*

*

*The second edition was dedicated to the late
Dr. James McGuire, friend and mentor*

*

The third edition is dedicated to Gwen

Contents

Chapter 15. Corticosteroids

Chapter 16. Osteoporosis Treatments

PART V. BEYOND MEDICATIONS: OTHER TREATMENTS

Chapter 17. Alternative and Complementary Therapies   283

PART VI. PRACTICAL MATTERS

Closing Thoughts   368

Preface

If you or someone close to you has rheumatoid arthritis, you probably have many questions about what that diagnosis means. This book is an attempt to answer those questions. *Living with Rheumatoid Arthritis* describes all aspects of this condition, from the physical and the emotional to the practical. I hope the book will help you not only to understand rheumatoid arthritis but also to deal constructively with the changes it may bring in your life.

This book will also let you know that you are not alone. It has been estimated that two to three million Americans have rheumatoid arthritis, and about 200,000 people are newly diagnosed each year. Worldwide, about 1 percent of the population has this condition, which affects people of all races and ethnic groups. People of all ages can develop rheumatoid arthritis, although it most commonly first affects people in their twenties, thirties, and forties. Three times more women than men have the condition.

Most people with rheumatoid arthritis lead highly productive, full, and satisfying lives. More than anything else, I hope that this book will provide you with the information that you need to lead as productive a life as possible.

This book is not intended to take the place of your physician. I hope, though, that it will help you to formulate questions about your own health which you can then discuss with your doctor.

People have many different ways of coping with the knowledge that they have a chronic illness. Some people, for example, cope by denying that they have an illness; others put blind faith in their physicians and don't ask any questions or make any decisions. Others go from doctor to doctor trying anything for a cure—whether it's a proven, prescribed treatment or unconventional therapies. Some people cope by giving up and letting the illness control them: they don't follow their physician's or therapist's advice because they think that nothing will help.

Studies have shown, however, that the people who cope best with a chronic illness are those who have an understanding of the disease process. This means that they learn everything they can about the illness so that they can take an active role in monitoring and caring for their own health.

What should you do when you learn that you have rheumatoid arthritis? First of all, educating yourself about rheumatoid arthritis and developing realistic expectations will help you overcome your fears and decrease your anxiety.

We know that fear of the unknown creates great anxiety, just as uncertainty creates stress. This is because, more often than not, our imaginations create scenarios that are much worse than the reality could ever be. The *truth*, therefore, can often be reassuring.

Second, once you understand rheumatoid arthritis, you will be able to communicate more effectively with health care professionals; the time you spend with your physician, nurse, or therapist will be more helpful to both of you. You know your body better than anyone else, and you can become an expert on *your* arthritis. Then you can work closely with your health care providers in developing a therapeutic program that is tailor-made for you and that addresses your specific needs.

Finally, what you know about your rheumatoid arthritis will help you cope more effectively with the challenges it poses. For example, you will better understand the value of medication, exercise, joint protection, diet, and other treatments. Understanding the rationale behind each of the components of your treatment program may make you a more active participant in that program.

You can't read away your arthritis, of course, but you can play an important part in making decisions if you understand it. For all the reasons mentioned above, please read on and take a major role in mastering your arthritis.

The first part of this book discusses the physical aspects of rheumatoid arthritis, including changes in the joints and other parts of the body. Part II describes techniques for coping with the challenges that rheumatoid arthritis poses, and Part III introduces a series of exercises that have proven beneficial for people with this condition. In Part IV, all aspects of drug therapy are discussed. Part V addresses other important forms of treatment including complementary therapies, nutrition, and surgery. Advice about practical matters from insurance to traveling is offered in Part VI. At the end of many chapters you'll find information about additional resources, including organizations and readings. At the back of the book there is a glossary of terms used in this book. Words that are defined in the glossary are set in **boldface** type at their first use in each chapter. Other important terms in the text are in *italic* type at first use in the book.

Acknowledgments

Many individuals participated in the previous editions of this book, and I remain indebted to each of them. With deepest gratitude, I acknowledge my previous co-author, the late Dr. James McGuire, who made *Living with Rheumatoid Arthritis* possible. I also recognize my aunt, Judith Nash, who painstakingly edited our first edition, enhancing content, style, and comprehensibility for our nonmedical readers. The spirit of her editing has persisted throughout the second and third editions. I am grateful to many medical professionals who have taught me along the way, but in particular to William Lages, Molly Fainstat, Thomas Bush, James McGuire, Elaine Lambert, and John Baum for the inspiration of their example and their teaching.

For the current edition I would like to thank my sister Sandy, a certified pedorthist, for her astute contributions to the rheumatoid foot care section. I would like to thank my mother, Carole, for reading the draft of this text and giving reinforcing feedback. I especially want to acknowledge my dearest friend and life-partner Gwen for her participation in this project. She has steadfastly listened with interest at the dinner table to my new insights and ideas about living better with RA. She has worked around my stacks of research papers, given up our shared time, and supported me throughout this endeavor. Most importantly, she has imparted to me a valued awareness of the sense of vulnerability, helplessness, and fear that people with chronic illness can sometimes suffer. Her support and understanding have made this venture possible.

I am grateful to the professional staff at Johns Hopkins University Press including Jacqueline Wehmueller for her continued guidance and support, Anne Whitmore for her meticulous and thoughtful copyediting, and to all the others who have contributed to the successful production of this edition. I would also like to thank Jacqueline Schaffer for her lovely medical illustrations that truly complement the text and enhance the understanding of complex medical descriptions.

I continue to be humbled by the many individuals with RA whom I have cared for since I first went into practice in 1991. In them I have witnessed the resilience of the human spirit. They remain my greatest teachers.

LIVING WITH RHEUMATOID ARTHRITIS

Introduction:
Defining Rheumatoid Arthritis

To most people arthritis means pain and stiffness in the joints. Indeed, if you trace the word *arthritis* to its Greek roots you will discover that it means inflammation (*itis*) of the joints (*arthron*). In practice the word is used to describe more than one hundred different joint disorders, many of which are not caused by inflammation at all.

There are several forms of arthritis which *do* begin as significant inflammation in the joints, and this inflammation causes damage to the joints. Rheumatoid arthritis (RA) is a form of **inflammatory arthritis.** With RA, inflammation plays a major role in causing joint problems. This inflammation can bring about warmth and swelling in the joints in addition to significant stiffness and pain.

It is believed that the inflammation of RA causes other problems, too. People with RA often have such symptoms as fatigue, low-grade fever, decreased appetite, depression, and muscle aches, along with pain and swelling in their joints. In fact, many people with RA say that they just don't feel well. These people are describing **malaise,** a vague feeling of illness. This overall feeling of illness is common with RA because the condition is **systemic,** meaning that it can affect more than one part of the body. RA is also a **chronic** illness, because it can last for months or years.

Which joints are involved in RA varies from one person to another. For example, some people have painful joints only in their hands, whereas others may experience pain in their knees or feet. One of the distinguishing characteristics of RA, however, is the particular pattern of specific joints that can potentially become affected. Those most commonly involved are finger joints, wrists, elbows, shoulders, some joints in the neck, jaw, hips, knees, ankles, and foot and toe joints (see Figure 1). RA most often affects the body symmetrically, meaning that the arthritis on one side of the body matches that on the other.

1

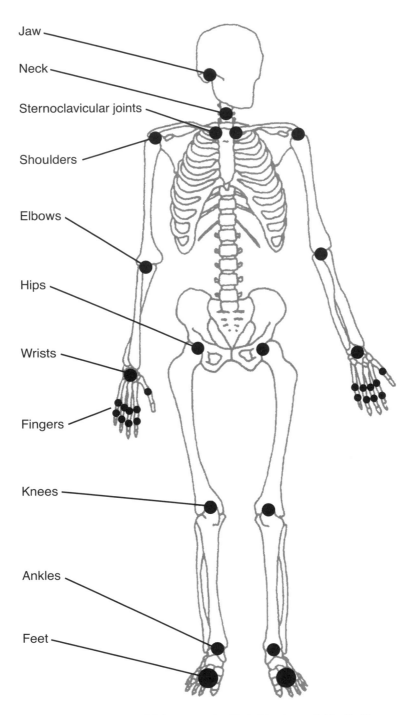

FIGURE 1. Joints commonly affected by rheumatoid arthritis

Jaw

Neck

Sternoclavicular joints

Shoulders

Elbows

Hips

Wrists

Fingers

Knees

Ankles

Feet

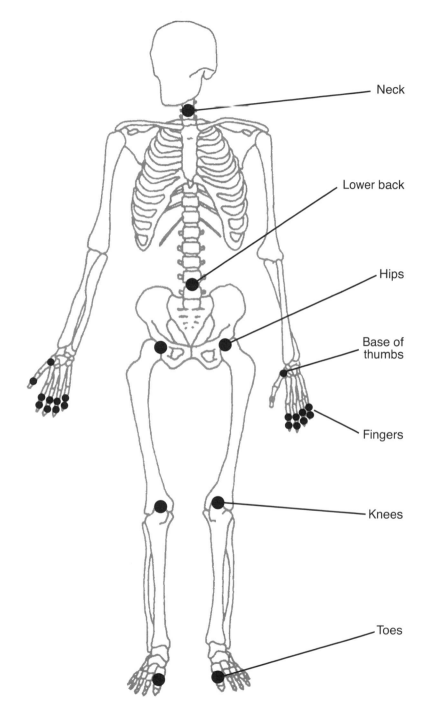

FIGURE 2. Joints commonly affected by osteoarthritis

One condition that is often confused with rheumatoid arthritis, by patients and physicians, is **osteoarthritis** (OA), also called *degenerative joint disease* (DJD). OA is quite different from RA. For one thing, OA is much more common, affecting an estimated 27 million people in the United States alone. In fact, nearly all of us will develop OA to some degree as we get older. The distribution pattern of joints affected by OA is different from that of RA, as you can see by comparing Figures 1 and 2, but some joints can be affected in both conditions. This is one of the causes of diagnostic confusion between these two forms of arthritis. Furthermore, some people have both OA and RA.

What causes rheumatoid arthritis? Researchers, physicians, historians, epidemiologists, theologians, and complementary practitioners have devoted an enormous amount of time and energy to trying to answer this question. We know that RA is not, for the most part, an ancient disease. It wasn't until 1800 that a French medical student, Augustin-Jacob Landre-Beauvais, in his doctoral thesis, conveyed the first medical reports describing RA. This was just after the start of the Industrial Revolution. Fifty years later, Sir Archibald Garrod coined the term *rheumatoid arthritis*. RA emerged during a period that was marked by an increase in pollution, dietary changes, and lifestyle transformations, and that raises the question of an environmental source triggering RA.

We have understood for some time that genetics plays a role in the development of RA. However, we also know that genes alone do not tell the whole story. Chapter 1 describes how genetic susceptibility to RA can be inherited but not necessarily result in the development of RA. This would, again, suggest that specific environmental factors might trigger the development of RA in individuals with a susceptible genetic code. And, we know that not everyone is exposed to the same set of environmental factors.

It has long been suspected that a virus, a bacterium, or another unknown microbe triggers the development of RA in people made susceptible by their genetic makeup. In 1912, Frank Billings proposed that RA was a response to chronic infection. Over the past century, scientists have searched for a link between hundreds of different infections and the development of RA. In the late 1920s tuberculosis was the suspected culprit. Other bacterial suspects along the way have included *Streptococcus* and *Mycoplasma*. In the late twentieth century, medical research focused heavily on viruses, such as Epstein-Barr virus, rubella, and parvovirus. Historically, we have focused on *external* pathogens (germs) in our search for the elusive microbe that prompts the development of RA. In the twenty-first century, we have introduced the notion that our own internal bacteria may be potential triggers for RA! You will read in Chapter 1 about how pathologic (bad) bacteria in our mouths and digestive tracts may be triggering an abnormal response in the **immune system** that contributes to the development of RA. In Chapter 18 you will read how our modern diet influences these bacteria.

People are often concerned about whether someone can "catch" RA from another person. In 1950, two investigators *tried* to transmit RA to volunteers, by injecting into their joints fluid taken from the joints of people with RA (Levinski and Lansbury, 1951). Thankfully, no volunteers developed RA. This was early evidence that RA did not appear to be a persistent *infection* of the joints. Currently, scientists are using sophisticated techniques to look for "footprints" of past and present microbes that we carry with us. Whether or not evidence of previous infection is found, we are quite convinced that RA is *not contagious*.

Scientists are looking at other, *nonmicrobial* environmental factors that contribute to the risk of developing RA. In the past 20 years, clear and convincing medical studies have suggested that smoking not only can increase the risk of developing RA but can contribute to its severity. Exposure to pollutants and chemicals has been implicated in some studies. You will read that even stress contributes to inflammation and increased symptoms of RA. The rise in obesity in recent years has also correlated with an increased risk for developing RA. Despite the presence of these factors, leading up to 1995, there was a four-decade decrease in the incidence of RA (Myasoedova et al., 2010). However, since that time, there has been a steady rise in the prevalence of RA in the United States that coincides with the epidemic increase in the prevalence of obesity here (Crowson et al., 2013). In the chapter on nutrition, you will read more about this as well as the ever-growing evidence that diet may be playing a role in the development of RA.

We are getting ever closer to more certain identification of several potential triggers for RA—microbial and nonmicrobial. In all likelihood, many of these triggers or exposures will be beyond our control. It is hoped, however, that at least some potential triggers may be preventable or remediable with lifestyle and diet modifications, which we will discuss throughout the book.

Perhaps the most groundbreaking of all research is our growing understanding in the field of **epigenetics,** where genetics and the environment meet. Although we are born with a given genetic heritage, the environment can have a direct role on which inherited genes are "expressed." In other words, we are not as captive to our genes as we once thought. Evidence is mounting that environmental factors, including diet, stress, lifestyle choices, weight, and even your thoughts, can alter how our DNA expresses itself! If this is true, we can intervene earlier in the course of RA with treatment and measures to prevent permanent damage. We will likely discover that there are several different conditions included in what we now call rheumatoid arthritis. New research on biomarkers in RA will open the door for "personalized medicine," allowing us to treat each person in an individualized way based on their own biological characteristics. In the meantime, healthy lifestyle choices, combined with cutting-edge medications, will improve the quality of life immensely for people with RA. With the advent of the **biologics,** we have already made astounding gains in reducing disability, hospitalizations, and surgeries in people with RA. Unraveling the complex series of events that causes the condition will give us new and exciting opportunities to treat, and one day cure, rheumatoid arthritis.

LEARNING ABOUT RHEUMATOID ARTHRITIS

The Joints and Rheumatoid Arthritis

The human body has more than one hundred joints. In the adult body many of these joints move very little or not at all, and we are mostly unaware of them. In this chapter we will describe the anatomy and function of the joints, before turning to a discussion of the joint in rheumatoid arthritis (RA).

THE JOINTS

The joints may be divided into three basic types according to the amount of motion each permits: rigid, slightly mobile, and freely movable. The different types of joints work in different ways to achieve different functions.

Rigid Joints

The joints that separate the bones in the skull and pelvis are examples of rigid, or fixed, joints. These joints are movable only during infancy, to allow for growth, or in special circumstances, such as pregnancy, to accommodate delivery. RA does not affect these joints.

Slightly Mobile Joints

Some joints, such as those between the vertebrae in the spine, normally move only slightly. The vertebrae (back and neck bones) are separated by a cushion of **cartilage** called a *disk*. In fact, when these joints move more than a very little bit, problems can arise. A "slipped disk," for example, occurs when the slightly mobile disk moves farther than it should. These joints are not affected in RA.

Freely Movable Joints

Freely movable joints, known as **synovial joints** or *disarthrodial joints*, are the kinds of joints most people think of when asked to name a joint. The shoulders, elbows, wrists, finger and toe joints, hips, knees, and ankles are all freely movable joints. Synovial joints can be affected by RA.

There are great differences among the various synovial joints in terms of structure and function. For instance, the knee and elbow joints permit motion primarily in one direction, because the contours of the bones on either side of these joints fit together like a hinge. The hip and shoulder joints, however, allow movement in many directions. To accommodate this wide range of motion, these are ball and socket joints.

Although different synovial joints function in different ways, all of them are composed of the same parts.

What Are the Parts of a Synovial Joint?

Synovial joints are composed of supportive structures, including the cartilage, tendon, ligament, and muscle, made up of various kinds of **tissue.** Each type of tissue in turn is made up of specialized **cells,** which give it one or more specific properties that allow the joint to function normally. The properties of the tissue in the different structures that contribute to proper joint function include resilience, elasticity, compressibility, and strength. (The major parts of a synovial joint are illustrated in Figure 3.)

The joint **capsule** is a fibrous wrapping that encloses the structures within the joint. Fibrous tissue is made up of slender, threadlike structures. This resilient tissue is similar to the "gristle" in a tough steak.

The synovial membrane, or **synovium,** is the lining inside the joint capsule. This smooth, fine membrane is normally composed of a thin layer of cells. It has a rich blood supply that allows nutrients to be delivered to the inside of the joints. The synovium and its cells produce a liquid called **synovial fluid** (or *joint fluid*), which both lubricates and helps nourish the joint. One component of this fluid is a lubricating substance called **hyaluronic acid,** which is secreted by the synovial lining cells. In a normal joint, a small amount of this fluid keeps the cartilage surface lubricated and reduces friction during movement of the joint.

Cartilage covers the ends of the bone. This tissue is made up of cells called **chondrocytes,** which are embedded in the surrounding material called *carti-*

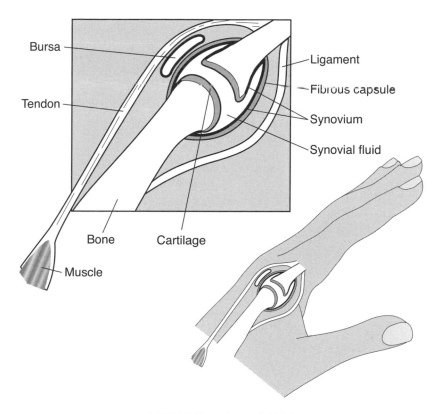

Bursa

Tendon

Ligament

Fibrous capsule

Synovium

Synovial fluid

Bone   Cartilage

Muscle

FIGURE 3. Normal synovial joint

lage matrix. Cartilage has a slippery surface that compresses easily and glides smoothly when the joint moves. The spongelike compressibility of cartilage allows it to soak up fluid and nutrients produced by the synovial membrane. A strong framework of connective tissue fibers called **collagen** holds the cartilage together and gives it durability. The sophisticated design of cartilage allows it to compress during impact while retaining its glossy surface to minimize friction. This provides a cushion for the bones. Unlike the synovial membrane, the cartilage has no direct blood supply; this may limit its ability to heal when injured.

Bone is found on both sides of a joint. Like cartilage, bone has living cells within its substance. Strong and durable, bone makes a suitable material for our body framework. Because of its rigidity, however, bone can fracture under mechanical stress, that is, physical pressure against it. The area of bone directly under the cartilage, known as the **subchondral bone,** is often damaged in RA.

Ligaments are the cordlike structures that attach one bone to another bone across a joint. These cords are much like sturdy guy wires, and they stabilize the joints so that the joints bend only in the direction in which they were intended to bend. For instance, the knee can either bend (**flexion**) or straighten out (**extension**). Ligaments on the sides of the knee prevent the joint from moving to either side when the knee is flexing. Other ligaments stop the knee from bending back on itself when the leg is fully extended.

Muscles are important contributors to joint function and stability. They serve as stabilizers and protectors of joints, in addition to being the source of power for all movement by the body. As you might expect, muscles provide the strength required to allow joints to move. Combinations of muscles acting in unison can result in a wide range of motions. This is how we can use the same joint (the shoulder) to reach behind our back, across our chest, and over our head. We do so by activating different muscle groups.

In addition to movement, the muscles provide stability for a joint, keeping it in a given position. For instance, if you raise your arms to comb your hair, certain muscle groups contract to lift your arms above your head. After your arms are raised, the muscles continue to work to keep your arms elevated while you use your hands and wrists to comb your hair. Similarly, when you are standing in a line without moving, your muscles remain contracted, to allow your body to stand erect, without collapsing at the hips or knees. Even without movement, then, muscles are critical: they allow us to retain stationary positions of our joints.

Lastly, muscles automatically protect the joints during movement, without requiring conscious thought on our part. As an illustration of this property of muscles, consider what happens if you unexpectedly missed a step while walking down a flight of stairs. Your muscles did not expect or prepare for the missed step, and so your knee or hip felt the jolt of movement without muscular support. If the step had been anticipated, the appropriate muscles would have contracted, acting much like a shock absorber on a car, to protect the joints during the step. This automatic protection function of the muscles results in a reduction of the impact on the joints in the course of daily living.

Muscles are attached to bone by **tendons,** which are similar to ligaments except that they connect muscle to bone instead of bone to bone. Because the tendons are located at the end of muscles, they move when muscles tighten, or contract. To demonstrate this to yourself, bend your arm at your elbow. At the same time, feel the area on the inside of your elbow for a ropelike structure at the end of the biceps muscle. This is a tendon.

The tendon is surrounded by an envelope known as the *tendon sheath*, in which the tendon slides back and forth. This sheath has a lining (similar to the synovial membrane) that permits easy gliding. When muscle tendons are in good health, they provide excellent support for the joint, much as ligaments do. Tendons and their sheaths can become inflamed, however, from overuse (producing a condition called *tendinitis*) or from RA (producing a condition called **tenosynovitis**).

Another structure located near the joints which helps the tendons and muscles move smoothly over bone is the **bursa.** Bursae are sacs, located between or under muscles, which help the muscles slide without resistance or friction. If these structures become inflamed they can become filled with fluid, a condition known as **bursitis.**

THE JOINTS IN RA

When considering how rheumatoid arthritis affects the joints and why it produces some of the symptoms it does, it is important to recognize that no two people with RA experience it exactly the same way. The severity of RA varies from person to person and joint to joint. Because of these differences, it is often difficult to assess precisely how much joint damage is present.

What Is Inflammation?

Our body has a natural defense mechanism for fighting off illness and disease. It is called the **immune system. Inflammation** is a common but complicated process that our bodies experience as a response to injury or infection. Inflammation is actually part of the body's immune system response to the injury or infection. Whenever we cut or burn ourselves, for example, inflammation occurs. It happens at the site of an infection (a person with bronchitis, for example, has inflamed bronchi, or airways). The symptoms and signs of inflammation are warmth, pain, redness, and swelling. The amount of inflammation is usually proportional to the severity of the injury or infection.

Under normal circumstances, unique immune cells, white blood cells called **lymphocytes, neutrophils,** and **macrophages,** strategically interact with one another to accomplish controlled inflammation. When the goal is fighting an infection, this team of cells works together to defend the body from the foreign invader causing the infection. They communicate with each other by chemical

messengers called **cytokines.** In the process of fighting infection, cells produce noxious substances that cause the symptoms of inflammation. Again,
under normal circumstances, after the infection is cleared, the cells retreat, and
inflammation subsides. In these situations inflammatory cells are extremely
useful in protecting and healing the body. After an injury, the goal of these
white blood cells is healing, and they work together to accomplish this goal.

Inflammation is usually self-limiting in that it goes away by itself after the
infection is cleared from the body. As the infection goes away or the wound is
healed and repaired, the signs of inflammation resolve as well.

How Is the Inflammation of RA Different from Normal Inflammation?

The inflammation that occurs in rheumatoid arthritis involves the immune cells
mentioned above, but the inciting event—the cause—of the inflammation, is
unknown. This trigger could be a virus or another foreign substance or **antigen**
(something that the body regards as foreign and reacts against). Normally, antigens are removed and destroyed by the body's immune system.

When a protective immune cell called the APC (antigen presenting cell)
hooks up to the antigen (the foreign invader), it starts the body's immune response. Soon there is an increase in the number of lymphocytes as well as other
inflammatory cells. Two types of lymphocytes, T and B cells, generally play an
integral but self-limited role in fighting infection. In RA these and other immune cells become chronically "overexcited," and this overexcited state works
to maintain inflammation in the joints. Unlike with normal inflammation,
the immune cells do not retreat. Continued inflammation produces the heat,
swelling, and pain of arthritis—and damage to joints.

In RA, the body launches a continuous immune response. Even when no
identified antigen is present or after it has left, the body appears to continue a
fight—against itself. Therefore, RA is often called an *autoimmune disease.* Immune cells mistakenly react against the body, causing **chronic** inflammation.
Now let's break down this RA inflammatory cascade further and see how it
affects the joints.

The Stages of RA: How Does Inflammation Affect the Joints?

Rheumatoid arthritis may be divided into five clinical stages. Each stage is characterized by the status of the *uncontrolled* inflammation present in the joints.

Stage 0 (normal). Although there isn't officially a stage 0, it is useful to consider the "before" conditions so that we can further understand the role that genetics plays in RA. In this pre-stage, people are normal in every way. Every person has an inherited genetic map that is passed down to him or her from both biological parents. It is presumed that people who later develop RA have a genetic susceptibility to the condition. Many familial studies have demonstrated that among people with RA there is an increased prevalence of RA in their first-degree relatives, that is, parents, siblings, and children. Several decades ago, a genetic marker, HLA-DRB1, was found to be more common in people with RA. The mapping of the human genome has allowed us to identify many other genes that are seen in higher frequencies in people with RA. However, not everyone with these identified genes goes on to develop RA. Hence, we know that genes alone do not tell the whole story. For instance, in patients with RA, the risk for identical twins to both develop the condition is about 15–30 percent and 5 percent among nonidentical twins (MacGregor et al., 2000). Since identical twins have indistinguishable genetic imprints, we know that simply inheriting the same set of genes is not enough for both to develop RA in the majority of cases. So, this suggests that, in most people, genetic predisposition alone does not absolutely predict the development of RA and that environmental factors probably play a larger role than genetics.

Because a vast majority of individuals with predisposing genes live their lives without acquiring RA, genetic testing is not recommended, or even available at the time of this writing. This does not preclude the possibility that, with continued technological advances, more sophisticated genetic testing or *genotyping* may be an option. Clearly, if having that information could indicate a useful prevention or treatment strategy for people at risk for RA, testing would become more commonplace. Even then, however, healthful lifestyle choices will be the cornerstone of any treatment strategy.

Stage 1 (preclinical RA). In this stage, people with RA still have no symptoms of arthritis, and their joints still appear normal (as in Figure 3). It is during this stage that the interplay of genetic and environmental factors takes place, in what is called a *gene-environment interaction*. New research has profoundly changed how we understand the gene-environment relationship. There is now powerful evidence that environmental factors can change the way our genes express our genetic code. This new area of scientific study is known as **epigenetics.** Lifestyle choices, diet, environmental toxins, and even chronic stress can determine whether parts of the genetic code are either expressed or suppressed. Parts of the code can be activated or deactivated by chemical switches that are triggered by various factors *outside* our bodies. The important message is that we are not captive to our genetic heritage and we may be empowered to control how our genes are expressed by our lifestyle choices. Next we will turn to the other side of the equation: the possible environmental triggers.

So, what is the environmental factor that provokes the gene-environment interaction that leads to an abnormal inflammatory response? Let's begin by saying that there are likely several potential triggers. In the introduction, we looked at the historical trail of microbes that have been considered through the decades as potential inciting factors for RA. Various organisms have been suggested, including viruses such Epstein-Barr virus, cytomegalovirus, and parvovirus B19. Numerous bacteria including *Streptococcus*, *Mycoplasma*, and *Escherichia coli* have also been considered. Many individuals with new onset RA can recall a recent infection. Also, blood samples have confirmed evidence of recent infection in approximately 10–20 percent of patients with newly diagnosed RA. However, no single infectious agent appears to be predominant. This suggests that, in all probability, there are several microbes that may act as triggers to start the inflammatory cascade.

Very new information seems to indicate that the offending microbe may even reside in our own bodies! In the past decade, there has been an intense, emerging interest in what has been termed the *microbiome*. This term encompasses our body's many microbes (good and bad), their genetics, and the interaction that they have with the human body. In 2007 the National Institutes of Health initiated the Human Microbiome Project in an effort to understand how changes in the microbiome can result in disease. Two areas have been directly linked to RA: the oral and the intestinal microbial environments.

There is a rapidly accumulating body of evidence that links periodontal disease (PD) to the development of RA. Periodontal disease is a disorder that is initiated by bacteria and causes inflammation and damage to the tissues that surround the teeth. One study found that patients with RA had an 8-fold increased likelihood of PD compared to those without RA (Pischon et al., 2008). Many studies have implicated the bacterium *Porphyromonas gingivalis* as a possible triggering factor for RA. Other bacteria are also under consideration (Scher et al., 2012). How do bacteria trigger RA? One theory is that these pathologic (bad) bacteria cause the formation of abnormal proteins, called *citrullinated peptides*. The immune systems of people with a genetic predisposition to

RA see these transformed proteins as foreign substances and make antibodies directed against them. **Antibodies**, also referred to as *immunoglobulins*, are distinctive proteins that the body normally produces to fight viruses and foreign bacteria, ones not normally present in the body. These specific antibodies are called anti-citrullinated protein antibodies (**ACPAs**). In this case, ACPA is considered an **autoantibody** since it is being directed against part of the body itself. You will read in Chapter 3 about blood tests for ACPA, which are highly specific tests for RA.

As an interesting aside, this connection of arthritis to dental problems is not new. Over 2000 years ago, Hippocrates recommended removal of a bad tooth to cure arthritis. In 1818, American physician and politician Benjamin Rush suggested extracting all natural teeth to cure rheumatism. Looking back even further may give us the most insight of all—why do we get periodontal disease? Researchers recently evaluated the calcified plaque from the teeth of prehistoric human skeletons and found very different bacteria. The dental plaque of skeletons preserves a detailed genetic record of the bacteria present in the oral cavity (Adler et al., 2013). Researchers have found that, as our diets changed over the past ten thousand years from a hunter-gatherer diet (meat, vegetables, nuts) to a diet rich in carbohydrates and sugar, so did our mouth bacteria. With the introduction of more extensive farming in the agricultural revolution, harmful bacteria that feed on carbohydrates became more dominant over healthy bacteria. With this change, the occurrence of periodontal disease increased considerably. We also know that RA is a relatively modern disease, not even mentioned in the medical literature until the nineteenth century. So, the changes in oral bacteria appear to parallel the historic occurrence of RA. You will read more about ancestral diets in Chapter 18 and the importance of good oral health in Chapter 5.

Besides our mouth bacteria, an enormous amount of evidence is pointing toward our own bowel bacteria as a potential trigger for abnormal inflammation in RA. Our gastrointestinal tract is colonized with beneficial and pathological (bad) bacteria. In a healthy person, there are important barriers that keep the contents of our bowel separate from the rest of our bodies. There is a growing understanding of how our bowel bacteria can favorably and unfavorably affect our immune system. Altering the healthy balance of bacteria appears to be a factor in the initiation and perpetuation of several inflammatory diseases, including RA. There is evidence that the types of bacteria in the bowel of people with RA are different from those of people without RA. Russian researchers recently analyzed the bacterial composition of stool samples and found that study subjects with RA had less good bacteria (like the *lactobacteria* and *bifidobacteria* species) and higher amounts of bad bacteria than did people without RA (Gul'neva and Noskov, 2011). When the pathogenic (disease-causing) bacteria overwhelm the beneficial bacteria, there is a decrease in the gut's immune defenses. This results in abnormal permeability of the bowel wall or what is called a "leaky gut." It is hypothesized that bacterial toxins are absorbed from the bowel into the bloodstream and set off an inflammatory reaction. The DNA of these bacteria has been found in the joint fluid of some people with RA (Van der Heijden et al., 2000). We will discuss in depth the importance of diet and its role in normalizing the intestinal bacteria in Chapter 18.

But, is the presumed trigger necessarily a germ or organism? Various nonmicrobial environmental triggers have been postulated over the years, including exposure to pollutants, silica dust, ultraviolet light, chemically altered diet, emotional stress, and changes in physical activity. The most powerful proven association has been between smoking and the development of RA. In the twenty-first century, medical studies have confirmed that a potent gene-environment interaction occurs between smoking and specific genes. There is a strong linkage between smoking, the HLA-DRB1 gene, and the production of ACPA. A study that looked at lung fluid samples from smokers found that a high percentage of the lung cells contained citrullinated peptides (Klareskog et al., 2006). Recall that these are the same type of abnormal proteins that provoke the production of ACPA in periodontal disease.

In a large study, smoking increased the risk of developing RA by more than 40 percent (Costenbader et al., 2006). This has been confirmed by several other studies. In people with specific genetic markers, the risk of developing RA increases more than 20-fold in smokers compared to nonsmokers (Klareskog et al., 2006). One group of researchers performed a nationwide study looking at identical twins where only one twin had RA. Then, they analyzed 13 of those pairs where only one of the twins was a smoker. The smoker was the twin with RA in 12 of those 13 pairs (Silman et al., 1996). Smoking not only triggers RA but also contributes to its severity and makes the RA more challenging to treat. In addition, smoking is a significant risk factor for periodontal disease, which further escalates the risk for RA.

Research has also suggested that obesity may be a trigger for rheumatoid arthritis. The exact mechanism for this has not been proven, but it is an area of rigorous research. It is known that fat cells (called adipose cells or adipocytes) can produce a type of cytokine called *adipokines*, which cause chronic inflammation. Abdominal fat made up of white adipose tissue appears to produce the most inflammatory cytokines. We will discuss this further in Chapter 18.

Remember that at stage 1, people have absolutely no symptoms and their joints are normal. It is during this stage that we have the highest likelihood of preventing the development of rheumatoid arthritis. Studies are under way to identify specific **biomarkers** that can reveal if a pivotal trigger is present in people with a strong genetic risk. A potential candidate is the blood test for ACPA, which was mentioned above. One study tested normal blood donors for ACPA. In those who tested positive for ACPA *and* had at least two close relatives with RA, the risk of developing RA within five years was 69 percent (Nielen et al., 2004). ACPA isn't present in all people with RA, as you will read in Chapter 3. However, if we can identify a panel of biomarkers like ACPA and test people with at-risk genotyping, we may be able to identify those individuals at high risk for developing RA. It goes without saying that a healthful lifestyle, including appropriate nutrition, exercise, and stress reduction, may be life altering. However, sometimes, despite the best efforts, a triggering event occurs that is beyond our control and RA develops. Fortunately, we have many avenues for successfully combatting RA.

Stage 2. In the previous stage, the correct genetic makeup and an RA trigger came together in a gene-environment interaction. The duration of time between the triggering event and when symptoms appear varies considerably. The time period between noting ACPA by blood test and later developing RA has been reported to be as long as 10 years (Nielen et al., 2004). It is in this stage that the symptoms of RA begin. The immune system acknowledges the presence of what it perceives as a foreign intruder or antigen by sending an *antigen-presenting cell* (*APC*) to confront the presumed invader. Several types of immune cells can act as antigen-presenting cells, but the most common among them is an immune cell called the macrophage, one of those white blood cells mentioned earlier. The APC grabs the antigen and "presents" it to the *T cell lymphocyte*. Recognizing the antigen as foreign, the T cell is activated and vigorously sends out a call for help to other members of the immune system, including B cells and other T cells (Figure 4). You will read in Chapter 14 how specific *biologics* called *T cell modulators* interfere with this "call to action" and so help control inflammation.

Early in the course of arthritis, lymphocytes migrate to the synovial lining, causing what is called **synovitis,** or inflammation of the synovium (see Figure 5). The macrophages and lymphocytes continue to promote inflammation by producing cytokines, delivering messages from one immune cell to another.

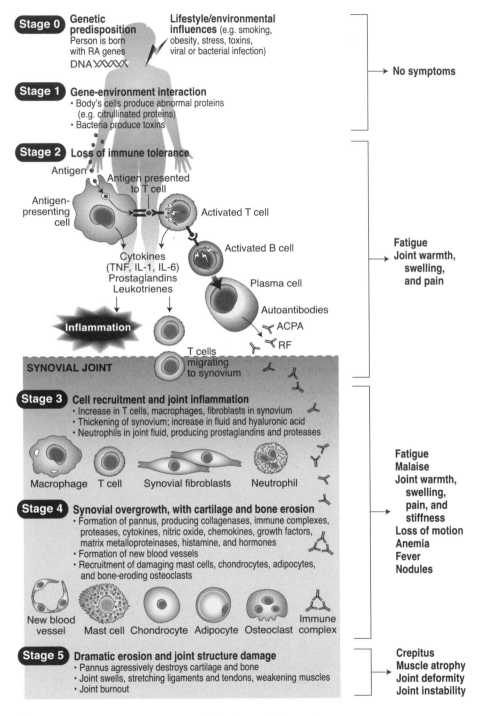

Stage 0 **Genetic predisposition**
Person is born with RA genes
DNA ✗✗✗✗✗

Lifestyle/environmental influences (e.g. smoking, obesity, stress, toxins, viral or bacterial infection)

→ No symptoms

Stage 1 **Gene-environment interaction**
• Body's cells produce abnormal proteins (e.g. citrullinated proteins)
• Bacteria produce toxins

Stage 2 **Loss of immune tolerance**
Antigen
Antigen presented to T cell
Antigen-presenting cell
Activated T cell
Activated B cell
Cytokines (TNF, IL-1, IL-6)
Prostaglandins
Leukotrienes
Plasma cell
Autoantibodies
ACPA
RF
Inflammation
T cells migrating to synovium

→ Fatigue
Joint warmth, swelling, and pain

SYNOVIAL JOINT

Stage 3 **Cell recruitment and joint inflammation**
• Increase in T cells, macrophages, fibroblasts in synovium
• Thickening of synovium; increase in fluid and hyaluronic acid
• Neutrophils in joint fluid, producing prostaglandins and proteases

Macrophage   T cell   Synovial fibroblasts   Neutrophil

Stage 4 **Synovial overgrowth, with cartilage and bone erosion**
• Formation of pannus, producing collagenases, immune complexes, proteases, cytokines, nitric oxide, chemokines, growth factors, matrix metalloproteinases, histamine, and hormones
• Formation of new blood vessels
• Recruitment of damaging mast cells, chondrocytes, adipocytes, and bone-eroding osteoclasts

New blood vessel   Mast cell   Chondrocyte   Adipocyte   Osteoclast   Immune complex

→ Fatigue
Malaise
Joint warmth, swelling, pain, and stiffness
Loss of motion
Anemia
Fever
Nodules

Stage 5 **Dramatic erosion and joint structure damage**
• Pannus agressively destroys cartilage and bone
• Joint swells, stretching ligaments and tendons, weakening muscles
• Joint burnout

→ Crepitus
Muscle atrophy
Joint deformity
Joint instability

FIGURE 4. The rheumatoid cascade

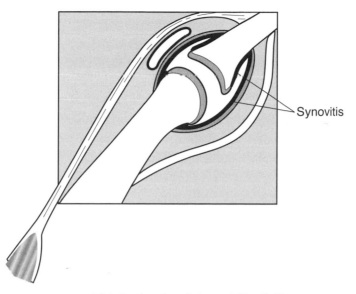

Synovitis

FIGURE 5. Joint showing stage 2 rheumatoid arthritis

Three specific cytokines, **tumor necrosis factor (TNF)**, **interleukin-1 (IL-1)**, and **interleukin-6 (IL-6)** have been identified as significantly increasing inflammation. People with RA have increased amounts of TNF, IL-1, and IL-6 in their joints. There are many other cytokines under study as well. Cytokines can induce an increase in the number of blood vessels going to the synovium, and with increased blood flow, the joints become warm. The leakage of cytokines into the bloodstream may also contribute to the fatigue that is so common in RA. Other cytokines are partially responsible for stimulating immune cells to produce **prostaglandins** and **leukotrienes,** both of which are potent producers of inflammation. Continued production of cytokines, prostaglandins, leukotrienes, and other substances leads to swelling, warmth, and pain in the joints. Chapter 14 describes how this knowledge about immune cells and cytokines translates into effective treatment options for controlling symptoms of RA.

It is also during stage 2 that B lymphocytes are transformed into another type of white blood cell, the **plasma cell,** which manufactures antibodies. In RA, for reasons that are unclear, the body appears to produce an excessive amount of antibodies, including autoantibodies, the type that are directed against our own body constituents. Two particular autoantibodies that are often found in the blood of people with RA are called **rheumatoid factor (RF)** and **anticitrullinated protein antibodies (ACPA).** (RF and ACPA are discussed in more detail in Chapter 3.)

But why doesn't the body go through the normal cycle of inflammation and turn itself off? There are many theories about this. One of them is that the disturbed immune system loses the ability to "ignore" antigens that are not overtly harmful. This very important function is called *immune tolerance.* So, why isn't the immune system getting the message that there is no need to fight? This appears to be in part due to the malfunction of a subset of T cell lymphocytes called *regulatory T cells.* These cells act as referees, determining what is foreign and what is not. Why these T cells lose their ability to tell the difference between harmless antigens and harmful antigens is an area of rigorous research.

Stage 3. In this stage there is a marked increase in the number of cells in the synovium, possibly stimulated by the presence of various cytokines. In addition to macrophages and lymphocytes, the synovium is also composed of resident cells called *synovial fibroblasts.* The synovium becomes much thicker, or **hypertrophied,** and this makes the joint feel doughy or spongy (see Figure 6). An increase in the amount of synovial fluid in the joint adds to the stiffness and limitation of motion of the joints. This accumulation of joint fluid is known as **joint effusion.**

With RA there is also an increase in **hyaluronic acid**, the lubricating substance in the synovial joint fluid. Many people believe that increased hyaluronic acid is responsible for morning stiffness (or morning **gelling**) and the stiffness

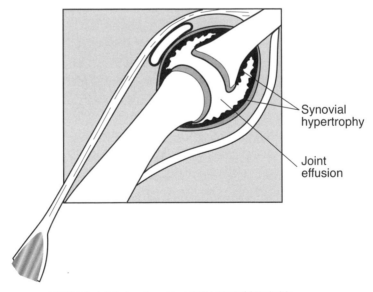

Synovial
hypertrophy

Joint
effusion

FIGURE 6. Joint showing stage 3 rheumatoid arthritis

experienced after sitting for a prolonged period of time without moving (gelling phenomenon).

Joint fluid contains inflammatory white blood cells, neutrophils (or polymorphonuclear leukocytes). Why the neutrophils appear in the synovial fluid and the lymphocytes reside in the synovial lining is not clear. In the joint affected by RA, neutrophils join lymphocytes in perpetuating the inflammatory process by producing prostaglandins, *proteases* (which break down proteins), and other damaging substances. In testing for RA, the physician may remove a sample of fluid from the joints to determine the relative proportions of these cells present. This helps the physician differentiate RA from other forms of arthritis.

A person in this stage of RA may experience significant joint symptoms, including pain, heat, swelling, stiffness, and loss of motion. Pro-inflammatory cytokines continue to escalate other inflammation symptoms, like fatigue, malaise, and often **anemia** (low red blood cell count). All of these inflammatory changes are still *potentially* reversible with proper medical therapy.

Stage 4. At this point, the inflamed synovium can grow (the **synovial cells** proliferate), spreading over the top of joint cartilage (Figure 7). This marked growth of synovial tissue is referred to as *synovial hyperplasia*. The synovium that has grown in this way is called **pannus**. Cells in the synovium, particularly the sy-

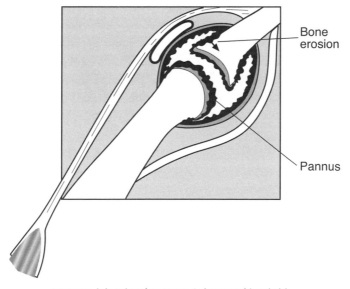

Bone erosion

Pannus

FIGURE 7. Joint showing stage 4 rheumatoid arthritis

novial fibroblasts, take on an aggressive character. Pannus produces **enzymes** called **collagenases**, which can destroy collagen, the cartilage proteins. Neutrophils in the joint fluid continue to release harmful enzymes. Although there are many beneficial enzymes in the body, these particular enzymes can break down, or degrade, the cartilage that protects the bone and joints.

The pannus continues to produce a wide range of inflammation and damage-inducing substances: cytokines, collagenases, proteases, *nitric oxide* (NO), *chemokines, matrix metalloproteinases* (*MMP*), *growth factors, immune complexes* (composed of autoantibodies), and many more (as illustrated in Figure 4). Other cells get recruited into the mayhem including *mast cells, endothelial cells* (blood vessel cells), *chondrocytes* (cartilage cells), and *adipocytes* (fat cells). Growth factors promote *angiogenesis* (the growth of new blood vessels). Resident bone cells called **osteoclasts** get activated and break down bone, resulting in the formation of tiny holes or **erosions.**

Stage 5. If the arthritis is left untreated, the pannus can further invade and erode cartilage and bone by producing more enzymes and other destructive substances. Any loss of cartilage reduces the amount of cushioning between the bones of the joint (Figure 8).

When erosions roughen cartilage, the ability to have smooth joint motion is lost. People with RA can feel a grating sensation in the joint during movement,

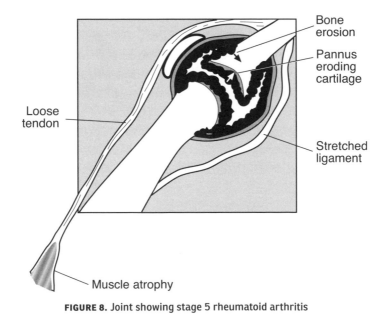

FIGURE 8. Joint showing stage 5 rheumatoid arthritis

and their physicians can feel the grating of the joint during physical examination. This grating is called *crepitus*. If the breakdown of cartilage is persistent, the cartilage can be totally eroded by pannus.

In stage 5 RA, uncontrolled swelling can cause ligaments and tendons to stretch, adding to the *instability* of the joint. Muscles become smaller (**atrophy**) and weaker because of disuse. Stretched ligaments and tendons and atrophied muscles interfere with the joint's ability to function properly, resulting in a joint that does not move as it was intended to. Inflammation and pannus can spread along the tendons in tenosynovitis, making the tendons weak and putting them at risk for rupture. When the cartilage is eroded and the supporting structures are loosened, other changes often occur which alter the shape and function of the joint. These mechanical changes are more a result of multiple abnormal forces occurring across the joint than of just ongoing inflammation in the joint itself.

Late in this stage, after the cartilage is totally eroded, the amount of inflammation and swelling often decreases, producing what is sometimes referred to as a *burned-out joint*. At this stage the stretched ligaments and tendons can actually become even looser, as the swelling pushing against them decreases. The looseness of these supporting structures can seriously affect the stability of the joint. (These changes and the prevention and treatment of them are discussed throughout this book.)

You can see that a complex array of cells and substances contribute to the cascade of inflammation and damage in RA. Believe it or not, the actual process is much more complicated than our description here! We have tried just to acquaint you with many of the major players in RA so that when you read about treatment options the terminology and science will be familiar.

SUMMARY

Of the three major types of joints in the body, only the synovial joints are affected by RA. All the parts of the joint play a role in normal function:

- The *capsule* encloses and protects the joint.
- The *synovium* provides lubrication and nutrition for the joint.
- *Cartilage* cushions and reduces friction during movement.
- *Bone* provides structure.
- *Ligaments* and *tendons* support the joint.

- *Muscles* provide joint movement, protection, and stability.
- *Bursae* decrease friction during movement.

Early symptoms of RA include pain, swelling, warmth, and stiffness (especially in the morning) in the joints, and mild restriction of motion. Joint symptoms and such generalized symptoms as fatigue are caused by a variety of inflammatory substances produced by different cells.

In RA, for unknown reasons, the normal cells of the joint lining and white blood cells become overactivated, resulting in uncontrolled inflammation in the joints.

In the early stages, RA is often reversible with timely medical therapy.

2

The Course and Prognosis of Rheumatoid Arthritis

For most people with rheumatoid arthritis (RA), questions about the future course of their condition are their major concern. Anyone who has been diagnosed with RA will naturally want and need answers to these questions to make plans for the future. Physicians and other health professionals will answer these questions as best as they can, given the present state of knowledge about the course of RA and what they know about the individual's specific condition.

Like many other chronic illnesses, however, RA is often unpredictable. The onset of RA may be gradual or sudden and may involve one or many joints. The course of arthritis is also varied, and it may even change over time in the same person. For these reasons, it is important to keep in mind that any prediction made by health care professionals about the future course of RA in any one individual is a guess—an educated guess, but a guess. Current research is investigating the use of **biomarkers** to provide more insight into the variations within rheumatoid arthritis and to give more accurate predictions of the course the condition might take, as well as which medications will work the best with each individual. (Read about biomarkers in Chapter 3.)

The questions people with RA most commonly ask about the future are presented in this chapter, along with the best answers the medical professional can provide at this time.

THE COURSE OF RA

How Does RA Usually Start?

Variability is the key ingredient in the answer to this question. Most commonly, RA starts gradually, with pain and stiffness in one or more of the joints noted in Figure 1. Usually, people first notice these symptoms in their hands. Early on, swelling may not be apparent, despite sensations of pain or stiffness. As the amount of pain slowly increases, however, swelling becomes obvious. Swelling in the joints usually appears within months of the onset of pain in the joints. Rarely, swelling does not appear until years after pain begins.

For seven out of ten people with RA, the symptoms of arthritis appear in matching joints, on both sides of the body; this is called *symmetrical arthritis*. For example, the left and right wrists may both be affected or the left and right knees. In addition to feeling pain in the joints, people experiencing the early symptoms of RA may feel very fatigued, as though they were recovering from a cold or the flu.

For some people, RA begins differently. These people may notice only increasing stiffness (particularly in the morning) without experiencing a great deal of pain. Others notice only progressively severe swelling, initially without pain. Still other people experience bouts of joint pain or swelling which appear suddenly and then disappear just as quickly. Someone who has these recurring attacks or flare-ups of arthritis that resolve quickly may be given a diagnosis of *palindromic rheumatism* before diagnostic evidence for RA develops.

Less commonly, RA can begin with only one or two tender, swollen joints in an asymmetrical pattern, that is, the joints affected on one side of the body are different from the joints affected on the other side of the body. Since this is an unusual way for RA to begin, health care providers may be hesitant about confirming a diagnosis of RA based on these symptoms. In time, about half of the people whose joint pain begins in an asymmetrical pattern will develop the more typical symmetrical pattern of RA.

RA sometimes begins as aching and stiff muscles, particularly in the shoulders and hips. This nonspecific aching may continue for weeks or months before the swelling of joints appears. Older individuals are more likely than younger people to have muscle aches and stiffness appear as the first sign of RA.

Finally, RA may appear as rapid onset arthritis, with swelling and pain in many joints as well as such systemic symptoms as severe fatigue, low-grade fever, loss of appetite, and weight loss seemingly developing overnight.

What Course of Arthritis Can I Expect?

After you have been diagnosed with RA, you will wonder what course or *natural history* your arthritis will follow. Will it continue in the same way it started, or will additional, or different, joints become involved in time? The answers to these questions are as different as the persons asking them. In some cases, the way arthritis starts allows physicians to predict the course it will follow, but this is not true in every case.

The following four general courses that RA can follow reflect the natural histories of *untreated* RA (Figure 9). Keep in mind that what follows are four *potential* courses. The actual course of any given individual's RA may be different from any of these four courses, and treatment will influence the course.

1. Spontaneous remission (Figure 9A). The person who develops signs and symptoms of RA and then, with little or no medication (generally only nonsteroidal anti-inflammatory medications, **NSAIDs**), becomes symptom-free is said to have gone into spontaneous **remission**. *Complete* remission of a disease is when there is no evidence of active disease or illness.

During remission from RA, blood tests, such as the **erythrocyte sedimentation rate (ESR)** or **C reactive protein (CRP)**, often produce normal results (discussed in Chapter 3). Generally it is estimated that 20 percent of all RA patients will have a spontaneous remission, but more than 50 percent of these

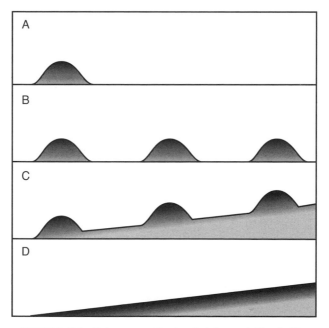

FIGURE 9. Potential courses of untreated rheumatoid arthritis

will have a recurrence of RA in the future. Thus, in reality, probably only 5 to 10 percent of untreated patients have a permanent remission. The majority of people with RA require continued treatment.

Patients and physicians often wonder how long they should wait for this potential spontaneous remission before starting stronger medications, (**DMARDs** [disease-modifying antirheumatic drugs] and/or **biologics**). The optimal time to start DMARDs or biologics varies from case to case, but most rheumatologists would begin them if they had concern for impending joint damage and certainly if joint damage was already visible on x-ray films, ultrasound, or MRI. (Read more about these tests in the next chapter.) When to start these medications is particularly important because it has now been proven that these drugs are most effective if taken early in the course of arthritis.

2. *Remitting (Figure 9B).* Some people with RA have a series of flare-ups of arthritis followed by returns to normal health between attacks. A person who has *remitting arthritis* may not need remission-inducing medications if there is no ongoing joint damage and if joint function returns to normal between flare-ups. The attacks themselves, when the arthritis is active, are commonly treated with NSAIDs. Attacks that occur very frequently or that are very lengthy may begin to affect the person's lifestyle, and then the person with RA and the physician may decide that DMARDs and/or biologics should be taken. Also, it is important to make certain that a small amount of damaging inflammation is not present in between flares. Many people can "get used to" the feeling of arthritis and believe that there isn't an issue when in fact there is still inflammation. People with RA can become very tolerant and stoical and may think that the disease is in remission when the symptoms are not as bad as they are during a flare-up. Blood tests and imaging techniques are important in these circumstances.

3. *Remitting progressive (Figure 9C).* The third possible course of RA is one in which the person experiences a pattern of flare-ups without a return to normal health between attacks. Joint damage over time is a distinct possibility in this course of RA, because some inflammation remains in the joints between attacks. In this case, DMARD and/or biologic therapy ought to be a serious consideration.

4. *Progressive (Figure 9D).* In this course, the person experiences a gradual increase in pain, swelling, and joint damage over time. Usually this progression occurs very slowly, but some people experience a rapid loss of function. Early

treatment with DMARD and/or biologic therapy in an effort to halt progression of arthritis is recommended.

Can a Remission Be Brought on with Medications?

DMARDs and/or biologics are used in an attempt to induce a remission of RA, and many people achieve improvement by taking one of these medications. (For more information about NSAIDs, DMARDS, and biologics, see Chapters 12, 13, and 14, respectively.) Unfortunately, it is not always possible to predict which of the many medications will bring about improvement for a specific individual. One drug may induce a remission in one person and not work very well for the next. For this reason, prescribing the proper medication often involves a trial-and-error approach coupled with close communication between the patient and the physician. As mentioned earlier, medical researchers are investigating the use of different biomarkers to help determine which medications will work best for which person.

Different medications have different potential side effects, all of which your doctor will discuss with you. (These are described in detail in Part IV.) It is very important to keep in mind that *no two people are alike in the way they respond to medications*; this means, among other things, that the risk for medication side effects and allergies varies from one person to the next. Therefore, when decisions are being made about which medication is best suited to you, *thoughtful, ongoing communication between you and your physician is essential*.

There are two principles that hold true for drugs that are intended to induce a remission. One is that early treatment is probably most effective. You must decide for yourself whether the potential benefits of early treatment, aimed at preventing permanent joint damage, outweigh possible medication toxicities. With your physician's guidance, you must balance risks, make informed decisions, and set realistic goals.

The second principle is that, by their nature, most DMARDs work slowly. In most cases inflammation did not develop instantaneously and it is unlikely to resolve rapidly, even with appropriate therapy. Improvement with a DMARD may take weeks to months. Most biologics have a faster response time than the older DMARDs, but they still often take weeks to produce results. For this reason, patience is required; you need to reserve judgment about the effectiveness of a medication until an adequate trial treatment period has elapsed.

NSAIDs are a group of medications aimed at reducing inflammation. They are effective drugs that often reduce pain and inflammation quickly (days to weeks). Nevertheless, however helpful they may be in controlling symptoms, NSAIDs probably have little effect on the course of RA.

We remain very optimistic about the effectiveness of our present medications and can assure you that many new medications are currently under intensive investigation. It is important to avoid becoming discouraged if one medicine fails, because very possibly the next medication you try will work for you. Also, there are many additional ways to help control pain, prevent joint damage, and improve function while waiting for the medications to take effect (these methods are discussed later in this book).

THE PROGNOSIS OF RA

Can Arthritis Be Cured?

Rheumatoid arthritis is generally a **chronic** condition in which true cures or permanent remissions are unusual with the medications *presently* available. This does not mean that most cases of arthritis cannot be controlled effectively, however. The majority of people with RA achieve good to excellent control with a treatment program consisting of medications, diet, therapeutic exercise, adequate rest, and proper joint protection. And most people with RA are able to continue with their normal activities, with some minor adjustments to accommodate joint changes that have occurred. The prognosis of RA has never been better and improves every year with the advent of new treatment options. With continued study and understanding of the science behind RA, we are optimistic that a cure may be a possibility at some future point.

Will Additional Joints Become Involved over Time?

Possibly. Most people initially develop pain in their hands and wrists, and it is likely that they will experience at the least some discomfort in other joints. But not all joints are affected equally by RA in all people. For instance, the person who is having significant pain and difficulties with finger joints will not necessarily experience the same degree of inflammation or pain in any other joints. Also, the many new medical options available today make it very possible to keep RA at bay, preventing progression to new joints.

Will I Become Disabled?

Today, treatment of RA begins earlier in the course of the condition, and treatment options are more varied and more effective. The currently available medications can be very effective, and many more are being explored. With the introduction of the biologics (Chapter 14), there has been a significant improvement in function in a vast majority of people with RA. Today, too, there is an appreciation of the value of therapeutic exercise, nutrition, and healthful lifestyle in improving function and avoiding disability. Even in the most challenging cases, in which arthritis persists despite the medical team's efforts, other options remain. Also, the many surgical procedures available today are infinitely more effective than those offered a few decades ago (see Chapter 19). On a happy note, studies have shown that the need for surgery has been cut in half in the new millennium.

Will you become disabled? Today, the odds against this are overwhelmingly in your favor, which is why it is best to avoid listening to a well-meaning friend's stories about her great-aunt who lives a wheelchairbound life because of RA. Remember, each person's case is different, and so much has changed in the approach to treating RA that comparisons are just not valid. The fact that you are reading a book about your condition and taking an active role in making decisions about treatment proves that you are different from the patients of a half-century ago.

Will you need to make some lifestyle changes? Yes, but that in no way means that you need to relinquish any of your life goals. If you have a good understanding of how to control the particular problems associated with your arthritis and if you remain open to learning new ways to make adjustments, you will succeed in living a normal, productive life. Will you be inconvenienced? Yes, definitely. Will you be disabled? Highly unlikely.

Does RA Shorten a Person's Life?

Statistically, RA, like most chronic illnesses, is associated with a very slight decrease in life span when *all* patients who have RA are compared with *all* people who are free of illness. This may not have any individual significance for you, because these statistics are derived from older studies with comparisons of large groups of people. In addition, with the advent of newer medications and better control of inflammation, these differences have been consistently shown to be decreasing since the mid-1990s. Also, the impact of making healthy lifestyle choices greatly improves the odds that you will live a full and long life.

A very small minority of people with severe RA (significantly less than 5 percent and decreasing) develop complications that make them very ill. These individuals have life-threatening conditions (discussed in Chapter 4). These unusual complications of severe RA are also well on the decline, as you will read.

SUMMARY

Rheumatoid arthritis begins in different ways and can follow a wide variety of potential courses.

RA responds best when treated early.

DMARDs, or disease-modifying antirheumatic drugs, and biologics can bring about an improvement in many people.

NSAIDs, or nonsteroidal anti-inflammatory drugs, can quickly ease the symptoms of inflammation and pain, but they are less effective than DMARDs and biologics in changing the course of RA.

The biologics work more quickly than traditional DMARDs.

Although true cures are unlikely at this time, excellent control of arthritis is possible with a comprehensive treatment program.

Most people with RA live normal, full lives with some minor lifestyle adjustments.

3

Diagnosing Rheumatoid Arthritis: Why So Many Tests?

You may be wondering why it took so long or was so difficult for your doctor to diagnose your rheumatoid arthritis (RA). It may have appeared at first that the physician was hedging on the diagnosis or refusing to provide you with a diagnosis on the spot. Because there are so many different ailments that can cause pain in the joints and so many different kinds of arthritis, the physician needed time to determine which was affecting you. And, as discussed in Chapter 2, the pain of RA begins a little differently in each person; there is no one set of symptoms by which the doctor can identify RA immediately.

It may be helpful to review the initial steps taken in reaching a diagnosis of RA: the clinical history, the physical examination, and a **differential diagnosis.** Early in the course of RA, diagnostic tests (for example, blood tests and x-rays) may not be much help in making a diagnosis of RA, although they can sometimes rule out other conditions whose symptoms resemble those of RA. Diagnostic tests *do* help confirm a diagnosis of RA in later stages.

CLINICAL HISTORY

The most valuable information you can provide to your doctor on an initial visit is your clinical history, the recounting of what symptoms you have been experiencing and when they began. Usually the doctor will ask you to describe your symptoms and then will ask you specific questions about your symptoms, such as:

- Which joints are painful or stiff?
- When is the pain or stiffness worse?

- What makes the symptoms better or worse?
- How long does the morning stiffness last?
- Do you feel tired much of the time?

Providing your physician with complete and accurate answers to these questions is one of the most important roles you can play in your own medical care. This is because the physician depends on an analysis of the clinical history to help identify the cause of your joint problems.

It's a good idea to prepare a written record of your symptoms as they occur. You can draw up a list of symptoms, including where you feel pain or stiffness or swelling and the time of day when it occurs or when it is the most bothersome; take this list with you to the doctor's office. The list will help you answer your doctor's questions accurately, because you will have a record of what you have been experiencing, written before your visit when you have time to recollect. Not everyone can remember *exactly* when pain or stiffness or swelling was *first* experienced or pinpoint the onset of changes in ability to perform a given task. Once you become aware of these changes, however, it is a good idea to keep a record of them.

PHYSICAL EXAMINATION

After the clinical history is taken, the physician will perform a physical examination. He or she will examine all of your joints, looking for evidence of tenderness, heat, swelling, and decreased motion. Your doctor will pay particular attention to the pattern of joint involvement, because one of the distinguishing characteristics of RA is the particular pattern of joints that can be affected. Often the physician will perform a *complete* physical examination (including taking your blood pressure; feeling your glands; examining your eyes, ears, nose, throat, and skin; listening to your heart and lungs; examining your abdomen; and checking your reflexes and muscle strength) to uncover clues that may help identify the type of arthritis you have.

Sometimes, in the early stages of RA, people find the results of the physical examination frustrating, because they are experiencing significant pain or stiffness in their joints and the physician may not be able to detect outward signs of joint inflammation. In these cases the physician has to proceed on the basis of the patient's description of the pain or stiffness he or she is experiencing. Again, the accuracy of the clinical history provided to the physician is extremely important.

DIFFERENTIAL DIAGNOSIS

After the physical examination, the physician will develop a differential diagnosis. This consists of a list of possible causes of your specific symptoms. The physician will order specific laboratory tests to rule out certain of the diagnoses and other tests in hope of confirming the proper diagnosis.

As we will see, blood tests and x-rays are seldom helpful in diagnosing RA in the very earliest stage. For this reason, your tests may not uncover any specific abnormalities. On the one hand, you'll probably be happy that the test results are normal; on the other hand, there's the frustration of knowing that something is wrong and not having a test result to prove it. Your physician may temporarily have to make an experienced best guess of the diagnosis. Effective treatment can be initiated before test results are diagnostically significant, however.

What Makes RA So Difficult to Diagnose?

Rheumatoid arthritis is the most common of the inflammatory forms of arthritis, and yet making an accurate diagnosis is often difficult. For this reason, your physician may have initially diagnosed your RA as another type of inflammatory arthritis, such as ankylosing spondylitis, reactive arthritis, arthritis associated with psoriasis or colitis, gout, pseudo-gout, or systemic lupus erythematosus (SLE). The symptoms of these forms of arthritis are similar to the symptoms of RA, and many excellent doctors initially misdiagnose RA as being another form of inflammatory arthritis (and vice versa). RA is also often diagnosed incorrectly as osteoarthritis, the most common form of arthritis.

A good clinical history, a thorough physical examination, some laboratory tests, and a good measure of time and patience are required to diagnose RA. A physician who is well acquainted with the pattern of joint involvement in RA is likely to have an easier time making an accurate diagnosis. Board-certified **rheumatologists** are specifically trained and experienced in making these difficult early diagnoses.

DIAGNOSTIC TESTS

Physicians rely on diagnostic tests to help them provide quality care to people with RA. Diagnostic tests can take the form of blood analyses, joint fluid analyses, urine analyses, and x-rays. (As might be expected, evaluation of blood and joint fluid requires that a needle be used to obtain specimens.) Diagnostic tests may be requested for any one (or more) of the following reasons:

- to make a diagnosis of RA
- to monitor disease activity in RA
- to rule out other types of arthritis
- to detect complications of RA
- to screen for potential side effects of a medication

In addition to laboratory analyses of body fluids and x-ray evaluation, physicians rely heavily on the patient history and physical examination to make a diagnosis of RA, as discussed above. In fact, early in the course of RA, when the results of diagnostic tests may be normal, the physician relies on an evaluation of each person's description of symptoms and the physical exam to make a diagnosis. When the findings from laboratory tests are inconclusive, making the diagnosis often requires a significant amount of observation time. Patience is required from both the physician and the patient in this case.

Your physician may request any of the tests described below. As you will see, many of the tests have more than one function. For example, a blood count may be ordered to look for complications of RA or to monitor for side effects of medications.

Many of the substances being tested for are examined by blood or urine analysis, which can be performed in a diagnostic laboratory or in the doctor's office, usually by the doctor's nurse or assistant. Some of the tests are more complicated, and only the skills of an experienced physician can ensure that they are performed safely and accurately. We will identify these procedures in the following section.

What Tests Are Used to Diagnose or Monitor Activity of RA?

Rheumatoid factor (RF), rheumatoid titer. Rheumatoid factor is an antibody found in the blood of 80 to 90 percent of people with RA. A blood test determines whether the antibody is present. The result is often expressed as a *titer*, which is a measurement reflecting the amount of a substance present. The presence of rheumatoid factor *usually* indicates that a diagnosis of RA is accurate, although a change in titer of rheumatoid factor does not necessarily reflect a change in the activity of arthritis.

Anti-citrullinated protein antibodies (ACPA), anti-cyclic citrullinated peptide antibodies (anti-CCP). These tests measure for the presence of specific autoantibodies that are frequently found in people with RA. Although these antibodies were first discovered in the 1970s, they did not become widely tested for until 2010 when ACPA became part of the official classification criteria for RA. The presence of these autoantibodies in the blood is now considered to be a more specific test for RA than rheumatoid factor. (There is more about ACPA in Chapter 1.)

Erythrocyte sedimentation rate (ESR), or "sed rate." The ESR is a test commonly ordered to monitor inflammation in the body. It is actually a measurement of how rapidly red blood cells settle (produce sedimentation) in a test tube. When inflammation is present in the body, certain proteins in blood make red blood cells (erythrocytes) settle faster, and this results in a high ESR. For people with RA, it is often useful to monitor the ESR, because changes in the sed rate can reflect changes in inflammation. A decrease in the ESR suggests that medical treatment has been effective. The ESR is not a specific diagnostic test for RA, however, because a high ESR can be caused by many other conditions, such as infections, that produce significant inflammation.

C reactive protein (CRP). CRP, like ESR, is a test frequently ordered to monitor inflammation level. CRP sometimes will be elevated when the ESR is not. Many clinicians prefer to look at both the ESR and the CRP, to get a more complete picture of the degree of inflammation. The CRP should be as low as possible. The therapies that lower it may also limit the damaging effects of RA. This test is also frequently ordered in people *without* RA to look for evidence of inflammation in other parts of the body. One reason is that the presence of inflammation may lead to increased risks of cardiovascular disease.

Synovial fluid studies. One of the most helpful tests in **rheumatology** involves the evaluation of synovial fluid (joint fluid). A rheumatologist, an **orthopedic surgeon,** or an experienced primary care physician can remove (aspirate) fluid from an inflamed or painful joint by needle with minimal discomfort. (The process of aspirating a joint is called *arthrocentesis*.) This test is extremely helpful in substantiating a diagnosis of inflammatory arthritis, because if the inflammatory white blood cells called **neutrophils** are found in large numbers, and if evidence of other forms of inflammatory arthritis (such as gout crystals) is absent, a diagnosis of RA is supported.

This test is also useful in ruling out other causes of joint swelling or arthritis. Doctors often examine the fluid for the presence of various crystals, which can be seen in the joint fluid of people with other types of arthritis (gout and pseudo-gout). Different types of crystals cause arthritis, **tendinitis,** and **bursitis.** The crystals that cause gout are composed of uric acid, whereas calcium-containing crystals are responsible for pseudo-gout. It is important to distinguish these conditions from RA, because treatment methods for the different conditions vary significantly.

Sampling of the synovial fluid from an inflamed joint is also necessary to look for the presence of infection. This is particularly important when the patient has a fever or is experiencing severe tenderness, swelling, or warmth in a single joint. Even people with established RA may need to be evaluated for infection if one joint is particularly hot and painful.

Diagnostic imaging. Several types of diagnostic tests can be used capture an image of the anatomy in people with RA. The standard x-ray is requested more often than any other kind of imaging method when evaluating for RA. Usually hand and foot x-rays are requested, but any symptomatic joint may warrant examination by x-ray. (Remember, it is common for x-rays to be completely normal in the early stages of RA, even for people with severe symptoms.)

The physician will examine the x-rays for signs of such abnormalities as mild thinning of bone (or decreased density) in the areas near the joints (called periarticular demineralization) and, later, the presence of tiny holes in the bones (erosions) and joint space narrowing. As explained in Chapter 1, erosions occur when **synovitis** has damaged **cartilage** and underlying bone. When cartilage has been eroded, the distance between bones (joint space) on x-rays appears smaller than normal. Since only bone can be seen on plain x-rays, and cartilage appears as black space, it is the black space between bones that is measured. Hence, *joint space narrowing* is actually a misnomer, in that the term really means loss of joint cartilage.

X-rays may also be used to rule out other causes of joint pain, including fractures, calcium deposits near the joints, and bone infection.

Standard x-rays of the chest are sometimes taken to rule out a problem in the lungs, a *rare* complication of RA. Also, some medications for RA (gold, methotrexate, and cyclophosphamide) can cause lung problems—but again, only *rarely*—and x-rays may be taken if symptoms of lung problems develop. Chest x-rays are occasionally scheduled to rule out other highly unusual causes of arthritis that have lung problems associated with them. Standard x-rays can be performed in a physician's office or in a radiology suite.

More sophisticated x-rays, requiring specialized equipment, are used in some situations. These imaging tests include the CAT (computerized axial tomography) scan, or CT scan, the MRI (magnetic resonance imaging), and the bone scan. Unlike standard x-rays, which produce images mostly of bone, CT scans and MRIs also show such tissues as muscle, cartilage, and other joint structures. The bone scan is generally performed to seek evidence of inflammation or infection within the bone. A bone scan can also show inflammation in the joints, but this would be an unusual test for that purpose. (A bone scan should not be confused with a DXA scan [called a "dexa scan"], which is used to look for osteoporosis; see below.)

In recent years, many rheumatologists have started performing *musculoskeletal ultrasound* in their offices. Ultrasound uses sound waves to look at structures inside the body. It has become a very useful tool to look for inflammation in joints, as well as evidence of erosions and other joint damage, and has the advantage of involving no radiation exposure.

Biopsy. When diagnosis is proving particularly difficult, a biopsy of the **synovium** (*joint lining*) is sometimes required. This procedure involves removing a small piece of the synovium from the joint with a special needle or, more commonly, an arthroscope (an instrument through which the physician can view the inside of the joint). Such a *needle biopsy* is performed in the office by some rheumatologists or orthopedic surgeons. The skin and tissues are numbed with local anesthetic (usually lidocaine). This procedure usually causes mild discomfort. *Arthroscopic biopsy* is performed in a surgical suite. After a local, spinal, or general anesthetic is administered, a small incision is made. A scope about the diameter of a pencil is then inserted into the joint through the incision. The tissue is generally removed with the same instrument. This procedure usually involves only mild discomfort. The tissue removed allows the doctor to verify the diagnosis of RA and to exclude other conditions.

Biopsy of other tissues in the body, including muscle, nerve, lung, and skin, is indicated in some of the rare complications of RA (discussed in Chapter 4). Successful execution of these biopsy procedures requires the special skills of physicians who have been trained to perform them.

HLA-DRB1. In some people this genetic marker is present on the surface of specific white blood cells. Many people with RA—about two-thirds of Caucasians with RA—have this genetic marker, and the presence of this gene indicates that the person *may* be susceptible to developing RA. However, since approximately

25 percent of people who do *not* have RA also have this marker, tests for HLA-DRB1 are not conclusive of the presence of RA or even a strong predisposition to develop it. Tests for genetic markers are not routinely available and are performed only in research settings or universities.

Biomarkers. The word *biomarker,* short for *biologic marker,* has different meanings in different fields. For our purposes, it refers to a laboratory test that can be objectively measured and that reflects some biological information about an individual that can help in their treatment plan. Although in its infancy, this area of research is expanding at an incredible rate. They don't exist yet, but some that would be relevant to RA would be:

- an early diagnostic biomarker, which would predict that you are at risk of developing RA
- a prognostic biomarker, which would identify more potentially damaging cases of RA that would warrant stronger medications
- a pharmacologic predictive biomarker, which would determine if a specific medication would work better than others
- a drug safety biomarker, which would determine if a treatment was safe for the individual
- a pharmacologic response biomarker, which would indicate how well a patient is responding to treatment

The availability of biomarkers like these would make an enormous difference in the lives of many people with RA. Some commercial ventures have developed a panel of biomarker tests (such as the Vectra DA) that look at several different biomarkers to give more information to your doctor about the status of your RA. Many research centers are investigating new biomarkers with the hope of finding tests that can individualize the treatment of your RA. The possibility of "personalized medicine" that relies on your body's own individual biology is very exciting.

What Tests Are Used to Rule Out Other Types of Arthritis?

HLA-B27. Blood testing can reveal the presence of another genetic marker, HLA-B27. This marker is often associated with one of several forms of inflammatory arthritis, called *spondylarthropathy,* which can affect the spine as well as tendons and ligaments. Reactive arthritis, ankylosing spondylitis, and psoriatic arthritis are all forms of spondylarthropathy. However, HLA-B27 is also present in about 5 percent of individuals who do not have spondylarthropathy, so it is not a good diagnostic test.

*Antinuclear antibody (ANA).*Testing for this antibody is often requested for people with newly manifested RA symptoms, in an attempt to exclude systemic lupus erythematosus as a diagnosis. Positive (abnormal) results may be an indication of lupus, but a positive result is often also obtained in people with RA. Other conditions associated with ANA include scleroderma, Sjögren's syndrome, and mixed connective tissue disease. In addition, ANA is present in many people without arthritic problems. This test, then, provides clues but not a definitive answer.

Gluten, wheat, and lectin intolerance testing. This is discussed in detail in Chapter 18.

What Tests Are Used to Screen for Complications of RA or Medication Side Effects?

Blood (cell) counts. Three types of blood cells circulate in the bloodstream: red blood cells, white blood cells, and platelets. When all three types of cells are checked through one test, that test is called a *complete blood count* or *CBC*. When information is required about the number and percentage of specific types of white blood cells, a CBC *with differential* is requested. This test is often used to screen for certain drug side effects and to search for evidence of infection.

Red blood cells help carry oxygen to tissues. An insufficiency of red blood cells is called *anemia*. When the number of red blood cells decreases, the delivery of oxygen to tissues decreases. This deficiency of oxygen can result in premature muscle fatigue, decreased stamina, and generalized fatigue and weakness.

Anemia frequently accompanies RA, and it may contribute to the fatigue which many people with RA experience. Anemia is most often a consequence of the **systemic** effects of inflammation on blood, and it often improves as arthritis is treated. However, some medications (such as nonsteroidal anti-inflammatory drugs, **NSAIDs**) can cause inflammation of the stomach lining and mild blood loss. In this situation, the anemia can be a side effect of medication. Finding the exact cause requires further evaluation. The tests used to diagnose and monitor anemia are the **hematocrit** and the **hemoglobin** level. Occasionally, a separate test called the reticulocyte count is indicated; this test reflects the rate at which new red blood cells (*reticulocytes*) are being produced.

The several types of white blood cells include lymphocytes, polymorpho-nuclear leukocytes ("polys" or neutrophils), monocytes, basophils, and eosin-ophils. An important function of white cells is to fight infection; in response to an infection, the body usually produces extra white blood cells, and a blood test would reveal a higher than normal number of them. Having too few white blood cells may interfere with the body's ability to fight infection. Thus, one side effect of any medication that causes a decrease in the number of white blood cells can be infection.

Platelets perform the clotting function in blood. The platelet count is often either high or low in RA. If the platelet count is too low (*thrombocytopenia*), the risk of excessive or spontaneous bleeding is increased. Because some medica-tions reduce the number of platelets in the blood, finding the exact cause of a lowered platelet count requires investigation. High platelet counts (*thrombocy-tosis*) can occur with chronic inflammation; they generally create no particular problems.

Complement studies. These blood studies, which include tests called C3, C4, and CH50, are used to determine whether a particular part of the immune system is activated. They are rarely performed for people who have an uncomplicated case of RA, but they can be helpful when a person has an unusual complication of RA called **vasculitis** (discussed in Chapter 4).

Liver function tests. Liver function or liver enzyme tests are blood tests that may reflect changes in the liver, such as inflammation and organ damage. Findings of minor abnormalities in these tests are common in RA. Interestingly, though, a change in liver function tests does not necessarily mean that the liver's func-tioning capacity has been altered. Elevated levels of liver enzymes generally suggest mild liver irritation or past damage. These tests are often used to search for evidence of pre-existing liver problems or to monitor the side effects of medications. Commonly ordered liver function tests include the SGOT (or AST), SGPT (or ALT), LDH, and alkaline phosphatase.

Urinalysis and kidney (renal) function tests. Examination of a urine specimen is an extremely useful test that most often is requested to screen for medication-induced complications affecting the kidneys. Rarely, patients with RA have minor abnormalities in the urine unrelated to medications.

The evaluation of kidney function is done by blood tests for *creatinine* and *blood urea nitrogen* (BUN). The levels of these substances present in the blood indicate how efficiently the kidney is filtering the body's toxins. Sometimes the physician will request a 24-hour urine collection to measure the excretion of creatinine along with a blood test for creatinine, to obtain an extremely accurate assessment of kidney function. Again, these tests are undertaken to monitor for medication side effects or to look for underlying kidney problems.

TB skin test, QuantiFERON-TB Gold, and T-Spot. Tuberculosis (TB) bacteria can be spread through the air from one person to another. When people get exposed to TB, they may get symptoms of infection in their lungs. Alternatively, the body may form a protective covering that surrounds the TB, and the bacteria become *latent* or inactive in the body. If that person starts taking a medication that suppresses the immune system, the TB bacteria can "awaken" or become activated, and this can cause an active TB infection. This is why, before treatment with **biologics**, people have to get tested for TB.

There are two kinds of tests used to determine if a person has been exposed to TB in the past: the tuberculin skin test and TB blood tests. The TB skin test is also called the *Mantoux tuberculin skin test* or the *PPD*. A small amount of fluid is injected under the skin in the lower part of the arm; 48–72 hours later, the person must have that area evaluated by a trained health professional to see if there is any redness or swelling. TB blood tests (also called interferon-gamma release assays or IGRAs) measure how the immune system reacts to the bacteria that cause TB. The two IGRAs available in the United States are the QuantiFERON-TB Gold In-Tube test and the T-Spot TB test.

Bone density testing or bone densitometry. Bone density testing is often performed to determine if a person is at risk for **osteoporosis,** a condition that is seen more frequently in patients with RA (see Chapter 16). There are several techniques of bone densitometry that can diagnose this condition. The most commonly used technique is called the DXA (dual-energy x-ray absorptiometry, or "dexa") scan. These tests are noninvasive and readily available. The density of bone in the lower spine and hip region, most commonly, but sometimes the forearm as well, is measured by minimal-radiation imaging. The test is very comfortable and does not require needles or medications. It takes approximately 15 minutes. The radiation exposure is very low, markedly less than a normal x-ray. Other measuring techniques include quantitative computed tomography (CT) and quantitative ultrasound.

SUMMARY

The steps taken in reaching a diagnosis of RA are the clinical history, the physical examination, a differential diagnosis, and diagnostic tests.

Standard x-rays and blood tests frequently produce normal results at the onset of arthritis.

At later stages, an evaluation of blood and joint fluid may be useful in the diagnosis of RA.

Once a diagnosis of RA is made, diagnostic tests may be useful in monitoring a person's condition: blood tests and x-rays or other diagnostic imaging can be performed to monitor disease activity and screen for complications of RA, and blood and urine tests are often ordered to screen for medication side effects.

Outside the Joints: Other Symptoms of Rheumatoid Arthritis

As a systemic illness, rheumatoid arthritis (RA) can affect more than one part of the body. That is why people with RA often have symptoms that are seemingly unrelated to joint stiffness or swelling. They may experience generalized fatigue, for example, or they may notice a decrease in appetite or run a low-grade fever.

Symptoms or changes occurring outside the joints are called extra-articular features of RA. Some extra-articular features, such as those mentioned above, are very common and cause only minor discomfort or inconvenience; others, such as swollen lymph nodes (an indication that **inflammation** is affecting other parts of the body), are less common; and still others are extremely rare and frequently serious. It is worth emphasizing that *significantly fewer than 5 percent* of persons with RA develop the most serious consequences of the condition. There is growing evidence that the incidence of these complications is becoming less and less with the introduction of new medications during the past one to two decades. In this chapter, the *less* common extra-articular features of RA are described. If you are experiencing any of these problems, *tell your doctor;* he or she needs to be aware of the situation and should be able to offer assistance.

BLOOD AND BLOOD VESSELS

How Does RA Affect the Blood?

Chapter 3 discussed the importance of testing the blood of a person with RA to determine if that person has *anemia.* This blood disorder, which affects between one-half and two-thirds of all individuals with RA, is the condition that results when the number of red blood cells decreases notably. Anemia may develop as one of the consequences of longstanding inflammation, and its severity often reflects the activity level of the arthritis. Called *anemia of chronic disease,* this type of anemia usually improves if the chronic disease is brought under control. In some situations, the drug *erythropoietin* (EPO) can be administered by a **subcutaneous** (under the skin) injection to increase red blood cell production temporarily. This medication can be used in a presurgical situation, when an individual wants to donate his own blood for a scheduled surgery.

Another kind of anemia, called *iron deficiency anemia,* may develop as a side effect of taking anti-inflammatory drugs, which can irritate the stomach lining and cause minor (or, rarely, major) loss of blood. Anyone who develops iron deficiency anemia needs to be evaluated to determine whether he or she is losing blood from the stomach. This may mean examining the stool for blood or investigating the stomach using other techniques (an endoscopy or upper gastrointestinal x-ray series). It may be necessary to discontinue nonsteroidal anti-inflammatory drug (NSAID) therapy and to begin a course of stomach-healing medication (more information about NSAIDs in Chapter 12).

Anemia may also develop as a component of an increasingly rare complication of RA known as Felty's syndrome. This syndrome, or pattern of symptoms, occurs in considerably fewer than one of one hundred people who have long-standing RA. In addition to having anemia and arthritis, people with Felty's syndrome develop an enlarged spleen and a decreased white blood cell count. A low white blood cell count means a reduction in the body's ability to fight infection and therefore means that infection is more likely to occur. Another complication of this syndrome is a decrease in the number of platelets in the blood, the blood cells involved in clotting. A low platelet count can be dangerous, because it carries the risk of excessive bleeding. Skin ulcerations and dark patches of skin are two other features of Felty's syndrome.

Treatment for Felty's syndrome generally involves use of disease-modifying antirheumatic drugs (**DMARDs**) including **biologics.** Rarely, however, when medication proves ineffective and the person with Felty's syndrome experiences recurrent infections, the person's spleen must be removed surgically.

As noted above, individuals with RA do, rarely, develop a low platelet count (*thrombocytopenia*) as a result of Felty's syndrome. On the other hand, people with RA often have a *high* platelet count (*thrombocytosis*), a condition that is generally harmless and resolves with treatment of the arthritis.

What About the Blood Vessels?

Vasculitis, inflammation of blood vessels, is a rare complication of RA which generally affects individuals who have high levels of **rheumatoid factor** in their blood (the presence and level of rheumatoid factor can be detected by a blood test; see Chapter 3). Blood vessels may become inflamed when too many **antibodies** are being produced by the **plasma cells** in the blood. The antibodies stick to each other and form complexes, and those floating immune complexes sometimes deposit themselves on a blood vessel wall, causing inflammation within the blood vessel and limiting the flow of blood.

Depending on the size and location of the blood vessels involved, vasculitis can be a relatively minor problem or a more significant one. When small blood vessels leading to the skin are involved (particularly the skin in the lower legs), skin ulcers may develop. Splinter-like lesions around and under the fingernails may result when small blood vessels in that area are affected. These ulcers and lesions generally require only meticulous skin care (in addition to treatment of the underlying arthritis) to prevent secondary infection of the skin. Gently washing several times a day with a mild antiseptic soap and then thoroughly rinsing and drying the skin and applying sterile bandages is usually effective for this. Occasionally the advice and services of a **plastic surgeon** or **dermatologist** are useful. There are also certified *wound care specialists* and even wound care centers that specialize in the treatment of skin ulcers as well as other slow-healing skin wounds.

When blood vessels leading to nerves are affected by vasculitis, numbness or weakness of a limb may result (this condition is known as *neuropathy*). More rarely, vasculitis involves the larger blood vessels that lead to internal organs. When nerves or internal organs are affected by vasculitis, very strong medications, including **corticosteroids** and cyclophosphamide, are used to treat the condition and prevent damage to nerves and organs.

EYES AND MOUTH

About 15 percent of people with RA develop *sicca syndrome*, which causes them to have a dry mouth, dry eyes, or both. This syndrome produces inflammation in the tear glands, which in turn causes the eyes to become uncomfortably dry. Eyes that are not being bathed by sufficient quantities of tears can feel itchy or gritty or it may feel as if there is something in them. Occasionally, the eyelids become red and irritated.

A dry, windy climate or exposure to air conditioning can aggravate the symptoms, as can medications; certain kinds of cold medications, sleep-inducing medications, tranquilizers, muscle relaxants, and narcotic analgesics can all increase eye dryness. If you are experiencing a problem with dry eyes, you may want to review your medications with your doctor. To help reduce the irritation of dry eyes, we also recommend the use of one of the many kinds of eye lubricants, or artificial tears, which are available both over the counter and by prescription.

Any other symptoms involving the eyes, such as pain, redness, or a change of vision, should immediately be brought to the attention of a physician. An **ophthalmologist** can examine the eyes to rule out the presence of two other conditions that can affect the eyes in RA. These rare conditions, called **scleritis** and **episcleritis,** may require treatment with corticosteroids in topical form (applied to the site of the problem) or occasionally with medications taken by mouth. These serious complications of RA need to be monitored closely by an ophthalmologist.

Dry mouth is another possible consequence of RA and is thought to be caused by inflammation of the salivary glands. Any of the medications mentioned above can exacerbate the problem of dry mouth, too.

For people who have a dry mouth, excellent oral hygiene is crucial, because a decrease in saliva can prompt tooth decay. Flossing the teeth and then gargling with an antiseptic mouthwash followed by thorough brushing with a tartar control toothpaste several times a day will help provide protection against decay. Ask your dentist what products are right for you, and find out from your dentist whether fluoride treatments might be a good idea. It is also important to avoid lozenges and candies that contain sugar. You have read in Chapter 1 about the possible relationship of **periodontal disease** to RA. This is another reason to maintain meticulous oral hygiene. Anyone who has a severe problem with mouth dryness or who experiences recurring swollen salivary glands should ask to be tested for primary *Sjögren's syndrome,* a condition that resembles RA.

Two treatments are available that stimulate the salivary glands to produce saliva. These two medications are pilocarpine (Salagen) and cevimeline (Evoxac). Possible side effects of these medications include sweating and palpitations.

Speak to your doctor if eye or mouth dryness is a severe problem for you.

NODULES UNDER THE SKIN

People generally first notice skin nodules while dressing or bathing. They appear beneath the skin as small knots called rheumatoid **nodules,** and they occur in approximately one-quarter of people with established RA. They are more likely to appear in people who have rheumatoid factor than in people who don't have it (see Chapter 3).

Skin nodules often form close to joints, overlying areas that are susceptible to trauma or pressure, such as tendons or bony protrusions like the elbows, knuckles, or Achilles tendon. They often come and go in a pattern that follows the pattern of arthritis.

Rheumatoid nodules are benign (harmless) lumps that should not be confused with enlarged lymph nodes or tumors (which may or may not be harmless). The nodules are only bothersome when they press against internal body structures, interfere with the motion of a joint or tendon, or become infected. Rheumatoid nodules are not painful unless they are positioned in an area that is frequently traumatized, such as the heel tendon, which is rubbed by the back of the shoe. Rheumatoid nodules rarely appear in places other than the skin. On occasion they do appear in the lungs, heart, eyes, and vocal cords, but even in these places they seldom produce symptoms. There is evidence that the incidence of nodules is decreasing with the decreasing severity of RA noticed over the past decades, thanks to the introduction of new classes of medication.

Rheumatoid nodules themselves do not merit special treatment unless they cause pain, decrease function, or become infected. Anyone who has rheumatoid nodules, however, should be considered for treatment with drugs that can produce remission, since the presence of nodules may indicate a more serious form of arthritis. Successful treatment with DMARDs and biologics can result in the resolution of nodules as well as improvement in arthritis. If a particular nodule is causing problems, surgical removal is an option. Although removal of rheumatoid nodules for cosmetic reasons is generally discouraged, surgery is occasionally performed to improve a person's appearance.

While it has been believed that *all* rheumatoid nodules are associated with having a more serious form of RA, there does appear to be an exception. A special form of rheumatoid nodule can occur in patients being treated with methotrexate. These nodules are sometimes referred to as *micro-nodules* because they are smaller than typical rheumatoid nodules. They most commonly form around the finger joints. About 8 percent of patients on methotrexate develop micro-nodules, though it is not clear why. The development of micro-nodules does *not* suggest that methotrexate is ineffective for your arthritis. If the micro-nodules are troubling, the addition of hydroxychloroquine (Plaquenil) can sometimes reduce their size.

NERVES

One form of neuropathy associated with RA, as described above, is a rare complication resulting from inflammation in blood vessels that lead to nerves. A more common form of neuropathy found in some people with RA is one in which the person develops numbness or a burning sensation in a "glove-and-stocking" distribution *without* any obvious blood vessel disturbance. In most cases, this second type of neuropathy improves with the effective treatment of the arthritis.

Inflammation can create localized pressure that squeezes or pinches a nerve and thereby causes numbness or weakness in the area served by that nerve. This *nerve compression* can also result from swelling or from structural changes occurring in the joint. Nerves that travel near joints in the elbows and feet are sometimes compressed in RA, the most commonly pinched nerve being the median nerve that runs through the wrist. When the wrist becomes swollen, pressure increases in the joint, and the nerve becomes compressed. This causes numbness and tingling in the middle three fingers, a condition known as *carpal tunnel syndrome.* Carpal tunnel syndrome can also develop if the nerve becomes bent or kinked. Chronic inflammation sometimes changes the alignment of the wrist and so causes the nerve to deviate from its normal path. People who don't have RA can also develop carpal tunnel syndrome. It occurs most commonly in people who keep their wrists bent in the same position for long periods of time (such as people who work at computer terminals).

Wrist splints often help decrease symptoms of carpal tunnel syndrome in RA patients. Other means of decreasing inflammation, such as anti-inflammatory medications or corticosteroid injections into the wrist, are also helpful. If the symptoms of carpal tunnel syndrome are severe or persistent, surgery may be required.

CHEST AND LUNGS

RA can produce breathing discomfort in two ways. The first occurs when the joints between the collar bones (*clavicles*) and breastbone (*sternum*) develop arthritis (see sternoclavicular joints in Figure 1). In this situation, experienced by about 30 percent of people with RA, pain can occur when deep breaths are taken or when the shoulders are moved. The condition improves with treatment of the arthritis.

Between 10 and 20 percent of people with RA may at some point develop the other source of breathing discomfort, pleurisy, which causes pain deep in the chest upon inhalation and results from inflammation in the lining around the lungs (*pleura*). A complication of this inflammation is pleural effusion, or fluid around the lungs, which less than 5 percent of people with RA develop. This fluid generally produces few symptoms, and its presence is determined by x-ray. Pleurisy and pleural effusion frequently improve with effective treatment of RA. If significant symptoms appear from pleural effusion, drainage of the fluid with a needle can be performed as an outpatient procedure. Temporary treatment with oral corticosteroids may be required. Both pleurisy and pleural effusions can have causes other than RA, so their presence may prompt further diagnostic evaluation by your physician.

Rarely, rheumatoid nodules develop in the lungs; these nodules are similar to those under the skin. They generally cause no symptoms and are diagnosed by x-ray. The greatest medical difficulty with such internal nodules is determining whether they are a result of RA or another, unrelated, condition. A biopsy of the nodule may be required to determine its cause.

In only 1 or 2 percent of individuals with RA, a more serious lung problem known as pneumonitis (also called interstitial lung disease) arises. Cough and shortness of breath are indications that this problem may exist. Because the lung tissue is inflamed in pneumonitis, anti-inflammatory medications are administered to decrease inflammation and prevent scarring (*fibrosis*).

Sometimes, but rarely, RA causes severe breathing difficulty, and the person requires hospitalization and urgent treatment to recover. If you ever experience difficulty breathing, be sure to consult your physician.

VOCAL CORDS

Another rare complication of RA is involvement of the joints of the vocal cords (*cricoarytenoid joints*). Usually there are no symptoms when this occurs, although some persons experience hoarseness, difficulty swallowing, a feeling of fullness in the throat, or pain radiating toward the ear. This complication is usually evaluated and treated by an ear, nose, and throat (ENT) doctor.

THE HEART AND CARDIOVASCULAR SYSTEM

The heart is seldom involved in RA, and when the heart is affected, most people experience no symptoms. When inflammation involves the membranous sac enclosing the heart (the pericardium), however, the person may experience symptoms similar to those of pleurisy (see above). This condition is called *pericarditis*. In very rare situations, a significant amount of fluid accumulates around the heart, a condition called *pericardial effusion*. This condition usually responds to corticosteroids (the fluid is reabsorbed by the body) and only seldom requires drainage of the fluid. Other parts of the heart are rarely involved in RA.

Of more concern, and a condition that occurs more commonly in people with RA, is cardiovascular disease, or plaque formation in the arteries of the heart (atherosclerosis, sometimes referred to as "hardening of the arteries"). This condition is common in Americans, with and without RA. There is increasing evidence that all forms of chronic inflammation can contribute to blood vessel atherosclerosis, which underscores the importance of getting inflammation under control. This is another reason for doctors to request the blood test C reactive protein (CRP) for RA patients. Equally important to controlling inflammation is improving any risk factors for heart disease that are in your control, such as high blood pressure, smoking, obesity, high cholesterol, chronic stress, and physical inactivity. We will be talking about how we can control most of these factors in several of the other chapters.

THE BONES

People with RA are at higher risk of developing osteoporosis than is the general population. *Osteoporosis* is "thinning" of the bones or decreased bone mass. Loss of bone density makes a person more likely to sustain fractures. Researchers have recently discovered that inflammation plays a major role in the development of osteoporosis, even early in the course of RA. Pro-inflammatory **cytokines** can stimulate the activity of a group of bone cells called osteoclasts. In the normal life of bone, osteoclasts break down bone, causing some bone loss on a daily basis in everyone. This breaking down is balanced, however, by other cells, called osteoblasts, which build bone. During skeletal growth or bone building, the osteoblasts work harder than the osteoclasts, and bone growth occurs. In situations such as RA and menopause, the balance favors the osteoclasts, so bone loss occurs. Monitoring bone loss by bone densitometry (see "Bone density testing" in Chapter 3) is increasingly being regarded as important, particularly since there are now medications available to put the system back into balance and help restore good bone strength.

Women are at higher risk for osteoporosis than men are, because they start with less bone mass, and at menopause bone loss speeds up considerably. Men with RA are at higher risk for osteoporosis than men without RA. In addition to the direct effects of RA on bone, other changes can occur. Men with RA can have low levels of testosterone, which can cause additional bone loss and osteoporosis (Stafford et al., 2000).

Some arthritis medications can increase the risk for osteoporosis. Corticosteroids are the most common cause of drug-induced bone loss. Lifestyle choices such as smoking and heavy alcohol use are toxic to bone. Also, being too sedentary and avoiding weight bearing exercises increase a person's risk of developing osteoporosis. A diet low in calcium and vitamin D also contributes to osteoporosis. (See Chapter 16 for osteoporosis treatments.)

SUMMARY

Nonspecific symptoms of RA, including decreased appetite, low-grade fever, minor weight loss, and swollen lymph nodes, are relatively common and are usually not serious.

Red blood cell, white blood cell, and platelet counts can be affected by RA.

People with RA may experience dry eyes and dry mouth.

Rheumatoid nodules can occur over areas that receive pressure.

Serious involvement of the lungs, heart, eyes, nerves, and blood vessels can occur in RA, but these complications are increasingly rare.

People with RA are at higher risk of developing osteoporosis.

Many of these conditions improve as the arthritis is brought under control, whereas others require separate pharmaceutical or surgical treatment.

COPING WITH
RHEUMATOID ARTHRITIS

5

Lifestyle and Coping Strategies

Life brings with it a series of changes, some of them predictable, others unpredictable. We encounter these changes, react to them, and adjust accordingly, often without being fully aware of what we're doing. Coping strategies that we develop along the way help us make effective adjustments so that we can grow with the resolution of each challenge and then move forward to face new experiences.

Because it brings a series of changes, life requires a series of adjustments. Those of you who are encountering the challenges posed by rheumatoid arthritis (RA) may know that physical, emotional, and financial changes may take place in your life during the coming years. You also know that there is no way to predict which changes will affect your life or when they will do so. Consider, though, that *now* may be the time to learn coping strategies that will enable you to adjust effectively to these changes, whatever they are and whenever they occur. We cannot control most of what happens to us, but we can control our reactions to those events. You can learn how to view change differently from a place of peaceful coexistence with reality. Stress is the inevitable result when we fail to adapt, and therefore failure to make adjustments can make life even harder.

Excessive stress is hard on anyone, but it has even larger ramifications for people with RA. New information has revealed that acute stress can actually *increase the signs inflammation* in the bloodstream. As part of our response to stress, the brain sends messages to the immune system which result in the release of **cytokines**, which worsen pain and swelling. This is probably not a surprise to many of you who have noticed that a flare-up of arthritis commonly follows a very stressful event. The results of chronic stress can have even larger ramifications. There are data suggesting that chronic stress can have an effect on your body's genetics. You have read about the growing field of **epigenetics** in Chapter 1. There is scientific evidence that exposing your genes to stress hormones over a long time can change the way the genes deliver information. Chronic stress can actually "switch on" parts of the genetic code that carry the potential for causing health problems. So, learning healthy coping mechanisms to deal with the unpredictable nature of life is crucial for our health.

How will you address each of the changes RA brings to your life? How can you effectively meet the challenges that lie before you? You can explore various coping strategies that have worked for other people and then develop and apply those that work best for you.

The coping strategies we will describe are neither complicated nor exotic. Most rely heavily on your own intuition and simply require you to draw them from within yourself in times of change. In fact, you have used them all of your life without realizing it. For example, consider that coping skills allowed you to make the transition from being a vulnerable youth to being a competent adult. You learned to cope with—and adjust to—being away from your family, earning your own money, buying groceries and preparing your own meals, and on and on.

To cope effectively with RA, you must try to recapture the openness of youth and temper it with the wisdom learned from experience. This involves developing new skills while improving upon old ones at the same time. With your wisdom, you give up the struggle to remain the same—recognizing its futility. Albert Einstein recognized this when he reasoned, "I must be willing to give up what I am in order to become what I will be." And what you can become has endless possibility. With the open heart of youth, you can continue to experience joy, enthusiasm, and the excitement that life offers us, with or without arthritis.

What's essential here is that you create a healthful lifestyle and develop strategies that are effective for *you*. It's been shown time and again that people benefit most from the strategies that they tailor for themselves, to fit their own needs. These strategies can be called into play over and over again as you approach each new challenge or crisis.

The coping strategies that we will discuss fit into two broad categories. The first involves creating a lifestyle and attitude aimed at wellness. There is no doubt that mastering a healthy lifestyle will empower you to cope with arthritis both mentally and physically. There is evidence that these lifestyle changes are an important component of improving your RA in a very tangible way. In addition to this, one cannot discount the enormous benefit of taking an active and positive stance in creating your own wellness. We know, however, that day-to-day obstacles do not disappear just because we are living well with a positive attitude. The second category of strategies will help you master methods of problem solving that will enable you to address those obstacles successfully.

The following guidelines may help you begin to design and adapt successful strategies for living well, even thriving, with RA, and help you cope with other aspects of your life, too. Here's a quick overview:

Creating a lifestyle and attitude aimed at wellness

- Kick bad habits.
- Eat right.
- Get fit.
- Get sleep.
- Think prevention.
- Go simple.
- Don't sweat the big stuff.
- Be your own best friend.

Developing success-driven methods of problem solving

- Define and assess the problem.
- Set realistic goals and expectations.
- Develop methods for problem solving and negotiating.
- Use all available resources.
- Modify negative thoughts and behaviors.
- Be willing to reassess.

In this chapter and the next two you will learn about powerful coping strategies such as creativity, humor, thinking positively, surrendering to events beyond your control, being proactive, and communicating your needs with grace and compassion. Successful coping involves a journey toward self-awareness. Finding or returning to one's core self is powerful and enriching.

In the remainder of this chapter we will provide general information about what's involved in each of these guidelines. In Chapter 6 we suggest ways in which the strategies developed from these guidelines may help you cope with pain and fatigue. Chapter 7 describes how these strategies might be applied to help you handle your emotions and other people's reactions to your illness— because people sometimes respond in a way that is patronizing or hurtful, often without meaning to.

CREATING A LIFESTYLE AND ATTITUDE AIMED AT WELLNESS

Kick Bad Habits

When first diagnosed with a chronic condition, you may feel like much is being taken away from you. But you have it in your power to create a healthful lifestyle and to give yourself something positive and rewarding. When you eliminate habits that limit your health, you will feel a sense of empowerment. We spoke in Chapter 1 about smoking and how it can possibly cause or worsen RA. None of us can change the past. However, let's look at the flip side. There is now compelling information that becoming smoke-free may lessen the severity of your RA as well as improve so many other aspects of your health. The need to make this change becomes an opportunity for wellness, and it is something that is within your power.

Will it be easy to stop smoking? Of course not. Smoking, for many, is like a reliable old friend that is always there to reach out for in times of stress—quite literally, an arm's length away. And isn't stopping smoking just giving up one more thing? Well, yes, but when we give up any toxic or dysfunctional relationship, in the end we are better for it. The first step is to decide to do it. We cannot emphasize that enough. Many people want to stop but that is not enough. You must *decide* to stop, and it has to come from you, not from your friends, family, or doctor. Once you've decided in your heart of hearts, the rest will follow. Ask for any help you need—from your doctor, from smoking cessation programs. Make a clean break of it. Dysfunctional friendships can't be reserved for special occasions, times of severe stress, or to be rewards for work well done. It will start with "just this one time" and soon that toxic old buddy will be hanging on for dear life! You will miss him, and you may grieve. But you will heal and open yourself to new health-enhancing habits. And, these habits will become friends worth keeping. But if you do slip, as we all will, show yourself compassion. Get up the next morning, escort your old friend to the curb, and don't look back. Every day is a new opportunity.

There are other unhealthful activities that people may use to self-soothe or to escape the sometimes difficult realities of our lives. Some of these habits include excessive alcohol or drug use, chronic overeating, and gambling. Regardless of what it may be, you will know that it is an unhealthful coping mechanism if it takes something away from your health, your self-esteem, or your relationships. When you walk away from these habits, you open the door for activities that can improve your health and well-being.

Eat Right

One of our most powerful prerogatives is the choice of what we put into our bodies. New data suggest that obesity can play a powerful role in promoting inflammation in RA. There is also new evidence that specific foods can promote inflammation. We discuss specific foods and diets as they relate to RA in Chapter 18. Here we are looking at diet as a lifestyle choice and a way to create health-enhancing coping skills. Clearly, one must rely on many skills in this arena. First, trying to learn what is best to eat with RA is a big task, given the enormous amount of information available and the ever-changing recommendations that we read in the scientific as well as the lay literature. So, the commitment to healthful eating requires a commitment to life-long learning. Hence, you will need to rely on the coping skills of curiosity, discerning investigation, flexibility, and a good deal of intuition. Regardless of changes in recommendations over time, we know that a healthful diet will be composed of fresh, whole (as found in nature) foods and avoidance of processed foods. Success will require a significant time investment for the purchasing and preparation of healthful meals. This will utilize the very important coping skills of forethought, planning, time management, and negotiation with yourself—no small feat. The reward will be healthful nutrition for you and your family and the knowledge that you are making that happen with your energy and resources. Mealtime will be an experience that you can have pride in, knowing that you have been proactive. And most importantly, well-planned meal choices may very well have a direct role in improving your RA.

Get Fit

Feeling strong and fit is one of the best coping mechanisms available. A consistent physical fitness program will help reduce anxiety, improve energy, and enhance your general health in many diverse ways. We cover exercise extensively in Chapters 9 and 10.

Get Sleep

Having a good night's sleep is important for all of us. There is no doubt that having joint pain can interfere with your sleep. Researchers have found that people with RA who do not get a full night's sleep most nights have more joint pain, as well as fatigue, and are more often depressed (Irwin et al., 2012). You can see how this can easily become a vicious cycle. Addressing sleep issues is very important in your journey to wellness. First of all, you must be *in your bed for enough time* to get enough sleep. This is a huge issue for people. You have to plan ahead in order to set aside a minimum of 8 hours for sleep; the requirement for people with RA is usually higher than for most people. I suggest adding, at least, another hour to that for "wind down time" before you try to sleep.

Stay away from stimulants, including alcohol, caffeine, nicotine, and sugar, in the evening. Review your medications and supplements with your doctor to make sure none are stimulants. Your physical comfort is paramount for a restful sleep and will take some planning. This may include taking sleep-inducing medications, applying heat patches to sore joints, or taking a warm shower or bath. Do what it takes to be pain-free at bedtime, and don't be afraid to ask your doctor for help. Your sleeping space should be dark, quiet, comfortable, and relaxing. Get rid of electronic devices and anything else that emits light (that includes televisions). Light disrupts the body's production of melatonin, a hormone that helps us sleep. Having the right mattress, pillow, blanket, and bedclothes is as important as taking the right medications. Taking the time to relax your mind as well as your body before bedtime is so important. Whether it is listening to music, breathing therapeutic aromas, meditating or praying, petting your dog or cat, or simply chatting quietly with your beloved, make the time to quietly exit your day with a peaceful mind. Never go to bed angry. If you have tasks you can't get off your mind, write down a "to do" list and resolve to let it go until morning.

Think Prevention

Staying well incorporates many important preventive behaviors. Clearly good nutrition, fitness initiatives, healthy habits, stress reduction, and adequate sleep are part of any prevention strategy. It is also important to manage other aspects of your health, such as blood pressure, blood sugar, and cholesterol. Staying up to date on mammograms, pelvic examinations, rectal examinations, prostate checks, colonoscopies, eye examinations, and routine vaccinations will help you to address issues before they can interfere with your good health.

There is another area of routine health maintenance that is particularly important in people with rheumatoid arthritis, and that is dental hygiene. You read in Chapter 1 about how a change in oral bacteria over the millennia likely contributed to the development of RA. And we know that *periodontal disease* (PD) is a very strong risk factor for developing RA in a person with the right genetic predisposition. We also know that people who already have RA have a higher than usual risk of developing gum disease. And research shows that people with persistent PD do not respond as well to RA treatment with TNF blockers, a biologic medication used to treat RA (see Chapter 14), as do those without PD (Savioli et al., 2012). For these reasons, preventing and treating periodontal disease is extremely important.

But, will changing the bacteria in our mouths to more healthful bacteria improve the outcome in RA? One study (Ortiz, 2009) confirmed that periodontal treatments, including scaling and root planing, and following oral hygiene recommendations, resulted in a decrease in RA symptoms, as well as an improvement in ESR results (an inflammation test; see Chapter 3) and levels of TNF (an inflammatory cytokine; see Chapter 1). It makes sense that, if we eliminate a potential trigger, there is the possibility that we may break part of the cycle of inflammation. The simple and inexpensive steps of frequent brushing, flossing, and routine dental care can make a significant difference in your RA and general health. Quitting smoking also improves oral health. Equally important is getting sugar out of your diet to the extent that it is possible. You will read much more about this in Chapter 18. You will also read about a thought-provoking ancient practice called "oil pulling" in Chapter 17.

Go Simple

Our lives are so much more complicated than they used to be. Technological advances are wonderful and have brought tremendous innovations into our reach, but in many ways they have rendered our lives more complex. If we are "successful," in others' estimation, we create and continuously build an infrastructure of our life. Then, we spend our vital resources—time, money, and energy—supporting the massive construction that we have created. Because we have no time, we reward ourselves and bribe our children with more stuff. No wonder that we feel drained and stressed!

Every one of us needs to take a hard look at this situation in our lives, whether or not we have a chronic disease. When you have RA, it is even more important to examine how you are spending your resources. You will need to spend your valuable energy on things that enrich your body and your spirit. This will mean taking a step back and objectively looking at your life. Eliminate things and activities that do not enhance your or your family's lives in a meaningful way. It is eye opening to see what you can thrive without. When you invest your valuable resources in things that really matter, the payback is impressive.

Don't Sweat the Big Stuff

When I was young, I loved spending time with my grandmother. She was beautiful, confident, joyous, and terribly funny. I felt happy, safe, and important just being near her. She had not had what many would call a blessed life. She had seen adversity many times including losing a young daughter and two husbands. I asked my mother why Granny did so well, given all that she had lost. Her answer was simple: "Granny never sweats the big stuff." I have thought about her answer so many times through the years. We all know how to not sweat the small stuff: we get past life's small hurdles by looking forward and seeing that they won't affect us in the long run, and that helps us cope. But what if the hurdles are big and they *do* affect us in the long run? What then?

How do you deal with a significant change like finding out that you have RA? How do you avoid fear, anxiety, anger, frustration, blame, and withdrawal? The answer is surprisingly simple. You choose to. You choose to accept change with quiet grace and without judgment. You choose to walk away from the futile struggle to remain the same. You choose to avoid the internal melodrama of reacting to what is beyond your control. And most importantly, you choose to keep your heart open. People who can view change as a natural course of life and continue to accept and offer love willingly and fully, without restriction, are a great inspiration to us. And, you can be your own inspiration every day. This doesn't mean that you shouldn't feel sad or take the time to work through a loss or bad news, which can temporarily cause anger and grief. It simply means that if you can find a way to accept change with an open heart, your inner energy will emerge to heal you mentally, emotionally, and physically. You will be nourished and healed by your own inner spirit. So make a choice to sidestep the battle, skip the melodrama, keep your heart open, and, like my grandmother, not sweat the big stuff.

Be Your Own Best Friend

As you tackle these new coping strategies, there will be days when you won't be at your best. You won't eat the right foods. You might be too tired to exercise or make the time for planning healthy meals. You may be late for work or yell at your kids for no good reason. You are human and have frailty. We all do. Show yourself the loving kindness that you would show a dear friend. Give yourself the grace of understanding. Don't breathe life into these misdemeanors. Get a good night's sleep that night. Quiet your mind. Tomorrow you can mend any transgressions and start again. No worries.

DEVELOPING SUCCESS-DRIVEN METHODS OF PROBLEM SOLVING

Define and Assess the Problem

To confront a problem, you first need to identify it. Although this may appear to be the obvious first step, it is a step that many people fail to take; and, once attempted, it is a step that often proves more difficult than people think. As an example, suppose you are frustrated because you are having difficulty removing lids from jars. It may be that the physical act of removing the lids is your problem, but consider that this is easily remedied by calling upon other people to help you or by purchasing one of the many assistive devices (discussed in Chapter 8). If you ask for and obtain assistance from someone else or if you purchase an assistive device and are pleased with the results, then the physical act *was* the problem, and it has been solved. If using these appliances or asking for assistance makes you feel dependent or inadequate, however, the problem is not your inability to remove the jar lids but your response to the need to seek assistance with a task that formerly you could perform easily on your own. In that case, identifying the problem becomes more difficult.

Before you can address it, you must recognize that a problem exists. Before you can solve a problem, you must *properly* identify it. As a general guideline, recognize that there will be times when you will need to think carefully about your own feelings to identify a problem properly.

Assessing a problem is different from identifying it. Assessment can best be carried out when you are as informed as possible about factual matters related to the problem. Being informed is particularly important if a physical limitation becomes a major problem, and that is one reason we recommend that you learn as much as you can about arthritis and its possible complications.

Consider this scenario: You have numbness in your fingers that wakes you up at night. Consequently, your sleep is disturbed, and you are constantly fatigued. If you think that feeling sleepy is your major problem, you are mistaken. The numbness—the cause of your restless nights—is the origin of your difficulties. Rather than taking sleeping pills as the first resort, a better course would be to pause to identify the problem properly and then to assess it. Seek more information. Dig deep. If you do, you will learn that inflammation in the wrists sometimes causes carpal tunnel syndrome, and you will also learn that wearing a wrist splint at night or getting an injection of a **corticosteroid** can make the numbness disappear, allowing more restful sleep. The combination of proper identification and appropriate information, then, can often lead to more appropriate treatment and a better resolution of a problem.

There will definitely be times when you'll need to consult more than one source of information to assess a problem. When you are consulting a physician, for example, you may want to obtain an opinion from a different physician (get a "second opinion") to satisfy yourself that you have enough information to assess and address the problem. Sometimes you'll want to talk with someone else just to get a fresh perspective on the problem. These are fine strategies, but a word of caution is in order here: it is important to avoid *overintellectualizing* a problem. If you spend all of your energy analyzing a problem, you will not move any closer to addressing it or solving it. It is easy to become obsessed with getting all the information, particularly with the availability of the Internet. Reading every available book and article on a subject or consulting numerous physicians ("doctor shopping") is an exaggerated version of a healthy analysis of a problem.

Set Realistic Goals and Expectations

For everyone, what is a realistic goal at one moment in our lives is not realistic at another time, and what would not have been a problem under different circumstances may now be presenting difficulties. When a problem is interfering with a goal, you might ask yourself whether the goal is realistic *at this particular time.* If you determine that the goal is unrealistic, you may find that what had seemed to be a problem no longer is, or that you needn't confront the problem you've been struggling with until later, when it may be more easily overcome. Or maybe, if you change your goal, you won't have to confront a particular problem at all or will be able to work around it. Do not let unrealistic expectations convince you that you are in a no-win situation.

For example, if you begin an exercise program and you decide you want to be able to walk three miles by the third day, you are setting an unreasonable goal. If your house is a mess and you are not feeling well and you set a goal of having the house spotless by sunset, you are setting an unreasonable goal. Setting unreasonable goals sets you up to be disappointed and discouraged, and discouragement may make you give up on your exercise program or put off yet again getting a start on household chores. On the other hand, you may succeed in meeting an unrealistic goal but pay too large a price in the days that follow.

A wiser plan is to divide goals into segments of small tasks that can be accomplished in steps. Not only will your ultimate goal stand a better chance of being accomplished (although perhaps in a week rather than a day or in four weeks rather than one), but also, encouraged by achievement of the smaller goals, you will gain confidence in your capability to reach the other goals you set for yourself.

It is often helpful to make a contract with yourself, composed of incremental assignments leading to the eventual goal. Success breeds success. Failure to attain an unrealistic expectation may make you resist trying again or afraid to try again. It may lower your confidence and self-esteem. On the other hand, when your self-expectations are in line with your capability, you are more likely to succeed.

A word about exercise plans (which are discussed in more detail in Chapters 9 and 10): If your goal is to improve your strength and endurance, don't be a weekend athlete. Instead, set daily exercise goals. Taking this approach will make it much more likely that you'll meet your goal.

Develop Methods for Problem Solving and Negotiating

You have identified a problem and established a reasonable goal. How do you proceed? How can you overcome barriers and reach your goal? You have several choices. You can

- eliminate the problem,
- circumvent it,
- work with the obstacle, or
- modify the goal.

Each of these methods is effective in different situations. This is where imagination and creativity come into play.

Eliminating the problem. After several weeks of having trouble rising from a chair because of arthritis in your knee, you discover that it is easier for you to get out of seats that are elevated. You then eliminate the problem by placing a firm, three-inch pillow in the seats of the chairs you regularly use. Your arthritis is still there, but the problem is solved.

A number of similar modifications can be made in your home and workplace environment to eliminate physical obstacles. In many ways, physical obstacles are the easiest to confront, but other kinds of challenges can also be resolved by eliminating the problem. Let your imagination expand the boundaries of your ideas.

Circumventing the problem. Problem solving often involves working around a problem by, for example, changing habits and schedules. A common dilemma for people with RA is a workday that begins early, when morning stiffness restricts movement. One way around this problem would be to start the workday later, if this could be arranged with your employer. Then, although morning stiffness will not disappear, no longer will it interfere with your work.

Working with the obstacle. People often find that working with an obstacle that cannot be modified poses a serious challenge. Imagine, for example, that you are a trained data-entry person and you have arthritis in your fingers. You must work at the computer, but prolonged typing causes your fingers to hurt and cramp up. You enjoy your job and don't want to change it. To solve this problem you must first accept the obstacle (arthritis in your finger joints) and then move on from there.

In this situation, numerous options are available to someone who has developed coping strategies. One might be to take frequent breaks at regular intervals, before fatigue and pain develop. During breaks from the computer, you can perform other tasks that you save for such times. You might want to keep a list of these tasks near the computer, so you will be reminded that you always have other work to turn to, and you will not feel as if you are wasting time while you are giving your hands a break.

You might use your creative resources to research technologies that are available to perform the needed tasks with less repetition. New technological advances appear every day, and one might be available to solve your problem.

You can also call upon two interpersonal skills, communication and negotiation, and discuss with your supervisor your wish to assume other job responsibilities to replace some of the time you formerly spent at the computer. Expanding your job description to include other useful, but less physically demanding, responsibilities will balance your day. While you are making changes, you may also want to diversify your skills. For example, you might want to enroll in some courses that would prepare you to take on new tasks.

Work toward becoming more organized and imaginative. You may find that your productivity (and value to your employer) actually increases when you stretch yourself and your horizons. Remember that your greatest attribute is your mind.

Modifying the goal. This is frequently a useful avenue for solving problems. Modifying the goal might involve changing your timetable for completion of a task or dividing the task into smaller goals, as discussed above. Once you have established that your goal is realistic, you'll still need to reassess it and modify it along the way. It is this fine-tuning that will allow you to succeed in your endeavors.

Developing skills such as effective communication, organization, and scheduling is a crucial part of problem solving. Using these skills should not be considered overcompensation. Rather, using them will allow you to make the most of your potential. Armed with these skills, people with arthritis often become more productive in every aspect of their lives.

Use All Available Resources

People are often surprised to discover how much inner strength they can muster when they are faced with adversity. The truth, however, is that we all depend on our inner resources to get through each day. Intangibles such as courage, optimism, and faith, as well as our creativity and skill in problem solving, are always at our disposal to help us overcome hurdles. Remember to look for them and put them to use.

You don't have to depend solely on your own inner strength, however. Family, friends, co-workers, health care professionals, arthritis support groups, religious groups, social service organizations, and vocational rehabilitation centers—any and all of these can be invaluable sources of support and encouragement. Although some of these people are trained and skilled in helping, others who are willing to help will need some guidance to know how they can be of assistance. Access to resources for people with rheumatoid arthritis has never been better.

Although you may be hesitant to seek outside help, you might consider that utilizing the special skills and support of other people benefits them as well as you. By helping you to help yourself, their assistance may allow you to retain your independence; and their lives will also be richer, since they have been able to contribute something to someone who needed their help.

Modify Negative Thoughts and Behaviors

When a new problem develops, it is tempting to indulge in negative thinking. After all, negative thinking is a part of human nature, and we all fall victim to it on occasion. Because RA is a chronic condition and the problems it poses can appear overwhelming, it is only natural that negative thoughts will occupy you from time to time.

It can be hard work to maintain a positive attitude. When we're in the middle of a thunderstorm, it is difficult to focus on the sun hidden behind the clouds. While acknowledging the difficulty of maintaining a positive attitude, let it be said: *Persistent negative thinking is harmful.* Persistent negative thinking can be our worst enemy. For one thing, negativism is often irrational in that it is based on emotions more than on facts. Focusing on negative thoughts usually makes us feel worse, and negative thoughts can lead us to take negative actions, alienating the people we love and need. Finally, negative thinking does not lead us to develop solutions to problems or help us to accomplish goals. In other words, it doesn't lead us to where we want to be.

Try to be vigilant about negative thinking: if negative thoughts go unchecked, they escalate. They tend to worsen and start distorting your perception of events and people. If you notice that negative thoughts are settling in to stay awhile, stop yourself immediately and redirect your thoughts. Tell yourself whatever will help you to stop these thoughts. For example, you might ask yourself, "How does this thought help me?" Or you can say to yourself, "Stop this useless garbage," "Enough of this negative thinking," "These ideas are getting me nowhere." Perhaps the words that work for you are as simple as "Cut that out" or just "Snap out of it."

Once you have focused your attention, step back, take a long deep breath, and get centered. After you have regained your lucid self, think objectively. What event or idea sent you down this negative path? Did this thought help you? Hurt you? Then, modify the thought into something constructive. This strategy, called *positive reappraisal*, can be an extremely useful tool in coping with any chronic illness.

Here are some examples of positive reappraisal:

Negative thought: "I can't do this."
Modified thought: "This will be a challenge, but I'll try to do it one step at a time."
Self-message: I am innovative and capable.

Negative thought: "I can't play ball with Billy like other fathers can with their kids."
Modified thought: "I'll show Billy the antique cars at the auction and we'll have a great time together."
Self-message: I have a lot to offer, and others enjoy my company.

Negative thought: "I'll just be in their way."
Modified thought: "We always have a good time together."
Self-message: They love me, not my joints.

Negative thought: "I don't even want to get out of bed."
Modified thought: "I'll feel so much better after my nice warm shower."
Self-message: I can help myself.

Negative thought: "My boss is a heartless jerk."
Modified thought: "I'll talk to my boss about ways that I can be more effective in my job."
Self-message: I am on the way to becoming a more valued employee.

Negative thought: "This is all my fault."
Modified thought: "I'd rather not have arthritis, but I will learn to work with it."
Self-message: Many good people have RA. I am a good person and I did not cause myself to have RA.

Negative thought: "I'll never get ahead."
Modified thought: "I am really becoming organized."
Self-message: I can develop skills I never had before.

Negative thought: "No one helps me; I'll just do it myself."
Modified thought: "I will develop a chore list for the kids and discuss why it's necessary that we work together as a family."
Self-message: Communication is essential; asking for help is okay.

Negative thought: "I will end up in a wheelchair."
Modified thought: "Most people with RA live normal lives, and I will too."
Self-message: Facts, not emotions, should control my thoughts.

Finally, it's important to remember that you only compound your troubles if you feel guilty about your negative thoughts. Everyone has them. You simply need to learn to redirect them and not let them control you. Once you experience the freedom of walking away from negative thoughts, it will be easier to avoid them in the future.

A good mental attitude is extremely powerful. It can't eliminate the arthritis, but it can definitely improve your ability to function, mentally and physically. Positive thoughts can provide you with sanctuary in even the most troublesome of situations. You can concentrate on treasuring each of your blessings rather than toting up all of your disappointments. This will fortify you and make you a person with whom people (including you!) will want to spend time.

Be Willing to Reassess

RA is unpredictable and often appears to follow a random and uncertain course. The frustration of this uncertainty can in itself be a significant impediment to effective coping. Why? Because you cannot predict when you will have a bad day, nor can you predict when you will have a good day. This makes planning ahead difficult, and it means that there will be times when plans made will become plans changed.

People with RA often feel as if they are on an emotional roller coaster: just when things appear to be under control, a flare-up of arthritis occurs and changes everything. A life that is full of ups and downs is difficult to deal with, but flexibility—learning to make *adjustments to changes*—can help you avoid becoming discouraged. You will need to remain flexible, and you will need to adjust your expectations and plans regularly.

The key to flexibility is expecting and accepting unpredictability. If you accept the unpredictable nature of RA, you won't feel quite so disappointed when your arthritis acts up. Ask yourself, "Am I better prepared to deal with this flare-up than I was a month ago?" Most likely you are. You will learn how to deal with each flare-up without allowing it to knock you down. Many people adjust to the unpredictability by backing up their scheduled plans with contingency arrangements. Many people use coping strategies to solve new problems as they occur. These people don't passively let life happen to them; they take steps to prepare themselves for what life brings their way. Learning and perfecting strategies for coping with change is the successful antidote for the unpredictability of RA.

6

Coping with Pain and Fatigue

For the person who has rheumatoid arthritis, pain and fatigue may be overwhelming at times, so much so that they leave the person feeling anxious and depressed as well as in pain and tired. But both the pain and the fatigue of RA come and go, and their severity changes as well. (In fact, pain and fatigue are often most limiting during the early stages of RA.)

There's no question that pain and fatigue are complicated symptoms that are frequently difficult to explain and understand. Like other aspects of RA, however, they are most effectively controlled when they are understood. For this reason, the person who makes the effort and takes the time to learn the causes, significance, and aggravating factors of his or her pain and fatigue is much more likely to be able to manage these symptoms.

PAIN

The pain of RA may be the most burdensome feature of the illness, especially when pain interferes with your ability to function as you once did. Because RA is a **chronic** condition, you may wonder whether you'll always suffer this much pain. The answer is, No!

What Is Pain?

A very simple explanation of pain is that it begins as a message from stimulated nerve endings (or pain receptors); this message is transmitted from the nerves to the spinal cord to the brain, where the message is interpreted as pain. Irritation, **inflammation,** or injury can activate the pain receptors. Even though the message causes pain, we have to be thankful for it, because it can prevent more severe injury. For example, when you accidentally touch a hot stove, stimulated pain receptors in your fingertips send a message to your brain that a dangerous situation exists—*tissue is being damaged.* After your brain interprets the signal, it quickly sends a message back to the hand: "That hurts. Pull away!" Pain can protect us!

The circuitry from the painful stimulus to the brain and back is incredibly intricate. In 1965 medical scientists Ronald Melzack and Patrick Wall proposed the *gate theory of pain,* which helps us understand just how complex pain perception is. They suggested that there is a "gate" located in the spinal cord which can be opened or closed under various situations. According to these researchers, when the gate is open, pain-related messages can pass through to the brain (although only a limited amount of sensory information can pass through the gate at one time). Interestingly enough, the body can send messages that compete with each other; one message can carry a pain-stimulating signal, and another can effectively close the gate to prevent that signal from being received.

If you have ever stubbed your toe or banged your elbow you have experienced this phenomenon. Once you begin rubbing the affected area (as most of us will do under the circumstances!) you send a message that competes with the pain message. This instinctive reaction to pain works because the sensation of rubbing is transmitted to the spinal cord through nerve fibers that are larger than the fibers through which pain messages travel to the spinal cord. The comforting message of rubbing is dispatched rapidly to the spinal cord, whereas the message of pain travels slowly, through small nerve fibers. Reaching the spinal cord before the pain message, the comforting message blocks out the slower, sharp pain signal and prevents it from reaching the brain. Without knowing it, you have closed the pain gate by your instinctive reaction.

The brain also appears to have its own mechanisms for decreasing acute pain; in times of need, the brain apparently has the capacity to send signals to close the gate. This capacity to close the gate is extremely powerful. We have all heard accounts of someone running into a burning building to save a child, for example. Although that person gets burned, he or she continues the quest to save a life. Or what about the football player who crosses the goal line on a broken or sprained limb? These individuals often relate that they felt very little pain during the experience. Why? The theory is that the body produces its own morphinelike substances, endorphins and enkephalins, and that these protective chemicals may be responsible for closing the pain gate in the situations described above. Stories such as these make us appreciate how powerful the brain can be in overcoming pain.

Chronic pain, which can be nearly continuous or unremitting, is very different from the transient and acute pain described in the examples above. It differs from acute pain both scientifically and emotionally. Chronic pain perception varies markedly among individuals. The brain and central nervous system can have a pivotal role in actually amplifying and maintaining chronic pain. The brain's involvement in chronic pain is demonstrated by the co-occurrence of other symptoms that originate in the brain, including fatigue, insomnia, memory disturbance, depression, and anxiety. The brain can also overcome chronic pain, although different processes are required for it to do so.

Pain and Your Emotions

Researchers, physicians, and patients all know that the degree of pain experienced from RA is not always proportional to the amount of inflammation present. From this fact we must infer that some people perceive pain more intensely than others do. How intensely you experience pain is linked *in part* to your emotions and to your understanding of what the pain *signifies*. What you believe influences your physical sensations!

Pain that follows war injuries is a well-documented example of how a person's perception of pain can be affected by the *meaning* that person attaches to it. In these instances, people who are severely wounded in battle often report feeling little or no pain after the injury. Perhaps this is because the injury signifies their freedom to return home. Or maybe their pain reminds them of the courage they displayed while fighting for a cause important to them. On the other hand, in a senseless and arbitrary automobile accident, a similar degree of injury will usually cause greater emotional and physical pain.

Because the pain of RA has different personal *significance* for each individual, it only follows that each person will experience the pain differently. The person for whom each twinge of pain symbolizes loss of function and control will probably vigilantly monitor and focus on his pain and may end up feeling that pain more intensely. In the medical world, we call this way of thinking "catastrophizing." On the other hand, someone who learns to view pain as a message alerting him to modify his actions and prevent joint damage will perceive less pain. Sometimes a positive attitude really can improve your condition. What you believe and how you emotionally respond to these beliefs has a direct effect on your brain and how it processes the pain message.

Emotions also play a remarkable role in the perception of pain. Does that

mean that the pain is all in your head? Certainly not! It is in our joints and muscles. But your emotions can intensify or lessen the perception of that painful
stimulus from the joints and muscles. People who feel confident, organized, and
in control often experience less pain. Those who are fearful or depressed suffer
much higher levels of pain. Your emotions function like a "volume control" on
how your nervous system processes sensory information (what you feel). When
you are stressed and afraid, the volume is turned up and there is an increase in
the neurotransmitters that facilitate the painful message, called substance P,
glutamate, EAA, and nerve growth factor. At the same time, the neurotransmitters that are known to block pain, like GABA, serotonin, norepinephrine,
and dopamine, are reduced.

Emotions can also increase pain directly. To illustrate this phenomenon,
consider one of the most common sources of pain in RA, muscle spasm. Muscles
that are continuously tight and do not relax adequately can be very painful.
Joint pain can often promote reflexive muscle spasm or tension. When the
muscle contracts and squeezes around painful joints, they become even more
painful. The connection between emotion and muscle pain makes sense when
we consider some other notorious sources of muscle tension:

- stress
- anxiety
- fear
- depression
- poor sleep patterns
- fatigue
- isolation

Do some of these conditions sound familiar? The truth is, we all encounter these
conditions in our day-to-day lives. Many of them are unavoidable. Depression,
fear, and other emotional reactions to life events (and to life in general) can
provoke muscle tension, as can poor sleep patterns. In RA, as in some other
disease conditions, these factors often trigger a vicious cycle of pain that is difficult to break.

What Is the Pain Message in RA?

We've stated that pain is caused by a signal or message. What exactly is that
message in the case of RA? In rheumatoid arthritis, inflammation that occurs
in the joints can irritate nerve endings in the joint lining (**synovium**), **capsule**,
and **ligaments**. This inflammation leads to swelling within the joints, which
causes these same structures to become stretched. Inflammation causes pain,

and swelling intensifies that pain. (You can tell a joint is inflamed, because it becomes warm, swollen, and tender.) Pain from joints that are highly inflamed sends the following messages: (1) Respect your pain. (2) Slow down, you're overdoing it. (3) Protect and rest your joints until the inflammation subsides.

Decreasing Pain

Just because pain is a valued signal doesn't mean you have to suffer through it without trying to decrease its intensity. After all, pain is exhausting! The first step in decreasing the intensity of pain is accepting that pain exists in your present life. This doesn't mean that you should surrender to a painful existence; it simply means that you must accept the fact that your joints are painful *today* and that you'll need to direct your energies toward getting through today. If you are filled with regrets about the past and fears of the future, you are fighting the presence of pain in your life. Regret and fear are wasteful emotions; they create feelings of guilt, blame, and anxiety, and these cause you further pain *today*. It is true but ironic that accepting pain is the first step in decreasing it.

Next, recognize pain as being a very personal experience. Understanding that each person has a unique awareness of his or her pain is critical, because effective strategies for combatting pain will differ for each person. You will need to take responsibility for your experience of pain, from how you perceive it to how you handle it. This does not mean accepting the blame for having RA. Rather, it means *not* viewing pain as an outside force that is directing you; don't allow your pain to have that much power! Instead, view pain as a force over which you can exert some control. This will mean assessing the source of your pain, the conditions that worsen it, your perception of it, and options that will allow *you* to direct *it*.

Once you have accepted the presence of pain in your life and taken responsibility for your unique experience of it, how can you begin to control it? You can select any or all of the following options.

Define and assess your problem. To use this coping tool (first discussed in Chapter 5), think about what is causing your pain. Trace your daily activities to determine whether some specific activity may be aggravating your unusually painful joints. If you identify such an activity, plan ahead to modify it in the future. The following examples may help you to find the cause of your pain and develop methods to alleviate and control it.

1. Pain in the morning. Morning stiffness and pain are usually related to inflammation. Setting your alarm clock to go off one hour before you need to get out of bed can help. Keep your medications at bedside, and take them when you wake up. An electric blanket can be useful in warming up the bed and your joints. Perform your gentle range of motion exercises in bed to loosen up your joints before getting up.

After you have risen, go directly from bed to a warm shower or bath (maybe someone else can draw the bath). In other words, ease into morning slowly, and give your joints ample time to loosen up.

2. Pain after sitting (called **gelling**). This pain is also caused by inflammation in the joints. Taking frequent stretch breaks during prolonged stationary periods can usually alleviate gelling.

3. Pain after exercise. If pain persists for more than two hours after exercising, you have overextended yourself. Analyze your exercise—distance walked, number of repetitions done, footwear worn, etc.—and review your exercise program with your doctor or therapist.

4. Pain with specific activities. Some activities that often cause problems: twisting off jar lids, getting into the shower, styling your hair, bending down to pick things up, carrying objects, making love. All of these activities can be modified to limit joint stress. (More about this later.)

The general approach here is to analyze painful activities, either by making mental notes or keeping a diary, and then to modify them.

Protect your inflamed joints. Protecting inflamed joints from excessive stress will decrease pain. In Chapter 8 we discuss the use of splints and describe techniques for avoiding stressful joint actions. Your **occupational therapist,** an expert in this area, will be an invaluable source of information to you. Strategies for protecting your joints require only a little extra time, and once you see how effective they are, you undoubtedly will make them an automatic part of your daily life.

Improve your muscle health. The two methods of improving your muscle health are to reduce muscle tension and to increase muscle strength. We have described how muscle tension contributes to joint pain. Certainly, warm baths or showers, warm compresses, relaxation techniques, gentle massage, imagery techniques, adequate rest and sleep, and tailored exercises will be of great value in reducing muscle tension. You can learn to do many of these treatments for yourself.

Increasing muscle strength is an excellent way to take stress (and thus pain) away from joints by providing increased structural support. A **physical therapist** trained in arthritis treatment can instruct you in exercise programs designed to increase muscle strength appropriately in people with RA. (Physical therapists can assist you with other techniques for effectively reducing pain; electrical stimulation, ultrasound, and hydrotherapy are examples.)

Close the pain gate. Emotional factors are as crucial as physical factors in creating your experience of pain. What methods can you employ to decrease the transmission of pain through the pain gate?

1. Utilize distraction. An enjoyable pastime is always an excellent means of distracting your mind from pain. Watching a favorite television show or DVD, going out to the theater to see a movie or play, reading a book, telephoning an old friend, taking a college course, exploring new hobbies—all of these activities can take your mind off your joints. Look for fun. Laughter is a great analgesic (pain reliever) and a muscle relaxant that has no adverse side effects. The prospect of having fun might seem inconceivable sometimes, because you feel so miserable, but if you pursue enjoyable activities, you *will* have fun.

2. Change your beliefs about pain. There are two ways to accomplish this. One is to view your pain scientifically as being a valued signal that provides a protective function for your joints. Viewed this way, pain is less likely to foster fear, anxiety, or depression.

Another technique is **imagery.** When your pain is overwhelming, try using visual imagery to change your view of it. Here are two examples you can experiment with. Begin each of them by sitting or lying down and then closing your eyes and taking a few long, deep breaths.

Example 1. Concentrate on your warm, painful joints, likening them to an uncomfortably hot, blazing fire. Imagine yourself slowly moving farther and farther from the flames, feeling less heat. Or imagine a cool, summer shower gently extinguishing the fire and the pain.

Example 2. Think of the pain throbbing in your joints as being like a team of horses, galloping out of control. Imagine yourself controlling the reins, slowing the horses down to a gentle pace. Then visualize a pleasant ride through the countryside, breathing in the fresh air, enjoying the surroundings.

In each of these examples, you are creating healing images to counteract the painful ones. If you can become involved in your images, your body will respond as if the imagined situations were real. Muscles will relax, heart rate and breathing rate will decrease, and pain can subside.

3. Address your stress, anxiety, depression, and fatigue. Remember that these symptoms and emotions lower your pain threshold by opening the pain gates, turning up the pain volume, and creating muscle tension.

Minimize inflammation. As mentioned above, learning to avoid activities that increase your joint inflammation is crucial, but if you do find that you have some post-activity inflammation, try applying cold packs to the warm joints for 20 minutes. Always wrap ice and other sources of extreme cold in a towel before placing them next to your skin.

There are several medical approaches to controlling inflammation. Most notably, your physician will prescribe medications for controlling inflammation. Nonsteroidal anti-inflammatory drugs (**NSAIDs**) are commonly used to decrease pain and inflammation over a period of days. Other medications, such as **DMARDs** and **biologics,** are intended to induce more sustained improvement; they work over weeks to months, by controlling the rheumatoid process.

Narcotic medications, such as codeine and hydrocodone, mask pain without changing the underlying condition, and so your physician may be reluctant to prescribe large amounts of these medications for you. This is not because he or she is heartless, but because totally masking pain would not be in your joints' best interest. Remember, pain can provide a valuable message; if you don't feel pain, you will not receive your body's warning signals, and you may overexert yourself and cause serious damage to your joints.

Another reason your physician will want to avoid having you use narcotics on a long-term basis is the addictive potential of these medications. If you develop a physical requirement for these medications, you may find that you have relinquished control over your body and given it to the prescribing physician. This places you in the uncomfortable position of having to convince your doctor that you are in severe pain so that he or she will continue to prescribe narcotics for you.

If you can use your mind's capacity to control pain, *you* will be in charge.

FATIGUE

You may find that fatigue is the most incapacitating feature of RA. Fatigue can limit your concentration and ability to function, so that even mustering sufficient energy to care for your family or to participate in social activities—much less to deal with the responsibilities of the workplace—can be difficult. The normal demands of everyday living can sometimes appear overwhelming to the person who is chronically tired.

Sometimes the fatigue and loss of energy that result from RA are severe. In fact, many people think that there must be something else wrong with them in addition to arthritis because they cannot believe that arthritis alone can affect their energy so drastically.

Fatigue may be unpredictable, and so it can interfere with plans you've made. You may feel exasperated or frightened by this loss of control over your energy level. Tiredness also contributes to depression, anxiety, and pain. Fatigue also increases pain in your joints. You need to know what you can do to alleviate this pervasive symptom.

Why Am I So Tired?

Fatigue or decreased energy in RA can be caused by the condition itself or by emotional upheaval, pain, lack of sleep, and general lack of physical fitness. Remember, RA is a systemic condition that can affect more than just the joints. The **anemia** that sometimes results from the condition, for example, can contribute to fatigue. Also, fatigue may be a consequence of inflammatory substances (**cytokines**) in the blood; fatigue from this cause may come on suddenly, early in the course of the disease, and may resemble the tiredness that accompanies a virus or flu. Effective control of RA through appropriate medications will lessen cytokine-induced fatigue.

Your emotions alone can exhaust you; think of how tired you feel after you've had a particularly emotional experience. Pain can be emotionally and physically exhausting, too; and when pain is combined with anxiety and tension, limited energy reserves can be depleted easily. Depression can cause or amplify fatigue. It's easy to see that effectively treating pain, anxiety, and depression is an important factor in controlling fatigue.

Obviously, fatigue can be the result of inadequate sleep. For people with RA, painful joints, tight muscles, fear, and anxiety frequently interfere with the ability to get a good night's sleep.

Finally, when people have had RA for a while, they may get out of condition. This loss of physical fitness may be a consequence of decreased activity, and it produces a different form of exhaustion.

Controlling Fatigue

Get adequate rest. Individuals with RA require more rest than they did before they developed the condition. Adequate rest takes many forms, including physical, emotional, and "local" rest (described below).

Getting adequate sleep is imperative, because sleep provides healing to the body and to the mind. A minimum of eight hours of sleep daily is recommended for people with RA, but more may be needed during periods when the arthritis is flaring up. If getting adequate sleep proves difficult, ask your doctor to recommend or prescribe pain or sleeping medications to help you.

Actual sleep is not the only way to rest physically and emotionally. Taking a fifteen- or twenty-minute break in the morning and afternoon can also make an incredible difference in productivity. Learning and performing stress reduction and relaxation techniques during tense times may be particularly beneficial (see Chapter 7). During these breaks, try to relax your mind and body. If you can lie down with your feet elevated, you'll increase the benefits of the break. Deep breathing exercises can also markedly reduce fatigue, particularly if combined with meditation. Taking prescribed breaks routinely each day may allow you to avoid the severe exhaustion that occurs when you become overly fatigued.

It's a good idea to reflect now and then on a typical day's activities. Think about what you do during the day and when you feel most tired. This review will allow you to schedule your rest breaks strategically, which will help you avoid becoming overtired. If necessary, discuss these recommendations with your employer; he or she will probably agree that this is time well spent. It is to everyone's benefit for you to retain your energy so you can be as efficient and productive as possible.

Local rest means resting specific parts of the body. Getting local rest will help you protect your joints from undue stress; this can be achieved by wearing splints, which can be fabricated to protect the wrists and hands, and by using techniques designed to reduce joint stress (these are discussed in detail in Chapter 8).

Set priorities. Your energy is most limited when your RA is flaring, and at these times it may not be possible for you to do everything you would like to do or even all you feel that you *should* do. At these times you need to be honest with yourself about what you can and cannot do. Start by setting priorities. Make lists of things to do, and then prioritize those things. Decide to do first what absolutely must be done, and save for a later date or eliminate everything that has the word *should* connected to it: "I *should* iron my dress." Instead, select a dress that doesn't need ironing, even if you just wore it last week. Being fashion conscious is a low priority if it costs energy that you don't have. "I should do some dusting tonight." The dust isn't going anywhere! Put that task aside until you have more energy, or consider assigning that task to someone else.

After you have thrown out the shoulds, divide the remaining tasks into steps. Discard the all-or-nothing philosophy. (Cleaning day—"I must do all my cleaning in one day so my whole house is clean at one time"—is an example of an all-or-nothing item you may find on your list.) Do a little each day; with strategic planning, you can stay on top of things.

Plan ahead. A little organization and planning will save you vast amounts of wasted energy. For example, an efficient work space is extremely important. In your place of employment, store all the equipment you generally need within easy reach and at a convenient height. Put things in their place, and know where things are kept. This way you won't waste energy looking for things or getting up frequently to retrieve something. Avoid clutter both at work and at home, and ask others to help you with this.

At home, store necessities for each task near the place where the task is performed. For example, store the laundry detergent near the laundry basket or the washer. (Incidentally, asking family members to bring their dirty clothes to—and collect their clean ones from—the laundry area means that each person expends a little energy rather than one person expending a lot.)

For you, effective planning might involve participating in more bulk activities. For instance, cooking bulk quantities on the weekend is a great idea. Making a large pan of lasagna or batch of chili and freezing portions for future use can save a lot of energy during a busy week. And if you wake up not feeling very well, you can take a package from the freezer for dinner later. Keeping convenience foods on hand for bad days is another good idea.

Bulk shopping can be useful, too. Once a month take someone with you and purchase staple items that you know you'll need for the month: sugar, flour, condiments, paper goods, cereal. That way you'll only need to shop more frequently for perishables, and your shopping load will be lighter. Avoid purchasing items in industrial size containers, however, because lifting and maneuvering these will put stress on your hands and wrists (or, if you prefer to buy goods in these large containers, make plans to divide them up into smaller portions, with someone's help, if needed).

What about energy for social outings? You may be avoiding all social events, fearing that you won't have enough energy or that you'll hold everyone else back. There are *some* activities you will temporarily need to avoid when your energy level is very low. These activities include all-or-none outings that don't allow time for adequate rest breaks (large group walking tours are notorious for this). You shouldn't have to push yourself in an effort to keep up. If you must decline a social invitation, be sure to let your friends know that you are still interested in future activities and want to be included. Your task will be to help organize activities with your family and friends that will allow for rest. Then remember to rest adequately the day before a planned activity. Only you know your own limitations. If you take an interest in outside activities, you'll find that loved ones can be extremely flexible. After all, it makes them feel bad when you can't participate. So, get involved.

Avoid wasting energy. We waste a lot of energy during the course of a day, so part of effective energy conservation involves asking questions such as, "Is there an easier way to accomplish this?" Simple changes, such as taking the elevator instead of walking the stairs, can save energy. Using carts to carry equipment or utensils even for small distances saves energy and wear and tear on hand and wrist joints. Sitting down to do activities that you usually perform standing can reduce knee and hip fatigue. Consider this: Do you *really* need to stand to wash dishes or shave or fix your hair? Break habits! Get a high stool, sit, and relax while you perform these necessary tasks.

You can also avoid wasting energy by establishing a step-by-step routine for tasks you undertake regularly. With proper planning, you can reduce the steps in some tasks and combine the steps in other tasks. Make each task as simple as possible.

Pace yourself. Pacing involves developing guidelines for energy expenditure. The amount of activity that precipitates fatigue varies greatly among individuals, so you are the only one who can set guidelines for yourself. As a general rule, however, it's a good idea to alternate energy-intensive activities with more relaxing ones throughout the day. Adding this kind of balance to your routine can prevent excessive fatigue.

Almost everyone with RA tries to "catch up" on days when they feel well, but using good days to their maximum has its drawbacks. Try not to overutilize those days, since doing so may result in a flare-up of your arthritis.

Divide the labor. Do not try to do everything by yourself. Instead, divide chores among several people to help lighten the workload. If you live with a partner or children, your job may be easier. If your children are old enough, set up schedules and jobs. It is simple to provide incentives to convince your children to help you, since there is always some small reward that they can earn. Helping with household chores is a great lesson in responsibility as well.

If you live alone, the challenge is greater, although not impossible. Meeting the challenge involves family, friends, and neighbors who might be willing to help you. If you can think of something that you can do for them in return, you won't be as reluctant to ask for assistance. For example, many young couples have difficulty finding affordable baby sitters whom they can depend on and trust. If you can present them with the opportunity for a free Saturday night, they will probably view your request that in exchange they mow your lawn or vacuum your carpets as a great bargain. Everyone wins! If you have special skills, use them in exchange for help. Obviously, many people will be happy to help you for nothing in return, and their presence might turn into a nice visit, providing socializing that can be therapeutic also. The important thing is for *you* to feel good about asking for help.

Get in shape. Being out of condition will almost always result in fatigue, and having RA means that it will be more difficult to stay in top condition. When your arthritis flares up, you have to rest your joints and muscles. This in turn can leave your body out of condition.

With appropriate medical therapy, the inflammation in your joints will eventually decrease. At this point you will need to get more involved in an exercise program. (See Chapter 10 for information about aerobic exercises that will increase your conditioning and help you get back in shape.)

Make use of medical therapy. Medications are useful in the long-term control of fatigue. As disease-modifying antirheumatic drugs (DMARDs) and/or biologics begin working to control your RA, fatigue will lessen. Anemia will also improve with the control of arthritis. Use the skills above to cope with fatigue until your arthritis is brought under control, then continue using them to make your life easier, more convenient, and more fun.

FOR MORE INFORMATION

Two helpful pamphlets, "Managing Your Fatigue" and "Managing Your Pain," are available from the Arthritis Foundation (1330 W. Peachtree St., Atlanta, Ga. 30309; 1-800-283-7800) or go to www.afstore.org.

Coping with Emotions— Yours and Everyone Else's

It is easy to see how having rheumatoid arthritis can affect the way you deal with yourself and with others. You may worry, at first, about how your friends and family will respond when they notice the changes in you. Or you may be surprised at the intensity of your own emotional responses to RA. Many of the emotions triggered by the disease are the kinds we would rather not experience. Eventually, however, you and all of the people around you will learn how to cope with RA, including its accompanying emotions.

The feelings we have about involuntary changes that take place in our lives are completely natural, but that doesn't mean we have to let them control us. For example, we know that a person who is plagued by negative thoughts and feelings is much more likely to feel tired than a person whose thoughts are optimistic. Persistent negative emotions drain human energies. If you are overcome by negativity, then you are reducing the amount of energy that is available to you for activities such as dining out, swimming, painting—all of the things you *like* to do. We also now understand that negative emotions create stress and provoke inflammation.

One of the emotions you may experience is grief; you may initially grieve because you have arthritis, and it represents to you a loss of control and ability. This is nothing to be ashamed of; everyone grieves over losses. Most people want others to share their grief, and they find that this helps them overcome their sense of loss. Learning to understand your feelings and cope with them will help you in all aspects of your life. On the other hand, if you let your feelings control you, they may affect your ability to cope with arthritis and every other aspect of your daily living. You can face these emotions head on and redirect your energy toward improving your condition.

ANGER

Why shouldn't you be angry? You probably have found it necessary to give up activities that you truly enjoy. Your days are more difficult and complicated than they used to be. It may seem that no one really understands the pain and frustration you're experiencing. You are frustrated with your doctor because your recovery is not as speedy as you would like it to be. These thoughts are all valid, and they would leave anyone feeling angry.

People respond to anger in several ways—and in different ways at different times. They may direct their anger inward, for example; people often blame themselves for their situation and suffer feelings of guilt as a result. Or they may direct their anger toward other people. Sometimes anger is suppressed entirely. Bottled up anger increases muscle tension and pain, provokes inflammation, and drains precious energy reserves.

Some people are angry and don't know it. Their anger is so well disguised that they fail to recognize it. Each of the following thoughts, or self-messages, contains a disguised element of anger:

"I'm just going to finish this project at my own pace, and if he doesn't like it, that's his problem."

"Why would I want to go golfing, anyway?"

"What does *she* know about arthritis?"

"He's just helping me because he feels guilty."

"I'm just not going to take that worthless pill."

"I should have stopped smoking and exercised more often."

People who make statements or have thoughts such as these are angry about their arthritic condition and the havoc it is creating in their lives. One of the dangers of unrecognized anger is that it is often turned against other people, in the form of casting blame, harboring resentment, or engaging in passive-aggressive behavior. This response hurts people who really care about you and only want to help you. And even more importantly, it hurts *you* mentally, emotionally, and physically.

Managing Anger

The first step in dealing with any emotion is to recognize it. Examine your thoughts and actions for signs of anger. Next, you have to acknowledge that nothing good will come from this kind of anger. If you recognize that you're angry and acknowledge that it is serving no good purpose, you'll have an easier time managing it. In addition to the coping strategies discussed in this chapter, those described in Chapter 5 can also help you deal with anger.

First, define and assess the source of anger. The people in the following stories have recognized that they are angry, and they have identified the source of their anger.

> Janice is angry because arthritis is interfering with her work. She's always been a competent and respected employee, and she hates the way her arthritis has changed her previously successful work routine.

> Margaret is angry because her family doesn't understand the emotional and physical chaos she is going through. She feels that there is a lack of help and encouragement in her home. She works all day and comes home feeling too tired to perform simple household tasks.

> Ken is frustrated and angry about the unfairness of having RA. He has always exercised, eaten right, and kept himself in excellent physical condition. He never smoked. He is angry that despite his good habits, he has arthritis. Friends who were not nearly as health conscious as he remain unscathed. "Why me? What did I do wrong?" he continues to ask himself.

Second, set realistic goals and expectations. Arthritis is interfering with Janice's work, and she's angry. Why? Is it possible that she's expecting too much from herself? Or are other people expecting more from her than she can provide at this time? It seems that Janice expects to be able to continue performing her job exactly as she's always done it, and she's frustrated because she can't. It also seems that she is stubbornly attached to her routine and has not accepted the changes in her capabilities. Janice needs to redefine her expectations. She needs to consider whether her routine is really that important and whether her schedules really need to be so rigidly defined.

Does Margaret expect her family to know automatically how she is feeling simply because they love her? Do they even have any idea of how they can best help her? Should they be able to sense that she is really angry about having arthritis, or are they receiving signals that she is angry at them? Are Margaret's expectations of her family reasonable?

No one with RA has knowingly brought this condition upon himself or herself, and so a person with RA might easily view the situation as being unfair.

Two facts are significant here. First, RA, like many other conditions, is neither fair nor just. Second, unfairness as a source of anger is difficult to resolve. It will never be possible for Ken to view his condition as being fair. He may try to "make things even" by making his friends feel as bad as he does about it, but he won't ever be able to make things fair in his own estimation. Any expectation of fairness is likely to result in frustration and anger. It seems that the only way around this, again, is to *change one's own expectations*. Don't expect things to be fair. Develop more realistic expectations.

Third, resolve your anger through problem solving and negotiation. Janice will have to break free of the ritual of doing things as she's always done them. She must give up the struggle to remain the same. She must be willing to accept changes in her capabilities, *at this time*, and adjust accordingly. Can she make changes in her work environment that will help her work more efficiently? Can she improve other skills to compensate for the increased time required to perform what were once easily completed tasks? Becoming more efficient and better organized and setting priorities will help Janice make it through her workday. Honest and open communication with her co-workers and employer will ease bad feelings. Being open to change and learning to adapt to her new physical limitations are the answers to Janice's dilemma.

How can Margaret get her family to understand the torment she is going through? Just expecting them to understand is unreasonable, particularly with all of the mixed messages she's sending to her family. She must talk candidly to them. She must learn ways to let them know her feelings before the anger and resentment build up and complicate what is already a difficult situation. Thoughtful communication—letting her family know how to help her—will settle Margaret's problem.

Ken must work around the obstacles that make him feel cheated. Moving forward through these problems will increase his feelings of strength and competence. Triumph over adversity will help eliminate his feelings of being victimized by RA. He must aim to overcome the inequities of having RA by using his energies to seek improvement. But most importantly, he must understand the indiscriminate nature of RA. Nothing he did or did not do caused his condition, and to view it as some form of punishment merely compounds the problem.

Finally, redirect negative energy by modifying negative thoughts and behaviors. If the energy spent on being angry is directed positively, it can be useful. Janice, for example, can direct her energies toward finding the *possibilities* instead of clinging to the *impossibilities*. Margaret can trade misdirected anger for her family's help and encouragement. And Ken can exchange resentment for the personal challenge of recovery. They all will feel relieved when they redirect their energy into constructive actions. When pent up anger is released, you can recharge your spiritual battery with your own inherently positive energy.

DEPRESSION

Depression is a common feature of RA. People with RA may be envisioning a life filled with pain or feeling old before their time. They may feel cheated. And self-esteem may waver when they find that they can't do some things they once did with ease. These are good reasons to feel sad, and prolonged or intense sadness can lead to depression. In addition, completely aside from emotional reactions to change, the physical process of inflammation itself can actually worsen depression, because of physiological changes that occur in the body that affect the brain and nervous system. So, getting your RA under control will help more than just your painful joints.

The following statements contain subtle cues that a person may be depressed:

"I'm too tired to visit the Bensons tonight."

"Nothing's wrong. I just don't have anything to say."

"It's Jimmy's birthday? I forgot."

"I feel okay. I'm just not hungry, that's all."

"I hardly shut my eyes all night."

"Honey, my joints are just too sore tonight."

Feeling melancholy is not the only symptom of depression. Loss of energy, decreased interest in previously enjoyed activities, forgetfulness, loss of appetite or excessive appetite, difficulty sleeping, and decreased libido can all be symptoms of depression. But these same symptoms can be caused by RA, so it's important to clarify their source.

There is a self-perpetuating cycle: depression results in further pain, poorer sleep patterns, added muscle tension, and increased fatigue—all of which can lead to deeper depression. This cycle needs to be broken. The primary motivating agent must be the person with RA, but there are plenty of strategies and people to help.

Managing Depression

Recognizing that you are depressed is very important, but it is only the first step. Depression often feels like a heavy veil that seems impossible to lift. It can be suffocating, leaving people feeling helpless and vulnerable. If you feel as though you are struggling beneath the weight of depression, you'll need to muster the fortitude that you still have but your depression has temporarily concealed. Do whatever it takes to retrieve your personal strengths.

Get the facts. What you tell yourself matters! What you *think* influences how you *feel*. Negative emotional reactions to your thoughts can affect your immune system and create *real* inflammation. What are you thinking that might be leading you to feel depressed? Is fact—or imagination—directing you? Are you fearful that you will always suffer this much pain? Or that arthritis will progress until you are eventually wheelchair bound? If so, fiction is dictating your feelings and your depression. Your inner voice is giving you harmful misinformation! You need to become objective enough to gather facts rather than succumbing to unfounded fears. If you can't be objective, consult someone who can, such as your physician.

Get help. There's no question that everyone can benefit from counseling from time to time. *Breaking free of depression is a difficult thing to do.* For this reason, anyone who is suffering from depression should feel free to use all available resources. For example, therapists—**psychologists** and **psychiatrists**—with expertise in chronic conditions can be very helpful to people who are in the process of adjusting to such life changes.

Frequently, depression is caused by a chemical imbalance. RA can often aggravate that imbalance. When this occurs or when the depression is so severe or chronic that the person is having a very hard time coming out of it, a physician may prescribe medications to help lift it.

With *mild* depression, talking openly to a good listener sometimes is all that is needed. Friends and loved ones will help you focus on what is important to you and what is worth looking forward to. Talking to people who are having the same experiences that you are having can make you feel less alone (the local chapter of the Arthritis Foundation can put you in touch with a support group in your area).

It's understandable if you feel that you're just not ready to face friends yet. You may need some time to arrange your thoughts and feelings. If being alone becomes a routine, however, you may want to consider seeking professional advice. Remember, this is a new experience for you, and you don't have to try to be your own expert.

Do not isolate yourself from others. Withdrawing from friends and activities because of depression will only increase your sense of loss and loneliness. At first it may seem easier to isolate yourself, because by doing so you can avoid questions, unwanted advice, and assorted comments from others. You may even convince yourself that it is your arthritis that is holding you back. You may be picturing yourself as a wet blanket—a person who is no longer any fun to be with—and make excuses to friends. These friends may begin to feel as if you don't want to see them. Be as honest with them about your feelings as you want to be, but don't avoid your friends. You will still enjoy their company, and they yours. Good friends are good medicine, and enjoying friendship combats depression. And, as your depression lifts, the symptoms of RA will be less burdensome.

Pursue something you enjoy doing. Think of activities that have lifted your spirits in the past. Getting involved in something that you once had fun doing is a good way to remind yourself of who you are, and enjoying an activity is a good way to take your mind off other troubles and to relieve stress. Write down twenty things that you enjoyed doing in the past, and then try doing some of them.

Focus on today. Learning and practicing stress reduction and relaxation techniques that focus on mindfulness of the present rather than regrets of the past or worries of the future may also be a tremendous help. There is more about mindfulness exercises in Chapter 17.

Focus on a positive attitude. Try to stand back and objectively listen to each negative thought as though someone else were expressing it. Allow yourself to see the impact of these negative thoughts, and then modify them into something positive. Sometimes focusing on a positive attitude can turn a half-step backward into two steps forward.

Improve self-esteem. Many people who are adjusting to having RA feel depressed about their physical appearance or changes in their capabilities. Keep in mind that not all of these changes need be negative. Appropriate exercise, often with new sports such as swimming, will improve your physical condition. Learning new skills, making new acquaintances, learning a new hobby, or attaining new goals will remind you that you are still a bright, innovative person, capable of growth and change. Do what it takes to remain a productive and fulfilled person whose self-esteem continues to grow and improve.

Help others. There is nothing more rewarding than helping another person. Focusing on someone else's problems can help you forget yours. When you view your life through their eyes, you will see that you have much to offer other people.

Exercise. Doing exercises as prescribed is an excellent way to relieve your mind of negative thoughts. People often feel better when they get regular exercise. Athletes have known this for a long time—they actually feel depressed when they don't exercise routinely. This is because exercise helps your body produce endorphins—natural body chemicals that boost your spirits. Don't leave exercise to chance; incorporate it into your routine.

Improve your diet. What you eat can influence your mental as well as physical health. Chapter 1 mentioned how the balance of bowel bacteria could positively and negatively affect inflammation. Our bowel has the second largest nervous system in the body (*the enteric nervous system*). Research reveals that the brain (central nervous system) and the gut (enteric nervous system) communicate both ways by neurotransmitters! The gut is constantly sending messages to the brain and vice versa. We have all felt "butterflies" in our stomach when we are nervous or excited, or sick to our stomach when we are upset or scared. There is now groundbreaking evidence that the function of the enteric nervous system relies heavily on a healthy balance of bowel bacteria (Burnett, 2012). Good bacteria in the bowel may direct the nervous system to produce neurotransmitters that reduce anxiety and depression. Our bowel bacteria may actually help us respond to stress! Researchers are trying to determine which bacteria strains promote the production of stress-reducing neurotransmitters. Studies are ongoing looking at the role of probiotics in depression, anxiety, Alzheimer's disease, autism, and several other central nervous system conditions. In the meantime, a healthful diet has a potent role in controlling the bacterial makeup of our digestive systems. In Chapter 18 you will read about nutritional suggestions, fermented foods, and probiotics.

ANXIETY, FEAR, AND STRESS

Anxiety

Generalized anxiety is a vague sense of unease or worry. It is usually not directed toward any one issue. Fear, on the other hand, has a definite direction. In RA, fear is usually directed toward immediate and future problems, such as pain and the possibility of disability, job loss, medication toxicities, loss of friends, and inability to meet financial obligations. Whenever anxiety and fear overwhelm our ability to cope, stress is the inevitable result.

Fear

What are you afraid of, and what is the basis of your fear? Fear of future adverse consequences associated with RA or its required medications is understandable, but do you assume that every possible complication or toxic reaction will happen to you? That situation is extremely unlikely. This form of worrying drains your energy and slows your progress.

Combat fear with facts. Learn to recognize the early signs of problems; then, if they do occur, you and your physician can act promptly and decisively to counteract them. If you arm yourself with facts you will feel better prepared, and if you remind yourself that you are not facing the future alone you will feel less frightened. Confronting each problem as it presents itself will make you feel stronger and better equipped to deal with future difficulties. Being adequately informed about RA and its course of treatment can be extremely reassuring.

Stress

Stress is a universal aspect of life—a predictable reaction to life's surprises. Our world is constantly changing and presenting us with new situations and environments. We are exposed to an enormous amount of information on a daily basis—much more than our ancestors were. We draw upon our resources to make adjustments to these changes. If the magnitude of the changes overwhelms our ability to adjust, we experience stress.

In our daily routines we are aware of the potential demands and know how to approach them, but when routines are altered—when change occurs—we may stumble. Stress associated with change is generally a result of our anxiety and fear of the unknown: we don't know what the future holds, and we may be afraid that we don't have what it takes to meet this unexpected challenge.

Uncontrolled stress has many negative repercussions. Stress changes the pain threshold by opening the pain gate (described in Chapter 6). Stress also causes physical and mental fatigue, which interferes with restful sleep, further increasing pain. Stress increases inflammation and can cause flare-ups of RA. It has even been shown that people without RA who endure chronic stress have high amounts of inflammatory cytokines in their bloodstream (see Chapter 1). And stress affects the body in other ways; it can result in increased heart rate and perspiration and in elevated blood pressure. It does this by revving our innate "fight or flight" response, which causes our bodies to pump out stress hormones like adrenaline.

Since RA is a change that has a great deal of unpredictability associated with it, stress can be a common response to it. In fact, the most stressful part of RA is its unpredictability. People with RA do not know what they need to prepare for. The course of the condition varies among individuals and varies over time in the same person. This results in having to make frequent adjustments, which in itself can be stressful. People with RA often say that if they only knew what to expect they might not feel so anxious, they might adjust more easily.

What if you could objectively accept the fact that unexpected events will happen? You can choose not to dwell on every potential or unexpected future consequence, such as medication toxicity, medical bills, pain, or future disability. What if you decided that when events occur in the future that are beyond your control, you would address them competently *at that time?* You and change can coexist peaceably without worry. Lessening your stress level will enable you to redirect your vital energy toward accessing resources and tackling change on an as-needed basis. When you can let go of worry, fear, and anxiety, you lessen stress.

But not all stress is harmful. Stress occurs with positive changes as well as negative ones. Consider how you felt when you graduated from school, bought a house, got married, or went on a long-anticipated vacation. We all know, too, that feeling a little stress can motivate us to get tasks accomplished. Everyone has experienced short-lived deadline pressure and responded to it with increased adrenaline and increased activity. When stress becomes a permanent part of your life, however, it can take its toll on you and your physical health. So, we must learn to harness the energy created by change and turn it into a positive force with which we can address change, head on and without the negative emotional reactions that drain vital resources.

You can use coping skills to approach negative stress. First, you must identify the source of stress (*define the problem*). This process includes figuring out which situations cause you stress at work and at home. Determine which of them can be modified and which cannot. By distinguishing between them, you can avoid the frustration of trying to change the unchangeable and set goals that can be accomplished.

To solve a stress-related dilemma (*solve the problem*), begin by appraising the situation. What are its demands? Are you reasonably able to meet them at this particular time? If necessary, modify as many of the demands as possible so that they are reasonable for you at this time. Then call on the following problem-solving empowerment tactics:

- Propose a reasonable long-term goal (reasonable expectations).
- Plan ahead (include short-term, attainable goals).
- Provide a supportive environment (foster communication).
- Promote your identified strengths (use all resources).
- Put priorities into perspective (does it need to be done now?).
- Prepare (get organized).
- Pace yourself (one step at a time).
- Place time slots in your schedule to allow for inevitable interruptions and rest breaks (expect the unexpected).
- Practice present-minded thinking (focus on the task at hand).
- Positively reappraise the situation and your abilities (modify negative thoughts and behaviors).
- Prove to yourself that you can do it (beginning can be half the battle).
- Praise yourself for a job well done (you know best what you've accomplished).

You can see almost any situation through by calling upon your imagination, and each time you overcome a stressful situation successfully you increase your ability to cope with stress. Each such experience will empower you! Remember, "A great part of courage is having done the thing before" (Ralph Waldo Emerson).

Relieving the Tension of Anxiety, Fear, and Stress

There are numerous techniques you can use to minimize anxiety, fear, and stress, ranging from the simple to the exotic. It's worth mentioning here that it is often difficult to separate emotional tension from muscle or physical tension. We know that decreasing tension in one area often relieves tension in the other area, so, as you'll see, many of these tactics for relieving emotional tension involve physical activities.

Simple tactics include taking short breaks during your workday to relax, away from noise, bustle, and demands on you. While you relax, collect yourself and consciously try to gather the energies that are being drained by stress. At home, a long bath combined with relaxing music can ease your mind and body of tension. Making a detour to the whirlpool or sauna on your way home from work is a good way to wind down from an exhausting day. Gentle muscle massage administered by a friend, spouse, or professional massage therapist can relax tired, tense muscles and decrease your level of stress.

Often, just relaxing your mind by engaging in an enjoyable task or talking with a friend can reduce emotional and physical tension. Taking slow, deep, and regular breaths (preferably from the diaphragm rather than the chest) is another simple but effective way to decrease muscle tension and stress.

One time-tested technique is a deep muscle relaxation method called **progressive relaxation.** Many people incorporate this technique into their daily and nighttime routines. Begin by finding a quiet place and getting into a comfortable position. Close your eyes. Strongly tense up (clench) your toe muscles for about five seconds. Then relax them, feeling the difference between tension and relaxation. Proceed by alternately tensing and relaxing all of the major muscle groups in your body, from toes to head. When done correctly (doing so takes practice) this technique will leave your body loose and relaxed. Dr. Edmund Jacobson, who first described this technique in 1929, discovered that it is physically impossible to feel nervous or anxious in any part of our body if our muscles are completely relaxed. This suggests that, if we are able to relax the muscles successfully, other features of anxiety will be eliminated. This is a wonderful example of the positive power of the mind-body connection.

Some individuals incorporate **imagery** into their relaxation techniques. Closing your eyes and imagining yourself in a pleasant, restful place may help you achieve a peaceful state.

Some people have found **biofeedback** to be helpful in controlling chronic tension and pain. This technique involves clinical measurement of involuntary body functions such as heart rate, blood pressure, skin temperature, and muscle tension with monitoring equipment that is painlessly attached to the skin. Information about the physical (biological) changes taking place in the body is directly *fed back* to the subject from the equipment. The person being monitored can use this feedback to identify behaviors that bring about pain or tension and can then modify thoughts that induce these changes. The ultimate goal of biofeedback is to achieve mental mastery of the body's responses.

Recognizing that the mind and the body are intimately connected opens other avenues to reduce mental as well as physical tension. Many mind-body therapies follow spiritual traditions of the East. **Meditation** is a fundamental element of many Indian and Chinese practices. A person can develop powers of concentration directed at calming the mind and thus the body.

There are several types of meditation. Most commonly, during meditation one focuses on a single thing: a word, sound, thought, image, or object. Many choose the breath as their focal point. It takes a lot of practice to disregard thoughts and push out the "clutter" that occupies valuable space in our mind. This form of meditation is called "concentration meditation." With practice and continued discipline, focusing thoughts becomes easier, and deep states of calmness can be achieved.

A second technique, called *"mindfulness"* or "insight" meditation, is completely different. It encourages you to attend to the present moment. When thoughts or emotions enter your mind, you observe them without judgment or analysis. You let the thoughts flow freely. As you witness your own thoughts, you bring clarity to what is really on your mind, without defensiveness, intellectualizing, or reaction. This nonjudgmental awareness of your own thoughts and emotions can help bring acceptance and insight. With this clarity of presence, you are free to take the next step.

Different techniques work for different people. The important point is that you must *make the time* in your schedule to give any technique a fair trial. How many of us have verbalized at one time or another that we "just need time to think"? Perhaps we should listen to what we are telling ourselves. Several studies confirm that some forms of meditation decrease the body's stress-related inflammation. This research has shown that meditation actually lowers the levels of inflammatory *cytokines* (see Chapter 1) and other measures of inflammation in the bloodstream. Meditation, imagery, and biofeedback can also affect the way pain and tension are *perceived* and may even affect the course of arthritis.

For many people, prayer and other spiritual activities provide a sense of order in the face of life's countless challenges. The belief in a greater power helps us to focus on what is truly significant in our daily lives. Studies have shown that many people are strongly influenced by activities such as prayer and worship. People who participate in these activities appear to recover faster from surgery, have reduced pain, and suffer less from stress. How each person exercises his or her spiritual self is an individual choice, but we know that the health of the spiritual self affects the health of the physical self.

People who are feeling anxious or afraid or who feel that their life or condition is controlling them can use any of these techniques and many more to help them manage tension. There is more about the mind-body connection and its role in healing, including a review of complementary therapies, in Chapter 17. The important message is that using tactics that sift out extraneous sources of stress will allow you to relax your mind and body so you can focus on what is really important for you and your loved ones.

DEALING WITH FRIENDS AND FAMILY

Your loved ones need to progress through these emotional changes with you. You will want their help and empathy (but not their pity). You will probably want them to acknowledge your limitations without viewing them as weaknesses. You will need the support of your loved ones, but you won't want them to hover or be oversolicitous. Achieving this balance will take communication.

From their perspective, your loved ones are also struggling with the changes that your having RA has introduced. They may be uncertain about how to approach you. Should they offer their help? Should they allow you to do what you can unassisted? Should they pretend that nothing's changed? They will need your guidance. You must set the tone and direction for your future interactions. Your messages to others should be clear and concise. You must communicate with them and not expect them to understand simply because they love you. Mixed messages result in misunderstandings and hurt feelings.

Asking for Help

It is difficult to ask for help with tasks that we once were able to do on our own, but we all need to do this from time to time. If you learn to ask for help in a way that lets you keep your sense of independence and confidence, you will be much more likely to ask for the help you need. Learn to ask clearly and without ambiguity, so that the person you're asking knows exactly how you need to be helped. Consider the following unproductive approaches:

"I'll just do it myself." (Martyrdom is overvalued.)

"Can't you see I'm in pain and can't do this?" (It does no good to try to induce guilt in someone else.)

"Wash the dishes or *else.*" (People who feel as if they are being punished for your arthritis will sooner or later come to resent your requests for assistance.)

"I *can* do it, but I think it's about time for you to do something around here." (Denial has the potential to develop into antagonism.)

Now consider the following requests, messages that preserve self-esteem while constructively conveying the need for assistance:

"Here's what I need help with. I know I can count on you." (Describe the task and show appreciation; the response will almost certainly be positive.)

"I'm certain I can do this part alone, but I could really use your help with the rest of it." (Be specific about your needs, including what you *don't* need help with.)

"I'll clean up the living room if you'll vacuum the rug." (Negotiation allows equal input from everyone.)

Remember, your attitude has a far greater effect on your personal interactions than your disabilities do. Everyone wins when you give your loved ones the opportunity to do the right thing.

The Special Case of Children

A parent who has rheumatoid arthritis may find the adventure of childrearing especially challenging. For one thing, children require structure and routine, and it's hard to maintain consistency when you have a condition that fluctuates. On good days you may not need help from your kids, or you may be able to participate in activities with them. On bad days you may require their help and understanding. Despite the unpredictable nature of your arthritis, you must try to be consistent in your interactions with your children and your response to them.

For example, if one week you say, "Jimmy, I want you to clean up your room. I don't feel well," and a week later, when you're feeling better, you say "Jimmy, why don't you go watch cartoons while I clean up your room?" it's not going to take too long for Jimmy to realize that he will have to do more when you are feeling bad and will be rewarded when you feel well. It's far better to separate Jimmy's responsibilities from your physical condition: "Jimmy, you're six years old now, and we think you're big enough to pick up your room."

Erase from your mind any feelings of guilt you may have for not doing everything for your children. Guilt provides no positive direction and provides an opportunity for your children to manipulate you. Redirect your energy toward teaching lessons in responsibility and independence that will last a lifetime. A final note: there's nothing to prevent you from rewarding children for taking on new responsibilities. This is another real-life lesson, because we frequently are rewarded for a job well done.

A second caution to parents is to avoid making promises like "We'll do this if I feel well." When something's coming up that is important to your child, develop a backup plan. This may entail something as simple as arranging for your child's other parent to participate in the activity, with or without you, or inviting a godparent or relative to share in the event and be ready to do so without you if necessary. If you are a single parent, think about asking the parents of your child's friends to help out if you are feeling ill. *Do not wait until the day of the occasion* to make alternate plans, as this may leave you feeling trapped and your child disappointed and potentially resentful. Again, the goal is not to link your child's hopes too closely to your level of health on a given day.

Love and Intimacy

At some time, nearly everyone's love life is affected by the daily stresses of living. Changes in energy, emotions, personal body image, and self-esteem directly affect how you feel as a sexual person. If you do not feel attractive, for example, you will not expect others to be attracted to you. To improve or renew your intimate relationships, you must first address the issues of energy, emotions, body image, and self-esteem in your life. When you start feeling strong and in control of your life, everything will change for you. With renewed confidence and self-esteem you will realize that you are a loving (and lovable) person capable of, and deserving of, an enduring and fulfilling relationship with your partner.

One key to a successful, loving relationship is communication, and this is particularly true when one partner has a health problem. It is not always easy for people to discuss their intimate concerns, however. Consider the following questions. If they are left unasked—and unanswered—they can seriously damage a relationship.

- Am I still attractive to my partner?
- Am I hurting her?
- Is he still interested?
- Why isn't he more concerned with my needs?

Misunderstandings over issues of intimacy can linger for months if they are not addressed. As a result, one or both partners may begin to avoid intimacy and even situations that may lead to intimacy. Once this pattern of aloofness is begun, it may be difficult to break. *Communication is the key.* Express your concerns to your partner:

- Do you still find me attractive?
- Am I hurting you?
- I want to make love but you seem distant. What's going on?
- Maybe you don't realize that sex first thing in the morning is often painful for me. Can we schedule a rendezvous for lunchtime?

Dr. Jackson Rainer of Webb University (Enliven Panel, 2000) believes that intimacy issues affected by RA are often ignored by the parties involved. He recommends working toward *intimacy* rather than placing too much emphasis on sexual intercourse. He believes that "the biggest sex organ is the skin, and the best sex organ is the brain." Couples should focus on "closeness, touch, pleasure, and contact" rather than the act of sex. He also makes the following suggestions:

- Talk about intimacy issues in a setting away from the bedroom.
- Be straightforward and concrete in your communication.
- Take small steps, and keep the dialogue going.
- Begin to court and date each other again.

People are appropriately becoming more comfortable talking with their doctors about problems with sexual function. Pain, fatigue, and medications can have an impact on libido as well as physical capabilities. In some men with RA, erectile dysfunction has been reported. If this is the case, we strongly encourage an evaluation by your physician. Low testosterone (male hormone) levels have been discovered in some men with RA. Therapy with testosterone in those individuals may make a difference in sexual function and interest. Testosterone replacement has been shown to have other positive effects in men with RA and low testosterone levels (Cutolo, 2000). Women can also be affected with sexual difficulties. Issues regarding body image and anxieties regarding health have been shown to affect many women and their sexuality (Gutweniger et al., 1999). Please do not ignore these issues. Help is available to work through these complicated concerns, but you need to ask for it.

As suggested earlier in this book, there may be times when physical limitations—fatigue, painful joints, and restricted motion—will interfere with your sex life. Creativity is *very* helpful in overcoming these obstacles. Upon request, the Arthritis Foundation will send you a free pamphlet called "Guide to Intimacy and Arthritis," which provides guidelines for comfortable physical intimacy. Here are some suggestions:

- Plan for sex at the time of day when you feel best.
- Take pain relief medicine ahead of time so that it takes effect before intercourse.
- Pace activities during the day to avoid becoming fatigued before sex.
- Perform range-of-motion exercises to relax your joints before sex.
- Take a warm bath or shower before sex to relax both you and your joints.

Planning for sexual activity may seem awkward and contrived when you first start doing it, but it need not be. With creativity and imagination, the preparation can become an exciting and stimulating addition to your relationship. It also sends a message to your partner that you desire to continue and expand your intimate relationship.

Friends and Relatives

Friends and relatives can be a wonderful source of support and inspiration for people with rheumatoid arthritis. Some of them will show great sensitivity and understanding and will provide help in trying times almost instinctively. Other people—most people, in fact—will look to the person with RA for direction. Let them know that you value their friendship and company, and show them how they can support you when times are hard. If you must decline a social invitation because of your arthritis, be sure to let people know that you want to be included in future get-togethers.

Friends and relatives can also be a tremendous source of irritation. Remember, there are many, many people who do not know much about RA. Although most people mean well, they may say the wrong thing. Maybe you will be able to center yourself and not be pulled into a defensive posture after an annoying comment. If you can answer with a gracious, thoughtful, and positive response, good for you! You are right where you need to be. If you are like most of us, your "knee jerk" reaction might be a comment that does not promote world peace. After all, you are human. A humorous approach—inside your own head—is one way to cope with the dumb comment or the thoughtless statement. Thinking a funny thought will help to defuse your irritation and give you a minute to find your balance and say something that preserves the peace between you and the comment maker. So, when someone makes an inappropriate remark, think about how you *wish you could* respond . . . then wait a few seconds . . . and instead make a constructive response to your friend or relative. The scenarios below apply this method to several common types of inappropriate comment:

The *should have* comment: "You *should have* exercised more; then you wouldn't have arthritis."

Think: "You *should have* gone to charm school."

Say: "That's an interesting hypothesis. Although exercise is important, its absence hasn't been shown to be cause rheumatoid arthritis."

The *should* comment: "You *should* drink six pints of apricot juice each day to cure your arthritis."

Think: "You *should* learn that silence is golden."

Say: "A balanced diet is very important for all people, including those with rheumatoid arthritis."

The *could have* comment: "You should feel lucky; you *could have* developed cancer."

Think: "I do feel lucky, you *could have* been someone whose opinion mattered to me."

Say: "I do feel good that I have a condition I can cope with successfully."

The *I know how you feel* comment: "I know how you feel. I have arthritis in my big toe, and it really limits my golf game."

Think: "Tiger Woods will sleep easier at night."

Say: "Did you know that there are more than one hundred types of arthritis? But it's really nice when people understand how challenging arthritis is at times."

The *I've got a relative* comment: "My third cousin twice removed has that
kind of arthritis and she's crippled."
Think: "I wish you were twice removed from me."
Say: "With early treatment and therapy, few people with arthritis today develop serious handicaps."

The *I've got a friend* comment: "My friend with RA tried daily artichoke ene-
mas and his RA is gone!"
Think: "I think we both know what you can do with that advice."
Say: "New and different alternative therapies are being studied every day.
It's great that researchers are really thinking outside the box."

The *brilliant observer:* "Did you know that your hands are swollen?"
Think: "You have excellent observation skills. I think I'll fire my doctor."
Say: "Yes, I did. Thank you for your concern."

The *doting relative:* "Serve your sister her dinner first! Can't you see she has
arthritis?"
Think: "Would you mind chewing and swallowing it for me, too?"
Say: "I appreciate your concern, but I can wait my turn. There will be things
I'll need assistance with in the future, and I'm glad that I can count on all
of you for your help."

Get the idea? You'll probably be surprised at the type of comment that will pop
into your head in these circumstances. Thinking silently of a humorous response is a good way to ventilate your annoyance without alienating the person
who makes a thoughtless remark. Most people are trying to be supportive. Be
patient and direct them in their efforts. Do not get angry or hurt. Use your energy to educate them about RA, so that they won't continue making senseless
comments.

FOR MORE INFORMATION

Two helpful pamphlets, "A Guide to Intimacy with Arthritis" and "Managing
Your Stress," are available from the Arthritis Foundation (1330 W. Peachtree St.,
Atlanta, Ga. 30309; 1-800-283-7800; or go to www.afstore.org).

EXERCISE AND REHABILITATION

Protecting Your Joints

Inflamed joints are more easily injured than joints that are not inflamed. Everyone who has rheumatoid arthritis (RA) must learn how to *protect* his or her joints, giving special attention to the joints in the hands and wrists, since these are particularly vulnerable to injury during daily activity.

Joint protection involves more than a list of things to do and not to do; it is a philosophy that should be incorporated into one's daily routine. At first the strategies may seem awkward or inefficient, and having to stop and think about how you move before you move can seem bothersome. With practice, however, these tactics will become routine. Joint protection will become second nature to you.

After your arthritis has improved, you should continue to follow the principles of joint protection. Your reward will be decreased pain and stiffness as well as preservation of the best possible joint function.

In this chapter each of the principles of joint protection is discussed along with examples of how these guidelines may be used. Try incorporating these guidelines into your daily life. An **occupational therapist** can help you understand these principles and apply them to your particular situation. Ask your physician to refer you to an occupational therapist, especially if you're having difficulty putting these principles into practice.

JOINT PROTECTION GUIDELINES

Respect your pain. Increased pain is a warning that you are overtaxing your joints. You should heed this warning and modify the activity. This principle is discussed in detail in Chapter 6; it is very important.

Balance rest with activity. Organizing your schedule so that you alternate energy-intensive activities with more restful ones will stretch your energy reserves and protect your joints as well. Conserving your energy by avoiding unnecessary tasks will leave you with more energy to exercise and do the necessary jobs.

Maintain your muscle strength. Strong muscles provide additional support to your joints and help protect them from undue stress. (Chapters 9 and 10 describe ways to build and maintain muscle strength.)

Avoid activities that cannot be interrupted for rest. Try to steer clear of prolonged activities that leave you no room or opportunity to rest. Consider that standing in a long line without being able to sit down will leave you fatigued. With some planning you can avoid peak hours and long lines at the post office, bank, and grocery store. Carrying a package for a long distance—across a large parking lot, for example—is another activity that can wear you out. Again, the best way to avoid this is to plan ahead: keep a portable or fold-up cart in your car. This will allow you to transport the object without exerting much energy. If it has a seat, it will also let you take small rest breaks during the trek if you need to.

Avoid positions that promote deformity. Sometimes ligaments and muscles become stretched with the inflammation of arthritis. This may cause unequal forces to be exerted across the joints, creating a situation in which the joints *drift*, or change their alignment. This is known as joint deformity. The word *deformity* is frightening for most people. The use of the word within this setting, however, merely describes a change in the normal positioning (and, sometimes, function) of joints. Later in this chapter we will describe positions that make deformity worse; these positions are to be avoided.

Utilize the largest joint and the strongest muscle available to complete a task. It makes good sense to call upon your most powerful joints and muscles to perform any given task. In this way you avoid putting stress upon smaller, less powerful joints and muscles. Consider the task of lifting a heavy book. If you pick the book up between your thumb and fingers, the fingers and wrist will have a great deal of stress placed on them. Instead, if you pick the book up by sliding your hands underneath the book, palms up, and then lifting it, your arm muscles and elbows will do the work, and you'll avoid putting extra stress on your wrists and fingers. As you apply this principle, you will learn to be observant and analytical about which joints and muscles are working and which joints are experiencing extra stress.

Avoid remaining in one position or using muscles in one stationary position for long periods of time. Remaining in one position for too long promotes stiffness or a **gelling** effect on inflamed joints. Muscles also become fatigued when you use them from the same position for long periods. (Think about how your muscles begin to cramp when you write for lengthy periods without stopping or readjusting the pencil or stylus.) Stiffness of joints and muscles can be avoided by changing to a different position every fifteen to twenty minutes. Frequent stretching also helps prevent joints from losing range of motion. Take frequent breaks, stretch, and change positions *before* muscle fatigue sets in.

Utilize splinting as needed. A splint is a fabricated support that is designed to stabilize inflamed joints. In RA, a splint may have any or all of three basic functions. It can be designed to (1) rest an inflamed joint by partially or completely immobilizing it, (2) protect a weakened joint from injury by supporting it, and (3) improve function of a damaged joint.

Splints should be used only if they decrease pain and inflammation or improve function. There is no good evidence available that splints prevent deformity. On the other hand, it has been proven that incorrect or prolonged use of splints can lead to increased stiffness, decreased strength, and decreased motion. If you believe that you are receiving no benefit from a prescribed splint, discuss this with your physician or occupational therapist.

Utilize assistive equipment as needed. There are numerous catalogues listing accessories that are useful for people who have arthritis—so many, in fact, that the choices may be overwhelming. Our advice is to use as little in the way of assistive equipment as possible, because these devices can actually *interfere* with your ability to function independently if you rely on them too heavily or if you use too many of them. This is not to say that there aren't many situations in which a specific item can help you considerably and spare your joints from excessive stress. More information about specific devices is given below.

PROTECTING SPECIFIC JOINTS

The following hints for protecting specific joints have proven to be quite effective. Please note that you needn't observe these principles or use these assistive devices for joints in which you have no arthritis; unaffected joints you can safely use normally and unaided. The discussion is organized by joint groups.

Hands and Wrists

Finger and wrist joints tend to slowly drift out of their natural alignment when there is chronic inflammation, as illustrated in Figures 10, 11, and 12. To avoid contributing to these deformities adhere to these principles.

- When stirring foods, hold the utensil with your thumb on top (as if you were stabbing a block of ice with an ice pick) and stir with shoulder motion.

- Avoid hanging a purse strap over your wrist or carrying heavy suitcases.

- Avoid supporting your body weight on your wrists and hands. For example, do not lean on your hands while standing against a table edge.

- Avoid stressful wringing and twisting motions. (Use an electric rather than a manual can opener. Roll hand-washed items in a towel rather than wringing them.)

- Do not wring your washcloth out; hang it where it can drip dry.

- Do not grip items tightly or hold onto them for long periods. Too tight a grip increases deforming pressures.

- Modify the size of articles that you grasp daily. You can cushion pressure points and enlarge the diameter of pencils, pens, toothbrushes, and other utensils by placing the handles inside a foam hair curler or wrapping them with soft foam rubber.

- Avoid actions that push your other fingers toward your little finger (as in Figure 11). When reading, don't hold a book in a way that puts weight on your fingers (use a book holder). Don't rest your chin on top of your fingers. Lift and carry objects with palms, not with your fingers. When getting up from a chair, use your palms rather than your fingers to push off.

- Open jars by putting pressure on the top with your palm and twisting from the shoulder rather than by gripping the lid with your fingers.

Remember to use the largest joint and the strongest muscle available to do the job. For example, shut doors with your hip or upper arm rather than your fingers.

Splints. The splints that are available today are made of lighter-weight materials and are smaller than they were in the past. They are also more comfortable and attractive than splints used to be. The ring splint illustrated in Figure 13 is an example of a modern splint that can be used by persons with swan neck (Figure 12B) or boutonnière (Figure 12C) deformity, if the splint improves function.

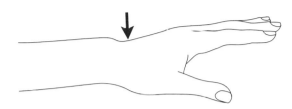

FIGURE 10. Wrist-deforming forces

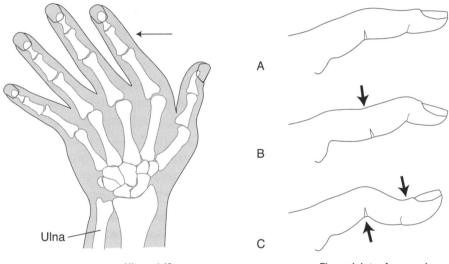

FIGURE 11. Ulnar drift

Ulna

FIGURE 12. Finger joints: A, normal;
B, swan neck; C, boutonnière

Hand and wrist splints can be either commercially fabricated (purchased over the counter) or custom fit by an occupational therapist or orthotist, in which case you will need a prescription from your doctor. Health insurance plans vary considerably in their coverage for such custom-made devices, so check with your insurer in advance. (An **orthotist** is an expert in the development and application of splints, braces, and other supports to improve function or decrease pain and inflammation.) The functional wrist splint illustrated in Figure 14 is useful because it allows some movement at the fingers while immobilizing the wrist. Some physicians prescribe a resting hand splint to be worn at night to rest finger and wrist joints. Remember, splints should be used only if they relieve pain or improve function.

Assistive equipment. People with hand and wrist problems may find use of the following equipment helpful:

- built-up handles
- faucet turners or levers
- key adaptors or levers
- button hook
- elastic shoelaces
- door opener
- car door opener or lever

- loop scissors
- luggage carrier
- mitt potholder
- padded wrist rest for computer keyboard
- battery-powered or plug-in electric toothbrush

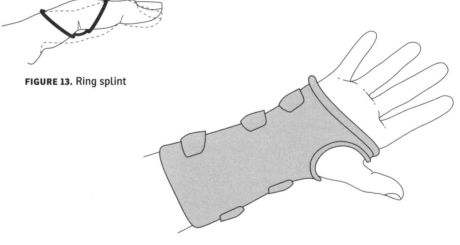

FIGURE 13. Ring splint

FIGURE 14. Functional wrist splint

Elbows and Shoulders

A position that can cause deformity in the elbow is illustrated in Figure 15A, in which use of the wrong kind of cane is shown putting stress on the elbow joint. Figure 15B illustrates a walking device that prevents stress on the elbow and cuts down on stress to the wrists, as well.

Here, as with hands and wrists, the principle is to avoid putting stress on the joint in a way that contributes to deformity. For example, when you are carrying heavy objects, keep them as close to your body as possible so that your spine can relieve some of the stress on your shoulders, elbows, and wrists.

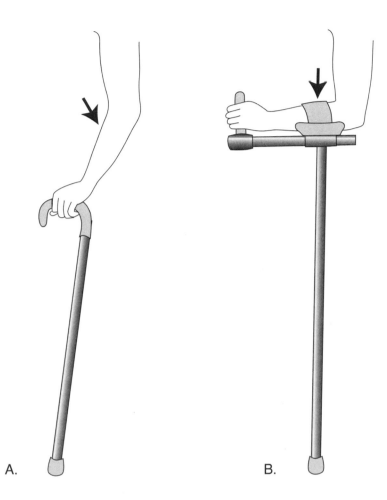

FIGURE 15. A, elbow-deforming forces; B, forearm cane

Assistive equipment. Assistive equipment to relieve stress on shoulders and elbows includes items that have extended handles or devices that extend handles and items that allow you to carry things without using your arms.

- extended handles on combs, hairbrushes, toothbrushes, utensils
- extended handle dustpan
- elbow crutch

- over-the-shoulder pouch
- knapsack
- small cart for carrying items (a folding shopping cart, for example)

Hips and Knees

People whose hips and knees are affected by arthritis need to make every effort to keep their weight down. This will limit the amount of pressure that is put on these joints.

One technique for avoiding putting undue pressure on hips and knees is to use your whole body to rise from a sitting position. Slide forward as far as you can in the seat and then lean forward over your knees and swing up. Try to push off with your forearms or palms (avoid using your fingers). Elevating yourself in the chair with a pillow will help.

Assistive equipment. People with arthritis in the hips and knees may find the following equipment helpful. Remember that these assistive devices should not be *overused*. For example, reaching is a good stretching exercise, and if reaching is not painful for you, you probably are better off *not* using a long-handled reacher.

- elevated seat with arm rests
- raised toilet seat
- stool
- shower bench

- extended shoehorn
- long-handled reacher
- tub grab bars
- walking aids (cane, walker)

Ankles and Feet

RA in the feet can cause swelling and stretched ligaments, and over time the foot often becomes broader and the toes higher than they were before. One of the best ways to protect your feet and ankles is to wear the proper footwear, because a shoe that fits poorly can injure sensitive toes and feet and cause further deformity.

Do not under any circumstances purchase a shoe that rubs or causes pressure and then expect to break it in. Any breaking in will only come to pass at the expense of your feet. The best advice really is, "If the shoe fits, wear it." Sandy Shlotzhauer-Turner, a certified pedorthist, recommends that you trace your foot while standing on a piece of hard cardboard. Cut out the foot tracing and bring it to the store. If possible, remove the inlay of the potential shoe and place it over the tracing. If the tracing goes outside of the inlay, the shoe will not accommodate your foot comfortably. If the inlay is not removable, you can see if the cardboard tracing inserts easily into the shoe without restriction. She also recommends looking for the following features in shoes:

- light weight
- deep enough toe box to clear top of toes; deeper if a cushioning insole or orthotic insert will be needed
- wide enough not to pinch toes together
- long enough that there is ⅜ to ½ inch between the end of the shoe and the *longest toe* (not always the big toe)
- breathable, supple uppers, like soft leathers and Lycra (materials that stretch to accommodate deformities)
- one inch or lower heel
- good shock absorption for soles and heels
- good support along the inside of the foot
- durable, stiff back for support

For the sake of your feet—the only pair you will ever have—always choose good fit over fashion. People with RA often have difficulty finding shoes that are comfortable, practical, and stylish. Proper fit may be complicated by deformities of the foot or toes. If the arthritis in your feet is mild, shoes that are deep and wide, such as good supportive walking shoes or athletic shoes, will usually suffice.

If you have deformities of the feet, you may require an insert, or orthosis, for your shoes. These shoe inserts (commonly referred to as "orthotics") can be purchased over the counter, or they can be specially designed for your feet by a **podiatrist** (foot doctor), **pedorthist** (footware modification specialist), or *orthotist/prosthetist* (orthotics and prosthetics specialist). For example, a certified pedorthist would take an impression of your foot by having you step into wax, plaster, foam, or other mold-making material. From these impressions, supports (called *accommodative orthoses*) can be designed that conform exactly to the contours of your feet and relieve pressure on sensitive areas by distributing the pressure to other areas of the foot. Other orthoses (called *functional orthoses*) are designed to correct foot and ankle function by altering forces and providing stabilization, thus improving biomechanics and gait. It is important to see an experienced practitioner who understands the nature of RA and its effects on the feet. Communities vary regarding how much expertise is available for these fittings. Ask your rheumatologist for suggestions. You will also need to purchase shoes that are wide and deep enough to accommodate the orthosis. There are several brand names available today that are considered "depth" shoes. These shoes can accommodate some deformities and allow enough space for inserts.

Sometimes an extra piece of rubber or leather (*metatarsal bar*) is applied externally to the sole of the shoe. This takes pressure off the ball of the foot, frequently an area of discomfort.

If you have severe foot damage or deformity you may require specially made shoes in addition to custom orthoses. Although expensive, custom shoes offer a precise fit for feet of all shapes. A casting of your foot provides an exact replica from which the shoes are fashioned. Some newer versions are more stylish than the classic orthopedic shoe. Your doctor, therapist, orthopedic surgeon, or podiatrist may be able to give you the name of the best provider of custom shoes in your area. This would generally be a certified orthotist, pedorthist, or prosthetist. These shoes are generally quite expensive, so the experience of the professional who makes them for you counts. It is important that you select a provider who is willing to make adjustments if the first pair feels uncomfortable to you. Also, find out whether a second pair can be purchased at a reduced fee.

Splints and more sophisticated ankle/foot orthoses (commonly called AFOs) are occasionally recommended for the back of the foot and the ankle. Your physician will tell you whether an AFO might be useful for you.

Finally, here is some excellent advice from Ms. Shlotzhauer-Turner about foot care for people with arthritis:

- Avoid walking barefoot.
- Keep your feet meticulously clean and dry to avoid skin breakdown and infection.
- Examine your feet often for signs of irritation.
- Look for blisters and pressure sores. If these signs of stress develop, change shoes and consider getting your feet measured and shoes fit by a certified professional.
- Avoid harsh chemical agents or cutting to remove calluses; they have formed for a reason. Find out what that reason is.
- Cut your toenails straight across slightly rounding the sharp edges with a small file.
- Elevate your feet and legs whenever possible to reduce swelling.
- Manage your weight.
- Do ankle and foot range of motion and stretching exercises for a few minutes before you get out of bed in the morning to reduce stiffness and discomfort upon arising.

FOR MORE INFORMATION

The Arthritis Foundation's Tips for Good Living with Arthritis has hundreds of joint protection tips as well as lists of resources. Order from the Arthritis Foundation Store, P.O. Box 932915, Atlanta, Ga. 31193-2915; by calling 1-800-283-7800; by email at afsorders@arthritis.org; or by going to www.afstore.org.

Living Better with Arthritis has been helping people with arthritis since 1979 with its catalogue of assistive devices for people with arthritis. Aids for Arthritis, Inc., 35 Wakefield Drive, Medford, N.J. 08055; 1-800-654-0707; www.aidsforarthritis.com.

9

Exercise and Rheumatoid Arthritis

Should you exercise or should you rest? The answer is, both, which at first must seem contradictory. In truth, though, both appropriate exercise *and* adequate rest are important in the treatment of rheumatoid arthritis (RA).

Appropriate exercise can only be managed through an *individualized* rehabilitation program, one that contains the right balance of exercise and rest *for you*. Devising such a program, of course, requires some knowledge of how RA is affecting *you*.

It wasn't so long ago that generalizations were made about patients with RA without regard for their degree of arthritis—but no longer. Now we know that a program that doesn't take the individual's needs into account is destined to be unsafe or unproductive, or both.

TRENDS IN THERAPEUTIC ADVICE

Proper treatment for RA, including the benefits of exercise, has been the subject of debate for decades. Understanding the historical change in attitude about exercise may help you understand the thinking behind what your physician or therapist is telling you now.

In the 1950s and 1960s, people with RA were routinely treated with bed rest. It was not uncommon, in fact, for a person with RA to be placed in the hospital for one or two months in an attempt to bring the arthritis under control. Since inflamed joints do improve with bed rest (when inflamed joints are splinted or immobilized, the swelling, pain, and heat decrease), the practice continued. In this same time period, exercises were rarely prescribed for *any* arthritis patient (regardless of how well controlled the arthritis was) for fear that the person's condition would worsen.

In time, some health care providers questioned the logic behind prolonged bed rest, which exerts negative effects on the body: muscles weaken, bones lose calcium and become more brittle, and overall fitness diminishes. Although joint inflammation improves with bed rest, people were getting out of shape—their general health was deteriorating—while their arthritis was coming under control.

Gradually, health care providers began prescribing exercises for their patients, and over time the amount of prescribed exercise has increased. Gentle range-of-motion exercises, aimed at preserving joint motion, and cautious muscle-strengthening exercises became essential components of an RA exercise regimen.

In the past thirty years, people have become much more exercise conscious, and trends in therapeutic advice for people with RA reflect this. In the 1970s and 1980s, for example, several inspired investigators decided to see what would happen if they increased the level of exercise in patients whose arthritis was under control. Marion Minor, a registered physical therapist at the University of Missouri-Columbia, as well as other researchers, reported interesting results. They discovered that some individuals with arthritis can perform more advanced strengthening exercises, as well as low-impact aerobic exercises, with positive effects. These people appeared to benefit from the exercise in numerous ways: they had improved stamina, less fatigue, and better ability to function, and they spent less time away from work and more time away from the hospital. Newer studies have confirmed that these exercises not only improve aerobic fitness and muscle strength, but even reduce inflammation (Cooney et al., 2011). This is a far cry from what we thought in prior years.

What physicians and others have learned from changes in treatment adds up to this: people with RA (like nearly everyone else) should exercise. Appropriate exercise can improve your energy and strength, increase joint stability, help prevent joint deformities, decrease pain, and allow you to function better. But exercise affects more than just the symptoms of arthritis; it helps build stronger bones, promotes self-esteem, improves the quality of sleep, and decreases muscle tension and anxiety. A fitness program faithfully adhered to will also benefit your lungs, your heart, and your circulation. By building muscle mass, exercise also increases your metabolic rate. This will help you to maintain a healthful weight.

The recommended amount and type of exercise depend on the degree of inflammation and the pattern of joint involvement a person is experiencing. This chapter and the next present a general guide to appropriate exercise and review some precautions as well as some commonly prescribed exercises. It is important to bear in mind that a book or Web site cannot perform the skilled evaluation that a physician and a physical therapist trained in arthritis can; nor can it give you individualized advice. By determining your specific needs, these health care professionals can prescribe an exercise program that will improve *your* function. You need to seek their advice before embarking on an exercise program.

TYPES OF EXERCISE

Three major forms of exercise are prescribed for people with RA: range of motion, muscle strengthening, and aerobic. Each of these three types of exercise is discussed below, and specific exercises are described in detail in the next chapter. Later in this chapter we discuss the more encompassing forms of exercise called mind-body exercises.

Range of Motion

Range of motion refers to the full range of movements that a joint can make. Range-of-motion exercises involve moving each joint as far as it can comfortably be moved in all directions. The goal of this form of exercise is to decrease stiffness and pain, maintain flexibility, and improve the function of the joints. As we have seen, inflammation and decreased use can impair function in the joints, and these exercises are designed to prevent that loss. No weights are used in range-of-motion exercises.

Stretching exercises are similar to range-of-motion exercises, but these exercises involve stretching the joint just beyond that which is comfortable. Joints should never be stretched to the point of excessive pain, however, and they should never be "bounced" in an effort to increase joint motion or range.

Range-of-motion and stretching exercises are fundamental to the warm-up stage for any exercise program. They should be performed once or twice per day and they can be performed whenever you need to decrease stiffness in the joints.

Strengthening

Strengthening exercises increase your muscle strength and muscle tone, allowing you to function with less muscle fatigue and more joint stability. Thus, muscles that are strengthened through exercise actually help protect the joints. Strengthening exercises are also needed by people with RA because muscles that are not used (generally because use causes pain) become smaller (atrophied), and this causes them to become weaker. Also, tendons and ligaments can stretch and loosen in response to swelling in and around the joints, decreasing joint stability; strengthening exercises can help the joints compensate for these changes caused by RA.

Isometric exercises involve simply tightening, or contracting, muscles (called *muscle setting*), an activity that helps maintain muscle strength. Isometric strengthening exercises involve *maximally* tightening your muscles by pushing or pulling against a fixed object, *without* moving your joints. *Moving your joints against high resistance should always be avoided.* One example of an isometric strengthening exercise is pushing against a wall without moving your shoulders, elbows, or wrists. With this exercise the arm muscles contract and get stronger but, since the joints are not moving, the joints are protected from increased stress.

Isometric strengthening exercises may also be performed by using *exercise bands*. These are elastic bands (or tubing) that stretch slightly but are very strong. They may be purchased commercially (Thera-Band and Thera-Tube are two name brands), or they may be fabricated from materials you may have at home (such as an elastic belt, bungee cords, rubber tubing, or garden hoses). Adjustable trouser belts that are somewhat stretchable work well, because you can adjust the size of the loop. You can also double over an elastic belt to decrease the amount of stretch or create a smaller loop. Several examples of isometric exercises using exercise bands are described in the next chapter.

One note of caution: Exercising with weights can stress an inflamed joint. You should avoid this kind of exercise (called *isotonic* strengthening exercises) unless your therapist or doctor instructs you otherwise.

Aerobic

Endurance or *aerobic exercises* are designed to increase overall fitness. They prepare your body to perform tasks over a period of time without becoming fatigued or exhausted. They improve your body's efficiency in using oxygen from the blood supply. Circulation, heart function, and respiration (breathing) improve, as well. New studies also show that aerobic exercise can even help reduce joint damage visible on x-rays (Scarvell and Elkins, 2011). Aerobic exercises compatible with RA include swimming, walking, bicycling, elliptical training, and even some forms of low-impact aerobics, depending on the extent of arthritic involvement of lower extremity joints. Aerobic exercise can also increase muscle strength.

STARTING AN EXERCISE PROGRAM

An exercise program is made up of three crucial components: warm-up, workout, and cool-down. Most people with RA find that an exercise program occupies about thirty minutes daily, usually ten minutes of warming up, fifteen minutes of working out, and five minutes of cooling down—but this may vary. You should never exercise to the point of extreme fatigue or exhaustion. Start low, go slow, and work your way up! In this way you can make progress without suffering setbacks.

People with RA need to schedule their exercise to coincide with the time of day when they are most rested and have the least pain.

Warm-up

A warm-up is necessary to allow the joints and muscles to loosen up slowly, in preparation for the workout. *Tight joints and muscles should not be exercised.* Warm up by doing range-of-motion and stretching exercises at a speed and intensity that are not uncomfortable, to prepare muscles for more intense exercise.

Workout

Which workout is best for you is determined by the degree of inflammation in your joints. Generally, unless your joints are very inflamed, a workout should include strengthening and aerobic exercises. When joints are very inflamed, the workout may consist of only range-of-motion exercises, done in ways that go only slightly beyond comfort, in an effort to maintain current range of movement.

Cool-down

The cool-down stage relaxes excited muscles and allows the heart rate and breathing rate to return to their before-workout levels. A cool-down also helps avoid postexercise pain or anxiety. Cool-down exercises can be range-of-motion exercises or aerobic exercises performed in slow motion.

EXERCISES THAT ARE RIGHT FOR YOU

Exercise recommendations for people with rheumatoid arthritis vary greatly, depending on the degree of arthritis activity present in the joints at the time. Before undertaking any exercise program, you should always review it with the physician or physical therapist who is most familiar with your specific situation. The key to developing and following an effective rehabilitation and exercise program is to know *your* arthritis.

You may already be aware that your arthritis can vary greatly over time. You may have experienced a severe flare-up of arthritis in the past after you overexerted yourself. If you know the pattern of your own arthritis well, you will be the best judge of which exercises will make you feel better and which ones will only make you feel worse.

In describing model exercise programs in the rest of this chapter, we have, for the sake of convenience, divided RA into three different levels of activity: very inflamed, moderately inflamed, and controlled. We recognize that this is an artificial division, however, and that few people fit neatly into any one of these categories all the time. Also, individuals have different exercise needs. Again, no one with RA should begin an exercise program without obtaining the advice of a health care professional who is familiar with that individual's needs.

For People with Very Inflamed Joints

A very inflamed joint is also known as an *acute joint* or a *highly active joint*. The joint will usually be warm, tender, and swollen. A joint is very inflamed if you experience significant discomfort when you move it through a gentle range-of-motion exercise. There is generally significant morning stiffness in very inflamed joints, as well. You may feel fatigue or muscle discomfort. This is often the level of arthritic activity people mean when they describe their arthritis as *flaring up.*

General exercise program guidelines for people with very inflamed joints include the following:

1. Move each *affected* joint through five repetitions of each range-of-motion exercise once or twice per day.

   Goal: Maintain motion and flexibility in joints.

   Precautions: Do not stretch joints beyond the point at which you feel increased pain. Do not push yourself to extreme fatigue.

2. Tighten each muscle *without moving the joint,* and maintain tension for six seconds once or twice per day.

Goal: Prevent muscle weakening.

Precautions: Do not use elastic bands or perform other forms of isometric strengthening if your joints are very inflamed. Simply flex and tighten the muscles.

For People with Moderately Inflamed Joints

Moderately inflamed joints are also known as *subacute* joints. Although the inflammation is moderate, these joints still cause some discomfort, and pain increases after the joint has been stressed. For example, you may not notice moderate inflammation in your shoulder until you attempt to retrieve an object from a high shelf. And moving moderately inflamed finger joints might not cause you any discomfort until you try to unscrew the lid of a jar. Subacute joints may have morning stiffness, but it does not last as long as it does in highly active joints.

General exercise program guidelines for people with moderately inflamed joints include the following:

1. Move joints through three, four, or five repetitions of each range-of-motion exercise. Do two or three stretches until you feel that you are at your maximum range of motion, then add one or two more stretches to be sure. Do this once or twice per day.

Goals: Maintain and slowly increase motion and flexibility. Increase muscle tone.

Precautions: Cut back the number of repetitions if increased swelling or pain occurs.

2. Incorporate isometric strengthening exercises into your regimen. Hold each contracted muscle against a fixed resistance (such as a stretched elastic exercise band) for six seconds without moving your joints. Use about three-quarters of your maximum strength (or less, if pain occurs). Do this one, two, or three times with each muscle group, taking a ten-second break between each contraction. Isometric strengthening exercises are usually performed only once daily.

Goal: Increase muscle strength.

Precautions: Your joints should be kept immobile during this form of therapy. Keep the tension in your muscles, not in your joints.

3. Gradual addition of endurance exercises may be appropriate at this stage. Adding a swimming program is often recommended, because the buoyancy of the water relieves stress on joints. Other forms of aerobic exercise may be recommended if your hips, knees, and feet are not inflamed. Before adding exercises such as walking and bicycling to your program, talk it over with your physician.

   Goal: Increase endurance and fitness.

   Precautions: Check with your doctor to see if you are ready for aerobic exercises.

For People with Controlled Joints

A *stable* or *inactive* joint is one that was previously inflamed but is now under satisfactory control. It is not necessarily a normal joint, because damage may have occurred in the past and changed its appearance and function.

Controlled or stable joints are generally not warm to the touch. They also display only minimal morning stiffness and tenderness. They may appear enlarged but are usually not filled with fluid.

Exercise recommendations for controlled joints depend on the amount of damage remaining as a consequence of past inflammation. General exercise guidelines include the following:

1. Continue daily range-of-motion exercises with a maximum of ten repetitions. You can decrease number of repetitions to two or three when maximal range of motion has been attained.

   Goal: Maintain and increase motion and flexibility.

   Precautions: Cut back repetitions if increased pain or swelling becomes evident.

2. Continue isometric strengthening exercises as with moderately inflamed joints. Once maximum strength is achieved you will be able to cut down on these exercises and devote more time to aerobic exercise. Your therapist may also suggest a form of isotonic exercise with small weights, if

your joints are under excellent control and do not show any sign of significant damage.

Goal: Increase strength.

Precautions: All strengthening exercise programs should be reviewed with your doctor or physical therapist. Placing inappropriate stress on damaged joints can result in increased deformity. Never use weights without checking first with your doctor or therapist.

3. Endurance exercises are most important in this stage, to help you regain aerobic conditioning lost when the arthritis was more active. Swimming is still the best form of aerobic exercise, but other forms of low-impact aerobics may be considered (for example, walking, bicycling, elliptical use, low-impact dancing). Half an hour of aerobic exercise three times weekly will increase your fitness. As you grow stronger and spend more time with endurance exercises, you can eliminate some of your strengthening exercises, although it is a good idea to continue range-of-motion exercises with affected joints. This will prevent shrinking or shortening of the muscle.

Goal: Increase endurance and fitness.

Precautions: Review all aerobic exercises with a physician who is familiar with your degree of joint damage and any other specific health problems that may interfere with doing aerobic exercise safely.

MIND-BODY EXERCISES

Many people enjoy participating in personal physical activities that engage both the mind and the body. These forms of exercise, which are performed with a strong mental focus, have become increasingly popular because of their proven benefits in flexibility, strength, and balance as well as stress reduction and mental focus. Many of these practices have their beginnings in ancient cultures.

Tai Chi

Tai chi is a traditional Chinese martial art that was developed in the thirteenth century. Since then, it has evolved into a relaxation technique, self-healing practice, and fitness activity. Its movements are slow, circular, rhythmic, flowing, and dancelike. It also encompasses elements of mental focus and breathing techniques to promote harmony of mind and body. It can promote flexibility, vitality, and increased power of attention. Western practitioners have shown that it can improve balance, decrease falls, promote relaxation, and decrease pain.

The practice of tai chi, with its controlled movements and graceful gestures, may prove very valuable to people with RA. A Norwegian study showed that patients with RA who performed tai chi experienced improved physical condition, greater confidence in moving, better balance, and less pain during exercise and in daily life (Uhlig et al., 2010). Tai chi is taught in several styles, variations, and techniques. It is always best to learn tai chi from an experienced instructor. A qualified teacher with knowledge about rheumatoid arthritis can determine if these techniques are appropriate for you or if modifications are possible. Review all movements with your doctor and follow our exercise precautions.

Qi-gong

Qi-gong is a self-healing art that dates back at least 3,000 years. *Qi* (pronounced "chi" and meaning "energy") and *gong* (skill) together literally mean "the skill of cultivating vital energy." Qi-gong, referred to as "the healing dance of life," combines the principles of movement, posture, breathing, relaxation, and visualization. Qi-gong involves gentle body movement and meditation with slow adjustments in body posture. Breath and movement are synchronized. Regular practice of Qi-gong can improve both balance and strength. With its relaxed motions, Qi-gong is less physically challenging than tai chi and may be more suitable for people with severe RA. Visualizations are used to guide the energy, enhance the mind-body connection, promote spiritual self-development, and promote healing. There are several variations on the practice of Qi-gong. As always, find an experienced teacher who understands RA.

Yoga

Yoga originated as the physical element of Ayurvedic healing practices, with origins in ancient India (see section on Ayurvedic healing in Chapter 17). There are several variations of yoga practice that have evolved over thousands of years. They have in common elements of stretching, postures, relaxation, meditation, and breathing techniques. Studies have shown that yoga can bring improvement in flexibility, strength, equilibrium, and stamina. There have been a few studies describing yoga benefits in RA. One recent study found that yoga participants had improved quality of life, general health, mood, fatigue, and the ability to accept and manage pain (Evans et al., 2013).

The focus on gentle stretching and strengthening is consistent with joint protection principles. Breath awareness and relaxation techniques in general help relieve stress and control pain. Yoga is best learned from an *experienced* teacher, because improper positioning can be harmful (to anyone). Let your instructor know which of your joints are inflamed; specific yoga postures can be modified for you, or supports can be used to take stress off inflamed joints. For instance, exercises can be performed while sitting in a chair rather than on the floor. Review yoga positions with your rheumatologist; individuals with significant joint damage or joint replacements may have limitations.

FOR MORE INFORMATION

A number of valuable exercise resources are available from the Arthritis Foundation, 1330 W. Peachtree St., Atlanta, Ga. 30309; 1-800-283-7800; Web site: http://www.arthritis.org; Web store: http://www.afstore.org.

The following brochures, pamphlets and guides are free by e-mail:

"Exercise and Your Arthritis"

"Arthritis Today Walking Guide"

"Range of Motion Exercises"

"Walking and Arthritis"

"Water Exercise: Pools, Spas and Arthritis"

The following exercise DVDs are available for purchase at the Arthritis Foundation Store:

"Arthritis-Friendly Yoga"

"Arthritis Water Exercise"

"Tai Chi for Arthritis"

"Take Control with Exercise"

Specific Exercises

The exercises described and illustrated below are examples of the three types of exercise prescribed for persons with rheumatoid arthritis (RA): range-of-motion, strengthening, and aerobic, or endurance. We have illustrated only one way to perform each exercise, but there are many possibilities for each one. For example, a majority of the exercises illustrated in a standing position can be performed while sitting or lying down. Many people even do their range-of-motion exercises before they get out of bed in the morning. This may be a good idea if your hips, knees, ankles, or feet are affected by arthritis. You may want to get a sense of how the exercise feels standing and then try to duplicate the motions while sitting or lying down. It is also possible to perform all your range-of-motion exercises in water. The benefits of buoyancy sometimes make it possible to perform exercises that would otherwise be too painful.

Strengthening exercises can also be performed in a variety of ways. You can do most of them sitting or lying. You may use an exercise band during strengthening exercises, but there are many ways to obtain the same type of resistance without using one. We have mentioned several alternatives in the text.

These exercises need not be performed in any particular order, although an exercise regimen should always begin with range-of-motion or stretching exercises. For instance, you may want to do several range-of-motion exercises first and then do some strengthening exercises. Or, you may want to perform exercises joint by joint (always beginning with some range-of-motion or stretching exercises). Some people like to do all of the floor exercises first and then move on to the sitting ones before performing the standing exercises last. Other people combine exercises. It's a good idea to try different approaches so you can discover a series of exercises that is comfortable for you.

If you do not have arthritis in some of the joints mentioned, you can bypass those exercises if you wish, although they can benefit anyone.

There are many range-of-motion, strengthening, and endurance exercises to choose from. Before you do any, please read Chapter 9, which provides guidelines about which types of exercises are best suited for your degree of **inflammation**. And keep the following guidelines and precautions in mind.

1. Review your exercise program with your physician or a **physical therapist** who is knowledgeable about RA. This is always important, but it is *crucial* if arthritis affects your neck or if your arthritis is severe. Take this book with you when you visit your doctor or therapist, and ask your doctor or therapist to check off the exercises that are best suited for your level of arthritis. You will also want the therapist or doctor to help you decide the number of repetitions of each exercise you should perform. There is a box (□) near each exercise heading to help you keep a record of the recommended ones, and blank lines (____) so you can write down the number of repetitions.

2. Make exercise a part of your daily routine.

3. Try to make exercise fun. Performing exercises with a friend or group can make exercise sessions more enjoyable. Your favorite music playing in the background can set the tone for exercising.

4. Exercise whenever you need to "get the kinks out." Doing a brief series of range-of-motion and stretching exercises is excellent in the morning, for example, or when you have been sitting for long periods. These exercises decrease stiffness in the joints.

5. A formal exercise program with range-of-motion (and strengthening and aerobic exercises if appropriate) should be done when your energy level is at its peak.

6. Balance your exercise program with adequate rest and sleep.

7. Always follow the rules of joint protection (see Chapter 8).

8. Be comfortable when you exercise:
   - Wear loose clothing.
   - Shower *before* exercising if you need to decrease pain and stiffness and increase flexibility.
   - Take arthritis medications in advance, timed to "kick in" during the exercise period.

9. Take deep, regular breaths while exercising. Muscles use more oxygen than usual during exercise.

10. Use smooth, flowing movement. Avoid jerking or bouncing motions.

11. To limit inflammation, apply cloth-wrapped ice packs to warm joints for twenty minutes following an exercise session.

12. *Never* try to perform an exercise that causes pain. If it hurts, do not do it. (Forget the "no pain, no gain" philosophy.)

13. *Never* exercise to the point of extreme muscle fatigue or weakness.

14. If you have pain in your *joints* for more than two hours after exercising or notice increased *joint* pain or swelling the next day, you are overdoing it. Cut back! On the other hand, some *muscle* soreness is expected when you first begin any exercise program.

15. If you have had joint replacements, always review exercises with your doctors, including your **orthopedic surgeon,** before proceeding.

16. Be adaptable to changes in your condition and modify your exercise routine accordingly.

17. Keep a log of exercises you have completed.

RANGE-OF-MOTION AND STRENGTHENING EXERCISES

If you have arthritis in your neck, consult your physician before attempting any of the following exercises. STOP IMMEDIATELY if you experience increased neck pain, dizziness, lightheadedness, numbness, or weakness in the arms or legs.

Neck Range-of-Motion Exercises

☐ *Exercise 1. Neck Stretch and Flexion*

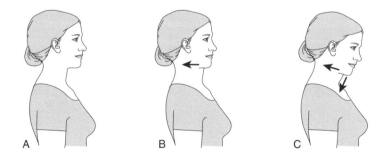

Starting position: Sitting upright in a chair with your shoulders straight (A).

Step 1: While you are facing straight ahead pull your chin back; hold your chin in place for two to three seconds (B); relax.

Step 2: With your chin tucked in, slowly tilt your head forward toward your chest until you feel the muscles tighten in the back of your neck (C). Do not let your head drop downward. Hold your neck flexed for two to three seconds.

Repeat this exercise _____ times, _____ times per day.

☐ *Exercise 2. Neck Lateral Flexion*

Starting position: Sitting or standing, facing forward.

Step 1: Remain facing forward as you tilt your head sideways toward your right shoulder. Do not lift your right shoulder. Hold for two to three seconds.

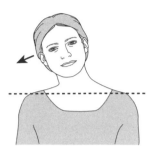

Step 2: Return to the starting position.

Step 3: Repeat, tilting to the left side.

Repeat this exercise ____ times, ____ times per day.

☐ *Exercise 3. Neck Rotation*

Starting position: Sitting or standing, facing forward.

Step 1: Turn your head as though you were looking over your left shoulder. Hold for two to three seconds. Hold your shoulders straight and do not let them turn with your head.

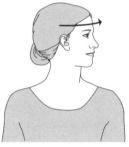

Step 2: Return to the center position.

Step 3: Repeat the exercise in the opposite direction.

Repeat this exercise ____ times, ____ times per day.

Neck Muscle-Strengthening Exercises

☐ *Exercise 4. Neck Extensor Strengthening*

Starting position: Standing or sitting with your back against a wall.

Step 1: Place the back of your head against the wall.

Step 2: Push your head back against the wall.

Step 3: Hold for six seconds and then relax.

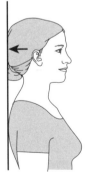

Repeat this exercise ____ times, ____ times per day.

☐ *Exercise 5. Neck Flexor Strengthening*

Starting position: Standing or sitting.

Step 1: Place the flat of your palm against your forehead.

Step 2: Push your head forward, opposing the resistance of your palm. Do not let your palm or your head move the other.

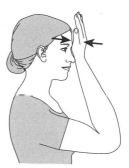

Step 3: Hold for six seconds and then relax.

Alternatives: If arthritis in your elbow, hand, or wrist presents a problem, wrap your arms around a beach ball or large, firm pillow and press your forehead into the ball or pillow, using your arms to make a resistance rather than your hands.

Repeat this exercise _____ times, _____ times per day.

☐ *Exercise 6. Neck Lateral Flexor Strengthening*

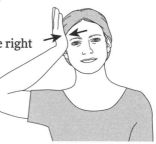

Starting position: Standing or sitting.

Step 1: Place the flat of your right palm against the right side of your head.

Step 2: Push your head sideways against your right hand, resisting any movement of either.

Step 3: Hold for six seconds and then relax.

Step 4: Repeat on left side.

Alternatives: If arthritis in your elbow, hand, or wrist presents a problem, use your upper arm, a beach ball, or a pillow as resistance against the tilting motion of your neck, similarly to the strategy described in the alternative at Exercise 5.

Repeat this exercise _____ times, _____ times per day.

Shoulder Range-of-Motion Exercises

☐ *Exercise 7. Shoulder Rotation*

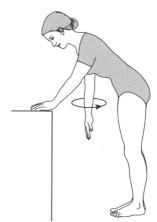

Starting position: Standing, leaning forward with one hand placed against a table for support.

Step 1: Swing your opposite arm in small circles, rotating from the shoulder.

Step 2: Slowly increase the size of the circles.

Step 3: Reverse arms.

Repeat this exercise _____ times, _____ times per day.

☐ *Exercise 8. Shoulder Abduction and Adduction*

Starting position: Standing or sitting with your arms at your sides.

Step 1: With your palms facing upward, swing your arms up along the side of your body until your hands touch above your head.

Step 2: Swing your arms back down to your sides.

Repeat this exercise _____ times, _____ times per day.

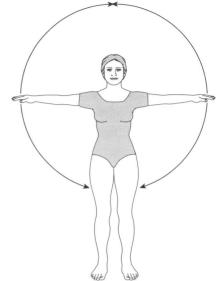

☐ *Exercise 9. Shoulder Flexion and Extension*

Starting position: Standing or sitting with your arms at your sides.

Step 1: Swing your left arm forward and your right arm backward simultaneously.

Step 2: Return your arms to your sides.

Step 3: Swing your right arm forward and your left arm backward.

Repeat this exercise _____ times, _____ times per day.

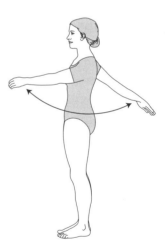

☐ *Exercise 10. Shoulder External Rotation and Scapular Adduction; Internal Rotation*

Starting position: Standing or sitting with your arms rotated out at your sides, palms facing forward.

Step 1: Bend your elbows so your fingers are pointing upward and palms turned forward, then pull your shoulders back, trying to squeeze your shoulder blades together (A); hold for two to three seconds.

Step 2: Keeping your elbows bent, bring your forearms to the front of your body, and try to make your hands and elbows meet (B).

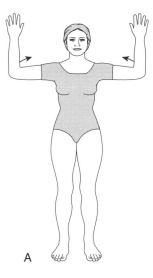 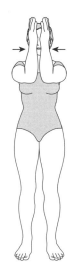

A   B

Repeat this exercise _____ times, _____ times per day.

☐ *Exercise 11. Wall Walk*

Starting position: Standing, facing a wall, an arm's length away.

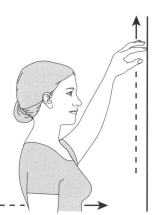

Step 1: Slowly walk the fingers of one hand up the wall, stepping closer to the wall as your fingers walk farther up it.

Step 2: At the maximal height, hold for three seconds, pushing your armpit toward the wall.

Step 3: Observe how close your feet are to the wall, so that you can monitor your progress.

Repeat this exercise _____ times, _____ times per day.

Elbow Range-of-Motion Exercises

☐ *Exercise 12. Elbow Extension and Flexion*

Starting position: Standing with your arms straight out from your sides, palms facing down.

Step 1: Hold your arms out, keeping your elbows straight (A).

Step 2: Bend your arms at the elbows, bringing your hands together in front of your body (B).

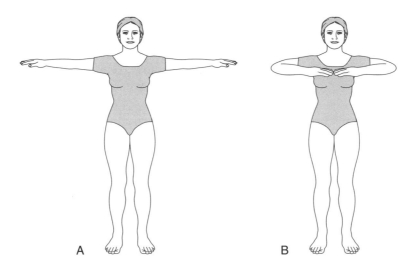

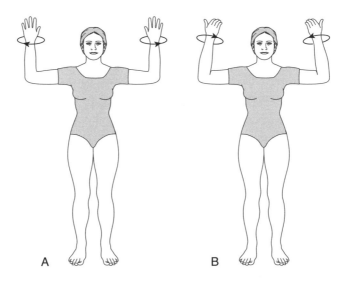

Repeat this exercise _____ times, _____ times per day.

☐ *Exercise 13. Elbow Pronation and Supination*

Starting position: Standing or sitting with your elbows bent, your hands up, and your fingers relaxed but pointing upward.

Step 1: Turn your palms to face forward (A).

Step 2: Turn your hands so that the palms face backward (B).

Alternatives: If this causes you shoulder discomfort, perform the exercise while you are sitting with elbows supported on a table. You can also do it with your arms held nearer to your body than is shown in the pictures.

Repeat this exercise ____ times, ____ times per day.

Shoulder and Elbow Muscle-Strengthening Exercises

☐ *Exercise 14. Shoulder Abductor Strengthening*

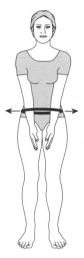

Starting position: Standing, with an exercise band encircling your forearms.

Step 1: Separate your arms slowly, until you feel a firm pressure from the band, tightening around your forearms.

Step 2: With your elbows straight, continue to push both arms out sideways against the band.

Step 3: Hold the muscle contraction for six seconds, then relax.

Alternatives: This exercise can be initiated with the band encircling your arms above the elbows. As your strength increases, the band can be lowered down your arm. Instead of an exercise band you can use a bungie cord or elastic belt.

Repeat this exercise ____ times, ____ times per day.

☐ *Exercise 15. Shoulder Flexor and Extensor Strengthening*

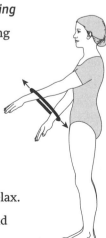

Starting position: Standing, with an exercise band encircling your forearms.

Step 1: Raise your left arm and lower your right arm simultaneously until you feel a firm pressure from the tightening band.

Step 2: Keeping your elbows straight, pull your left arm upward and push your right arm downward, resisting the pressure of the band.

Step 3: Hold the muscle contraction for six seconds then relax.

Step 4: Repeat steps 1 through 3, raising your right arm and lowering your left arm.

Repeat this exercise ____ times, ____ times per day.

☐ *Exercise 16. Shoulder External Rotator Strengthening*

Starting position: Standing, with an exercise band encircling your forearms.

Step 1: Keeping your elbows pressed to your sides, move your hands away from each other until you feel the band tighten around your forearms.

Step 2: Push outward with both forearms (keeping your elbows pressed tightly against your sides), resisting the pressure of the band.

Step 3: Hold the contraction for six seconds then relax.

Repeat this exercise _____ times, _____ times per day.

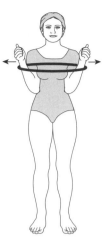

☐ *Exercise 17. Shoulder Internal Rotator Strengthening*

Starting position: Stand with your elbows bent at your sides, with your forearms against your chest.

Step 1: Press your forearms against your chest while holding your elbows in position.

Step 2: Hold the muscle contraction for six seconds, then relax.

Repeat this exercise _____ times, _____ times per day.

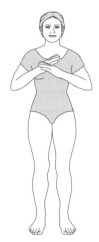

☐ *Exercise 18. Elbow Flexor and Extensor Strengthening*

Starting position: Standing, with an exercise band encircling your forearms. (If you are using an elastic trouser belt, you may have to double it up for this exercise.)

Step 1: With your elbows bent, move your left forearm upward and your right arm downward until you feel the band tighten firmly around your forearms.

Step 2: Pull your left forearm upward and push your right downward, resisting the pressure of the band.

Step 3: Hold the muscle contraction for six seconds then relax.

Step 4: Repeat steps 1 through 3, raising your right arm and lowering your left arm.

Repeat this exercise _____ times, _____ times per day.

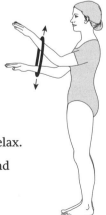

Wrist and Finger Range-of-Motion Exercises

☐ *Exercise 19. Wrist Extension and Flexion*

Step 1: Bend your wrist up as though you were waving to someone (A).

Step 2: Bend your wrist downward as far as you comfortably can (B).

Repeat this exercise ____ times, ____ times per day with each hand.

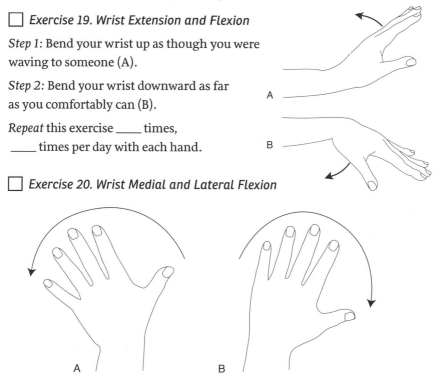

☐ *Exercise 20. Wrist Medial and Lateral Flexion*

Step 1: With elbows bent and palms facing inward or forward, bend both wrists sideways in the direction of your little finger (A).

Step 2: Bend both wrists sideways in the direction of your thumb (B).

Repeat this exercise ____ times, ____ times per day.

☐ *Exercise 21. Finger Walk*

Step 1: Touch your thumb to your index finger (A).

Step 2: Touch your thumb to your middle finger (B).

Step 3: Touch your thumb to your ring finger (C).

Step 4: Touch your thumb to your little finger (D).

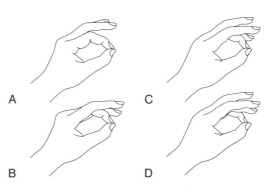

Repeat this exercise ____ times, ____ times per day with each hand.

☐ *Exercise 22. Finger Flexion and Extension*

Starting position: Begin by warming up with a finger walk (Exercise 21).

Step 1: Slowly curl your fingers, beginning at the tips and progressing down the knuckles until you form a loose fist (A).

Step 2: Slowly uncurl your fingers, completely straightening and then spreading them (B).

Repeat this exercise _____ times, _____ times per day.

Hip Range-of-Motion Exercises

☐ *Exercise 23. Hip Flexion and Extension*

Starting position: Standing, with right hand placed on a counter or table for balance.

Step 1: Swing your left leg forward, keeping your knee as straight as possible.

Step 2: Swing your left leg backward.

Step 3: Slowly increase the length of the swing until slight discomfort occurs. Do not let your leg's acceleration swing it beyond the painful limit.

Step 4: Turn around, place left hand on surface, and repeat with your right leg.

Repeat this exercise _____ times, _____ times per day.

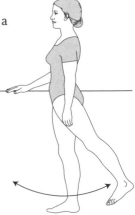

☐ *Exercise 24. Hip Abduction*

Starting position: Standing, with your right hand resting on a counter for balance.

Step 1: Slowly swing your left leg outward and return it to the starting position for the prescribed number of repetitions.

Step 2: Turn around, place left hand on counter, and repeat with your right leg for the prescribed number of repetitions.

Repeat this exercise _____ times, _____ times per day.

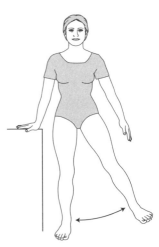

☐ *Exercise 25. Hip Rotation*

Starting position: Standing, with right hand placed against a support.

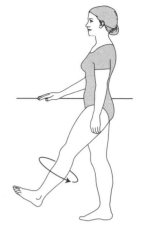

Step 1: Move your left leg forward, holding your knee straight, and make small circles in either direction with the whole leg, rotating from the hip.

Step 2: Gradually increase the size of the circles.

Step 3: Turn around, support with left hand, and repeat steps 1 and 2 with your right leg.

Repeat this exercise ____ times, ____ times per day.

☐ *Exercise 26. Hip External and Internal Rotation*

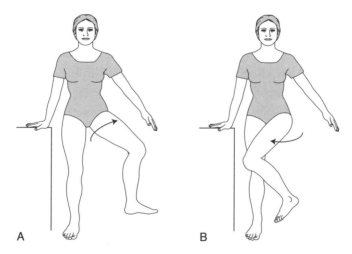

A   B

Starting position: Standing, with right hand resting on a support.

Step 1: With your left knee bent and lifted, turn your left leg outward (A).

Step 2: Turn your left leg inward, bringing it in front of your right leg (B).

Step 3: Turn around, support with left hand, and repeat with your right leg.

Alternatives: Similar movements can be performed while you are sitting or lying on your back.

Repeat this exercise ____ times, ____ times per day.

☐ *Exercise 27. Hip Flexion with Hip and Knee Muscle Strengthening*

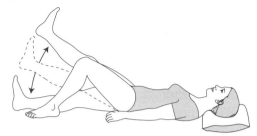

This exercise is more advanced than other range-of-motion exercises. Be sure to start slowly at first. Cut back on repetitions or discontinue this exercise if knee or hip discomfort occurs.

Starting position: Lying flat on your back.

Step 1: With left leg bent, lift your right leg slowly upward, keeping the knee straight. Don't lift higher than left knee.

Step 2: Lower your leg, slowly if you want maximum strengthening.

Step 3: Straighten left leg, bend right leg, and repeat, lifting left leg.

Step 4: You can increase the height of leg elevation gradually if lifting the straight leg to the height of the other knee is uncomfortable at first.

Repeat this exercise _____ times, _____ times per day.

Knee Range-of-Motion Exercises

☐ *Exercise 28. Knee Flexion*

Starting position: Standing, resting your hands on a support.

Step 1: Bending your left knee, raise your left heel upward behind you.

Step 2: Lower your left heel slowly.

Step 3: Repeat with your right leg.

Alternatives: You can perform knee flexion while sitting down (depending on the type of chair you are in) or lying on your stomach.

Repeat this exercise _____ times, _____ times per day.

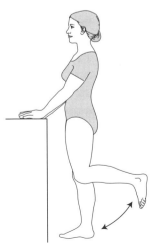

☐ *Exercise 29. Knee Extension*

Starting position: Sitting in a chair, with your feet flat on the floor, arms at your side with hands facing downward on the seat or resting on the arms of the chair.

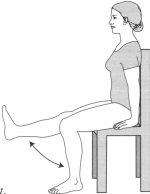

Step 1: Slowly raise your left lower leg to a horizontal position.

Step 2: Slowly lower your left leg.

Step 3: Repeat with your right leg.

Repeat this exercise _____ times, _____ times per day.

Hip and Knee Muscle-Strengthening Exercises

☐ *Exercise 30. Hip and Knee Muscle Strengthening*

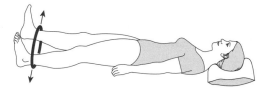

Starting position: Lying on your back, with an exercise band encircling your lower legs.

Step 1: Lift your right leg without bending your knee until you feel the band tighten around your lower legs. If you have lifted your leg more than six inches, the circle made by the band is too large in diameter.

Step 2: Elevate your right leg while resisting the motion by pushing down with your left leg on the floor or bed.

Step 3: Hold the muscle contraction for six seconds, then lower your right leg.

Step 4: Repeat steps 1 through 3, raising your left leg.

Repeat this exercise _____ times, _____ times per day.

☐ *Exercise 31. Hip Abductor Strengthening*

Starting position: Lying on your back, with an exercise band encircling lower legs.

Step 1: Slowly spread your legs apart until you feel a firm pressure from the band around your legs.

Step 2: Push each leg outward, resisting pull of the opposite leg.

Step 3: Hold the muscle contraction for six seconds then relax.

Repeat this exercise _____ times, _____ times per day.

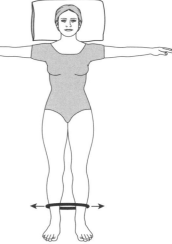

☐ *Exercise 32. Knee Extensor and Flexor Strengthening*

Starting position: Sitting in a chair with your back held straight, feet on the floor, with an exercise band encircling your lower legs (legs far enough apart to hold the band in place but not farther than hip width).

Step 1: Slowly raise your left lower leg, pushing upward against the resistance of the band.

Step 2: Hold the muscle contraction for six seconds, then return left leg to earlier position.

Step 3: Repeat steps 1 and 2 with other leg.

Repeat this exercise _____ times, _____ times per day.

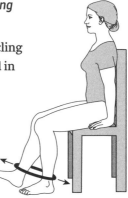

Ankle Range-of-Motion Exercises

☐ *Exercise 33. Ankle Flexion and Extension*

Starting position: Sitting on a stool or bed or other surface high enough that your feet do not touch the floor.

Step 1: Bend both ankles by pulling your toes toward your body; hold for two to three seconds; relax.

Step 2: Straighten your ankles by pointing your toes away from you; hold for two to three seconds.

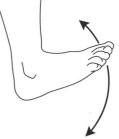

Alternatives: This exercise may also be performed while lying down.

Repeat this exercise _____ times, _____ times per day.

☐ *Exercise 34. Ankle Rotation*

Starting position: Sitting, with your feet dangling.

Step 1: Draw an imaginary circle with the toes of each foot, either both feet at the same time or alternating.

Step 2: Gradually increase the size of the circle.

Step 3: Rotate the feet the opposite way, drawing the circle in the other direction.

Alternatives: This exercise may also be performed while lying down.

Repeat this exercise _____ times, _____ times per day.

AEROBIC OR ENDURANCE EXERCISES

It is essential that you consult your doctor before beginning any aerobic exercise program.

When your arthritis is controlled and your joint flexibility is at its optimum and your muscles are strengthened, you are ready to begin improving your stamina. Aerobic exercise will enhance your fitness by improving your heart and lung function as well as your circulation.

To gain the most aerobic benefits from your exercise, you must (1) raise your heart rate (beats per minute) to a conditioning level, your *target heart rate;* (2) maintain your target heart rate for fifteen to thirty minutes in each aerobic session; (3) perform your aerobic program at least three times each week.

These three principles are your *goal*, not where you will be at the start. Also, some deviations from these principles, discussed below, might be helpful for you. However, even with variations, benefits can be gained from an aerobic program from the very beginning. If aerobic exercise is new to you, begin your program slowly. In time you will be fit enough to satisfy all three of the principles.

Trying to perform too much aerobic exercise too soon is counterproductive. You may experience extreme fatigue, shortness of breath, dizziness, and increased joint pain. People with RA often have aerobic capacity that is 20 to 30 percent lower than others' aerobic capacity because of their loss of physical activity and the effects of inflammation (Cooney et al., 2011). You have some catching up to do, but there is no hurry. So, be patient. *Don't overdo it.*

What Is Your Target Heart Rate?

Your *target heart rate* is the number of beats per minute required for exercise to produce cardiovascular benefits for you. It is based primarily on your age. Determining your target heart rate requires some calculation, with your *maximal heart rate* being the first computation. (This is the highest heart rate that is safe for individuals of your age.) Your *target* heart rate is calculated to be 70 percent of your *maximal* rate. **Warning: Do *not* exercise at your *maximal* heart rate.**

To calculate your *maximal* heart rate, use the following formula: 220 minus your age equals your maximal heart rate. To calculate your *target* heart rate, multiply the maximal heart rate by 0.70 (which represents 70 percent). By way of example, suppose you are 60 years old. You would calculate your target heart rate in the following way:

$$220 - 60 = 160 \text{ (maximal heart rate)}$$
$$160 \times 0.70 = 112 \text{ (target heart rate)}$$

Hence, the target heart rate for someone who is 60 years of age would be 112.

In considering aerobic fitness for people with RA, a lower target heart rate may still be helpful and will probably be safer. Studies have shown that target heart rates as low as 50 percent of maximal heart rate can still give benefit (Scarvell and Elkins, 2011). If you are a beginner, start with these lesser targets. Using the same type of calculation, for an out-of-condition 60 year old with RA, figure your target rate this way:

$$220 - 60 = 160 \text{ (maximal heart rate)}$$
$$160 \times 0.50 = 80 \text{ (beginner's target heart rate)}$$

IMPORTANT: If you are taking medications called beta blockers or calcium channel blockers, these formulas will not work for you. These medications can lower the heart rate. If you are on one of these medications, discuss your target heart rate with your doctor.

Taking Your Pulse

To find out what your *heart rate* is at any time, you must take your pulse. Turn over your left hand so that you are looking at the palm (Figure 16). Use the tips of your right index, middle, and ring fingers to feel for the pulse. Place your fingertips at the base of your thumb on the bone at the edge of your wrist. Then, slowly slide your fingertips toward the middle of the wrist, feeling for a pulsation. (If you feel **tendons,** you have gone too far.) You'll need practice to learn how much pressure to exert. Too much pressure will stop the pulse. Not enough pressure will prevent you from feeling it. Practice by using different degrees of firmness. You may also take your pulse in your right arm using the fingers of your left hand.

Once you find the pulse, you will need to count the pulsations to get your heart rate. Look at a watch or clock that measures seconds. Count the number of pulsations occurring in a fifteen-second period. Then, multiply that number by four. This will give you your actual heart rate in beats per minute.

For your convenience, the following chart lists some target heart rates and beginners' target heart rates for various ages as well as the number of pulsations you will feel at your wrist in a fifteen-second period if you have reached your target heart rate. If you like, select the row that is closest to your age and use that number as your target rate.

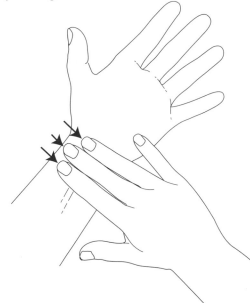

FIGURE 16. Taking a pulse

AGE (YEARS)	TARGET HEART RATE (BEATS PER MINUTE)	BEGINNER'S TARGET HEART RATE	TARGET WRIST PULSE (BEATS IN 15 SECONDS)	BEGINNER'S TARGET WRIST PULSE
20	140	100	35	25
25	137	98	34	24
30	133	95	33	24
35	130	93	32	23
40	126	90	31	22
45	122	88	30	22
50	119	85	30	21
55	116	83	29	21
60	112	80	28	20
65	108	78	27	20
70	105	75	26	19
75	101	73	25	18

Beginning Your Aerobic Exercise Program

The form of aerobic exercise you select depends on several factors: convenience, time constraints, the joints that are affected with arthritis, and, most important, the type of exercise you enjoy. Possibilities include brisk walking, swimming, stationary bicycling, using an elliptical machine, low-impact aerobics or dancing, cross-country skiing, and rowing. After you have chosen a program and your doctor has approved it, we recommend that you follow these guidelines when beginning:

- Always warm up for five to ten minutes with range-of-motion and stretching exercises.

- Start slowly. Try five minutes of aerobic exercise the first day, checking your pulse before and after. If your pulse exceeds the target rate, slow down.

- Increase the time spent doing aerobic exercise by small increments each session. Alternating five-minute spurts of high-intensity exercise with low-intensity rest periods is a good way to increase the duration of aerobic exercise. As you get in better condition, shorten and then eliminate the rest periods until you can do fifteen to thirty minutes of uninterrupted aerobic exercise. In the beginning you should check your pulse at least every five minutes. If longer sessions are not possible for you because of joint pain or significant fatigue, it is perfectly okay to have two or three mini-sessions of ten minutes each throughout the course of the day. New research shows that these aerobic mini-sessions still add up to improved fitness and cardiovascular health.

- *STOP IMMEDIATELY if you develop chest pain, palpitations, dizziness, shortness of breath, extreme fatigue, weakness, or increased joint pain.*

- If you have pain for more than two hours after exercise or experience increased joint pain or swelling the following day, modify the program.

- Always follow aerobic exercise with at least five minutes of cool-down exercise, allowing your heart rate and breathing to return to normal.

Guidelines for Specific Aerobic Exercise

Swimming or aquatic therapy. Your local chapter of the Arthritis Foundation may be able to recommend an arthritis aquatic program close to you. Roxanne McNeal, of the Aquatic Therapy Services in Abingdon, Maryland, has the following advice:

- Pool temperatures of 92° to 98° F are suitable for range-of-motion and stretching exercises but *not* for active aerobics. (Contact the management at the pool where you plan to exercise and ask what the temperature range of their pool is.)

- Pool temperatures of 82° to 86° F are best for aerobic exercise. Doing aerobics in higher pool temperatures can cause the body temperature to increase and blood vessels to dilate, resulting in lightheadedness.

- Avoid pool therapy if you have an open wound, a fever, severe low or high blood pressure, or a history of uncontrolled seizures.

- Breathe regularly from the diaphragm throughout the exercise.

Bicycling
- Adjust your seat height so that your legs almost fully straighten out when pedaling.

- Do not ride a bike with the handlebars too far away from the seat. This increases stress on the lower back, shoulders, elbows, and wrists.

- If you can adjust the pedal tension, keep it at the lowest level, to limit stress on your knees.

- Indoor cycles with arm motion attachments can decrease stress on the knees and still provide a good aerobic workout.

- Try out various models of stationary bikes, including recumbent bicycles, (at a gym) or outdoor bicycles (at a bicycle shop) before purchasing one.

- Cooling down with light pedaling can be substituted for a range-of-motion cool-down.

Walking

- If you have severe arthritis of the knees or hips, walking may not be for you. Consider swimming or biking.

- Soak your feet in warm water, doing some gentle foot range-of-motion exercises as you soak, before walking, to loosen up joints.

- Perform hip and knee range-of-motion exercises to stretch muscles in preparation for walking.

- Walk on a flat, level, relatively firm surface.

- Wear supportive walking shoes or athletic sneakers with good shock absorption capability.

- Swing your arms for balance while walking.

- In inclement weather, walk in a shopping mall or on an indoor track. Many malls have walking clubs you can join.

- If your feet are warm after walking, soak them in cool water for ten minutes.

FOR MORE INFORMATION

The Arthritis Foundation sponsors the following exercise programs: Walk with Ease, Tai Chi, Exercise, and Aquatics. Contact your local Arthritis Foundation for more information.

MEDICATIONS

Medications Past,
Present, Future

Taking medications can be inconvenient, and few medications are free of potential side effects. In the treatment of rheumatoid arthritis (RA), however, the benefits of medication almost always outweigh their inconvenience and risk. Medications decrease **inflammation** and prevent the permanent damage that can occur when RA is not brought under control. They can also help control pain. In short, medications are an *essential* ingredient in the treatment of RA.

This chapter looks at how approaches to treatment, especially pharmaceutical treatment, have changed in response to new information emerging from medical research and experience. Then Chapters 12, 13, 14, and 15 describe the three major groups of medications used today for treating RA and discuss how to take them, when to take them, when *not* to take them, and what their benefits and potential side effects are. Chapter 16 addresses the prevention and treatment of **osteoporosis.**

THE PAST: THE CONSERVATIVE APPROACH

Traditionally, medical therapy for RA was outlined as a pyramid approach (Figure 17). Treatment options started at the base of the pyramid. Doctors would begin conservatively, by prescribing what was thought to be the safest medication. From the 1940s through the 1960s, this first-line medical therapy took the form of large doses of aspirin. In the 1970s and 1980s, many new nonsteroidal anti-inflammatory drugs (**NSAIDs**) became available. Because they are convenient and often well tolerated (patients notice few side effects), NSAIDs have gradually replaced aspirin as the first line of therapy.

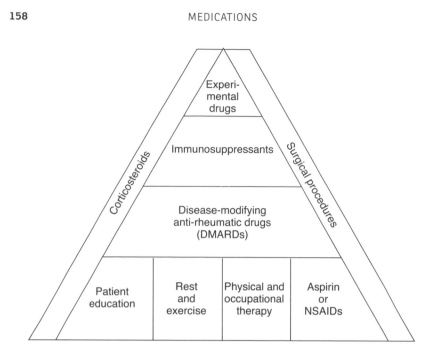

FIGURE 17. The traditional therapeutic pyramid

Also located on the base of the pyramid were other conservative forms of treatment, such as rest, physical therapy, and diet. Because *early* RA was thought to be a purely inflammatory and reversible condition, doctors believed that anti-inflammatory therapy *alone* was justified. Before doctors moved up to the next tier of treatment and prescribed second-line therapy, actual *damage* would need to be apparent by physical examination or x-ray. This was consistent with the theory of the time, which held that the early phase, the *inflammatory phase*, of RA was only *infrequently* followed by a more damaging *proliferative phase*. In this later phase, the **synovium** would become thicker and destructive. Doctors often waited one to three years for evidence of this damage before prescribing disease-modifying drugs (drugs that attempt to induce a remission by stopping the proliferative phase). These disease-modifying antirheumatic drugs (**DMARDs**), or *remittive* (causing **remission**) drugs, were thought to be unnecessary and too dangerous for early use.

THE PRESENT: MORE AGGRESSIVE APPROACHES TO THERAPY

The treatment of RA has changed dramatically in the past thirty years. Several important pieces of information have altered how we treat RA. First, it has been widely acknowledged that irreversible damage *can* take place during the first two years of RA, even before such damage is observable by standard x-rays. Second, we now know that, despite their effectiveness in decreasing inflammation, NSAIDs and **COX-2 inhibitors** do not change the course of RA, because they do not affect the damaging proliferation, or overgrowth, of the synovium. Finally, we have discovered that DMARDs and **biologics** (described below) appear to be most effective in *preventing* damage if they are used *early.* Hence, the old pyramid strategy, which postponed the more powerful medications until after damage was visible, has been abandoned by most **rheumatologists** for a more aggressive approach. In this modern strategy, commonly known among rheumatologists as "inverting the pyramid," disease-modifying medications (DMARDs) are initiated as soon as it is clear that a person has RA. The challenge today is to determine how early in the course of RA we should use our most powerful new biologic response modifiers.

In late 1998, we took a giant step into the modern era of rheumatoid arthritis treatment. After years of research, the first biogenetically engineered drug, Enbrel (etanercept) was made available to people with RA (more about this drug in Chapter 14). Etanercept was the first in a class of drugs called the biologics. These medications are designed to target very specific parts of the immune system. Since 1998, other biologics—Remicade, Kineret, Humira, Simponi, Orencia, Actemra, Rituxan, and Cimzia—have been introduced, and more are on the way.

Most of our current biologic therapies are directed against one of three inflammatory **cytokines: tumor necrosis factor (TNF), interleukin-1 (IL-1),** and **interleukin-6 (IL-6)** (see Chapter 14). Cytokine-directed biologics have allowed us to make huge gains in our war against inflammation and its potential damage. Scientists have identified several other inflammatory cytokines as targets for treatment (among them, IL-12, IL-15, IL-17, and IL-20). And studies are under way to determine the benefits of blocking these and other cytokines.

Two of our current biologics focus on redirecting immune cells that have gone awry in RA. Two immune cells, in particular, the T cell and the B cell, are critical players in the misdirected inflammatory reaction that occurs in RA. In Chapter 14, you will learn how our two current cell-directed biologics work in an effort to rebalance the immune system. Other immune cell "modulators" are in clinical trials at this time.

In 2012, Xeljanz, the first oral medication with biologic-like effects, became available. Xeljanz is in the category of medications called the **kinase inhibitors.** Although officially an oral DMARD, it works more like a biologic in that its effects are very focused at specific functions of the immune system. These exciting new agents work on the "inner mechanics" within the immune cells in an effort to disrupt the passage of inflammatory signals. Similar drugs are in clinical trials.

THE FUTURE

The future will clearly bring efforts to identify other pivotal components of the immune system that have gone awry in RA. Potential treatments aimed at these specific elements of the misdirected immune system will increase our arsenal for fighting inflammation. If these treatments are effective, we will have more options to prevent the damaging effects of RA on the bones and joints. Pharmaceutical and biotechnology companies are looking at dozens of different targets in the cascade of events responsible for RA.

The success of the Human Genome Project has made it possible to trace genes that may be linked to RA, and the future undoubtedly will bring novel drugs that exploit this new information. New research in the field of **epigenetics** (see Chapter 1) will help us determine how to avoid triggers that "switch on" the parts of genes that can lead to conditions like RA.

Medical researchers are becoming more interested in the effects of diet on RA (discussed in Chapter 18). There is an expanding scientific rationale for dietary management as an adjunct to traditional RA therapies. As we learn more about nutrition effects, we may begin to make dietary recommendations that can work in tandem with pharmaceuticals, biologics, and other therapies. All of this new information about RA makes us more hopeful about the future than ever before.

CURRENT TREATMENTS: NSAIDS, DMARDS, BIOLOGICS, KINASE INHIBITORS, AND CORTICOSTEROIDS

The five major groups of medications prescribed for the treatment of RA are:

1. NSAIDs. Nonsteroidal anti-inflammatory drugs are used to reduce inflammation quickly. This category also includes the COX-2 inhibitors. (See Chapter 12.)

2. DMARDs. Disease-modifying antirheumatic drugs are used in an attempt to induce a remission. This category contains traditional DMARDs and immunosuppressants. (See Chapter 13.)

3. Biologics. These drugs, which form a subset of DMARDs, are biogenetically engineered and usually given by injection or IV infusion. (See Chapter 14.)

4. Kinase inhibitors. Another subset of DMARDS, kinase inhibitors have effects similar to biologics but they are taken by mouth. (See Chapter 14.)

5. Corticosteroids. Steroidal anti-inflammatory medications are used to reduce inflammation, but work by a mechanism different from that of NSAIDs. (See Chapter 15.)

All of these medicines can sometimes cause unwanted side effects. Being aware of the potential side effects of medications you are taking will help you recognize the symptoms early and will help ensure that you obtain prompt treatment if a negative side effect does occur. Do not focus too intently on the potential side effects of medications, however. Doing so can cause unnecessary worry and stress. A proper balance is to be found somewhere between being aware of the symptoms of side effects and constantly watching for the occurrence of them. Keep in mind that severe and irreversible side effects rarely happen.

As stated above, new medications become available frequently. For this reason some drugs that are in use by the time you read this book may not be included in the following chapters. In any case, please consult your doctor for more information about medications.

A final note: It is a good idea to use only one pharmacy to fill all of your prescriptions, if possible. This allows the pharmacist to monitor the medications you are taking (possibly prescribed by more than one physician) and caution you and your physicians about potentially harmful drug interactions.

FOR MORE INFORMATION

The Arthritis Foundation offers free brochures about most drugs used in the treatment of rheumatoid arthritis. To order brochures, call 1-800-283-7800.

Aspirin, Nonsteroidal Anti-inflammatory Drugs (NSAIDs), and COX-2 Inhibitors

Nonsteroidal anti-inflammatory drugs (**NSAIDs**) are among the most commonly prescribed drugs worldwide. These medications are classified as *anti-inflammatory* because they reduce pain and swelling quickly. They are classified as *nonsteroidal* because they are not included in the corticosteroid (cortisone) family of medications (see Chapter 13), which are also anti-inflammatory agents.

Aspirin and NSAIDs (pronounced *en'-seds* or *en'-sayds*) are used to treat a wide variety of inflammatory and painful conditions. With few exceptions, these medications work by arresting the production of the inflammatory substances known as **prostaglandins** (discussed in Chapter 1). Aspirin and NSAIDs can reduce pain, swelling, and stiffness in the joints by limiting the production of these chemicals.

These medications usually produce results within one to three weeks of first use, and therefore they are termed *fast-acting* or *rapid-acting* antiarthritic drugs. They are generally the first line of treatment for rheumatoid arthritis (RA). Despite their effectiveness in controlling *symptoms*, these drugs do not appear to alter the course of the disease itself. In other words, they do *not* induce a remission of RA. Given this fact, your doctor may prescribe one or more second-line drugs along with anti-inflammatory medication, in an effort to induce a remission. (These slower-acting, disease-modifying drugs are described in Chapter 13.)

Several types and brands of anti-inflammatory drugs are now available, and more are currently being tested. Finding the medication that will benefit you the most may take some time and experimentation. One may give you little relief, while another may be extremely effective. One may produce unpleasant side effects (such as indigestion), while another does not. Sometimes, only by trying several medications, one at a time, can you and your doctor determine which anti-inflammatory medication will help you the most. The last addition to the NSAID family was the COX-2 inhibitor subset of anti-inflammatory drugs. COX-2 inhibitors appear to be better tolerated, causing less stomach irritation and ulceration. However, you will read below about other issues with them that may be of concern.

Anti-inflammatory medications vary widely in cost as well as in effectiveness. A difference in cost is always found between two forms of the same drug: these two forms are the *generic*, or non–brand name drug, and the brand name drug. The generic version will be the less expensive. Generic medications contain the same active ingredients found in brand name drugs, but the inactive ingredients may differ. Although these drugs are often as effective as their brand name counterpart, the quality in the production of brand name drugs has traditionally been more closely controlled, and therefore brand name drugs tend to be more consistent in their effectiveness. There is no evidence that generic arthritis drugs have more side effects than brand name medications, however; and if the expense of medications is a critical factor for you, you might want to consult your physician or pharmacist regarding the advisability of selecting a generic version or a similar but less expensive medication.

ASPIRIN

Aspirin (acetylsalicylic acid) is an extraordinarily effective medication that is often underestimated by patients and physicians alike. It is actually the standard against which all other anti-inflammatory drugs are compared. We underrate its value because it is inexpensive, available without a prescription, easily obtained, and has been around a long time. In addition to decreasing inflammation, aspirin also decreases pain and fever. Few medications can boast as amazing a profile and successful a track record as aspirin.

Different doses of aspirin work differently: low doses of aspirin (one "baby aspirin" a day) provide some protection for people with heart problems, whereas one or two tablets taken every four to six hours can relieve a fever or headache. For treating RA, we are interested in the anti-inflammatory effects of aspirin, which occur only with very large doses.

It is not uncommon for doctors to prescribe 10 to 20 regular-strength aspirin tablets per day to control inflammation. Such large doses, called *high-dose aspirin therapy,* must be accompanied by routine monitoring of blood salicylate levels. The salicylate level in your blood must be adequate to control inflammation without being so high that it causes side effects such as ringing in the ears (tinnitus). *Do not take large doses of aspirin unless you are under the supervision of a physician.*

Aspirin is available in several forms that span a wide price range. Every formulation contains the same active ingredient: acetylsalicylic acid. One aspirin product is no more effective than another as long as the dose and absorption are adequate, but differences in the formulations of aspirin products do affect the convenience of aspirin use and may have some bearing on the side effects produced as well.

Plain Aspirin

Over-the-counter brand name examples: Empirin, Norwich

This is the most economical form. Although aspirin is aspirin as far as effectiveness is concerned, aspirin that dissolves easily is less likely to settle near the stomach lining and irritate it. Hence, a very hard, compact tablet may not be as safe as a more powdery variety. Aspirin that smells like vinegar is old and should not be used.

Buffered Aspirin

Over-the-counter brand name examples: Arthritis Pain Formula, Ascriptin,
  Bufferin

Buffered aspirin contains an ingredient that partially neutralizes stomach acids. This form of aspirin may cause less stomach upset or indigestion than other forms, but it does not decrease the risk of developing **gastritis** or a stomach ulcer from aspirin use.

Film-Coated Aspirin

Over-the-counter brand name examples: Anacin, Bayer

A film or coating on the tablet makes it easier to swallow. This coating is not an enteric coating, nor does it protect the stomach in any way.

Enteric-Coated Aspirin

Over-the-counter brand name examples: Ecotrin Entab-650
Prescription brand name example: Easprin

An enteric coating on any medication causes tablets to pass through the stomach and into the small intestine before dissolving. There is evidence that this decreases the risk of stomach upset and direct irritation. The risk for gastritis and ulcers, although present, is slightly decreased with this formulation.

The slowly dissolving coating sometimes interferes with the body's ability to absorb this type of aspirin. There have also been reports that enteric aspirin is retained in the stomach of patients with sluggish digestive systems. If this form proves ineffective for you, your doctor may want to check the salicylate levels in your blood to determine whether you are adequately absorbing your medication.

Timed-Release Aspirin

Over-the-counter brand name example: Eight-hour Bayer Timed-Release
Prescription brand name examples: Encaprin, Zorprin

This controlled-release preparation gradually releases the aspirin. Because much of the aspirin is released after the tablet or capsule reaches the intestines (rather than in the stomach), this form may decrease stomach upset and indigestion. It does not eliminate the risks of gastritis or ulcer. Because it is taken fewer times during the day, it is more convenient, but it is significantly more expensive than regular aspirin.

Side Effects of Aspirin Therapy

For a list of side effects of aspirin, their frequency, and what can be done about them, see Table 1. The most common side effect of high-dose aspirin therapy is stomach distress, the symptoms of which are usually minor and can be relieved by taking the aspirin with meals.

Another common side effect is blood passed in tiny amounts daily in the stool. This is usually not dangerous, but over the long term it can lead to **anemia.**

Some people on high-dose aspirin therapy develop serious stomach problems, such as gastritis and stomach ulcer. Fortunately, bleeding ulcers are infrequent. Anyone developing one of these problems needs to stop taking aspirin and begin treatment with special stomach medications. The medication *miso-prostol* (Cytotec) helps prevent these side effects. (See the end of this chapter for details about available stomach medications.)

Cautionary Notes

Before starting aspirin therapy, discuss the following with your physician:

- Any history of allergy to aspirin or other anti-inflammatory medications. Symptoms of allergy include rash, hives, and swollen lips or eyelids. Wheezing and difficulty with breathing are rare but serious allergic responses.

- A history of asthma, nasal polyps, stomach ulcer, bleeding problems, colitis, or kidney or liver problems.

- Any medications that you are presently taking. Of particular importance are blood thinners, diabetes medication, blood pressure pills, seizure medication, and other over-the-counter pain medications.

TABLE 1. Side Effects of Aspirin

SIDE EFFECTS	INCIDENCE	SIDE EFFECT THERAPY
Nuisance		
Increased bleeding from cuts or tendency to bruise easily	Common	Unnecessary
Ear ringing or temporary changes in hearing	Common	Discontinue aspirin or reduce dosage
Nausea, indigestion, or heartburn	5–25%	Take aspirin with food, reduce dosage, or change medication
Serious		
Gastritis or stomach ulcers	Occasional	Discontinue aspirin and take stomach medication
Bleeding ulcers	Infrequent	Obtain prompt medical evaluation, discontinue aspirin, and take stomach medication
Abnormal liver tests	5%	Discontinue aspirin if markedly abnormal

While taking aspirin:

- Contact your physician promptly if you notice dark or tar-colored bowel movements, persistent indigestion or nausea, or stomach pain that is relieved by eating.

- Never take more than one anti-inflammatory drug at a time (aspirin counts as a drug). If your doctor prescribes a new NSAID, he or she will almost certainly take you off high-dose aspirin; if he or she fails to discuss this with you, you should ask about it. *Do not take over-the-counter anti-inflammatory medications such as ibuprofen or naproxen while you are taking high doses of aspirin.* If your physician approves, *acetaminophen* (such as Tylenol) may be taken while you are taking aspirin. Unless you are instructed otherwise, you should take aspirin at mealtime, to reduce indigestion and stomach irritation.

- Inform your dentist, surgeon, and anyone else performing health care procedures that you are on aspirin therapy. Because aspirin increases the tendency to bleed, these practitioners may need to alter their procedures to account for this condition.

- Avoid drinking alcohol and smoking, because these practices increase your risk of developing a stomach ulcer.

- Your doctor may periodically request blood tests for blood cell counts, kidney and liver tests, and tests for electrolyte (sodium and potassium) levels, and may examine your stool for blood.

Pregnancy and breastfeeding. Aspirin should be avoided during pregnancy, particularly during the last trimester, unless specifically prescribed by your doctor. Aspirin therapy may affect the fetus or cause complications during labor and delivery.

Salicylates are excreted in breast milk, and therefore large doses of aspirin should be avoided while nursing.

TRADITIONAL NSAIDS

Like high doses of aspirin, NSAIDs can decrease pain, stiffness, and swelling in the joints. NSAIDs are generally more convenient to take than most forms of aspirin, and they generally cause less stomach upset. Since the first modern

NSAID (indomethacin) was marketed in 1965, many more have become available; you probably are familiar with one or more of them (see Table 2).

Dosages of NSAIDs are not equivalent; 1 milligram of one NSAID is not necessarily equal to 1 milligram of another NSAID. For example, one 800-milligram tablet of ibuprofen is nearly equivalent to a 75-milligram tablet of ketoprofen. *Dosages of NSAIDs should be determined and monitored by your physician.*

TABLE 2. Nonsteroidal Anti-inflammatory Drugs (NSAIDs)

DRUG	BRAND NAME	GENERIC AVAILABLE?
Diclofenac sodium	Voltaren	yes
	Voltaren XR	yes
Diclofenac potassium	Cataflam	yes
	Cambia	no
	Zipsor	no
Diclofenac	Zorvolex	no
Diclofenac/misoprostol	Arthrotec	no
Diclofenac topical	Voltaren Gel	no
	Pennsaid	no
	Flector Patch	no
Diflunisal	Dolobid[b]	yes
Etodolac	Lodine[b]	yes
	Lodine XL[b]	yes
Fenoprofen	Nalfon	yes
Flurbiprofen	Ansaid	yes
Ibuprofen	Advil[a]	yes
	Medipren[a]	yes
	Midol[a]	yes
	Motrin IB[a]	yes
	Motrin	yes
Ibuprofen/famotidine	Duexis	no
Indomethacin	Indocin	yes
Ketoprofen	Orudis[b]	yes
	Oruvail[b]	yes
Magnesium choline trisalicylate	Trilisate[b]	yes
Meclofenamate	Meclomen[b]	yes
Meloxicam	Mobic	yes
Nabumetone	Relafen[b]	yes

TABLE 2. *Continued*

DRUG	BRAND NAME	GENERIC AVAILABLE?
Naproxen	Naprosyn	yes
Naproxen sodium	Naprelan	yes
	Anaprox	yes
	Anaprox DS	yes
	Aleve[a]	yes
Naproxen/esomeprazole	Vimovo	no
Oxaprozin	Daypro	yes
Piroxicam	Feldene	yes
Salsalate	Disalcid[b]	yes
Sulindac	Clinoril	yes
Tolmetin	Tolectin[b]	yes

Note: Unless noted otherwise, these NSAIDs are available by prescription only.
[a] Available over the counter, without prescription.
[b] Brand no longer available in the United States.

The NSAIDs listed below are commonly used in the treatment of RA. With the exception of ibuprofen and naproxen, the NSAIDs described here are available only by prescription. (The scientific name of the drug is given first; the names in parentheses are proprietary brand names.) One or more side effects of individual drugs may be mentioned in the descriptions, but not all are given there. Side effects of NSAIDs in general are discussed following this listing and are summarized in Table 3.

Diclofenac Sodium (Voltaren, Voltaren XR)

Tablet size: 25, 50, 75 mg
Extended-release tablet size: 100 mg

Diclofenac Potassium (Cataflam, Zipsor, Cambia)

Tablet size: 25, 50 mg
Available in powder packet for dissolving as a solution

Diclofenac (Zorvolex)

Capsule size: 18, 35 mg

Diclofenac is available in three chemical forms and is usually taken two or three times daily, depending on the dose size. Extended-release diclofenac is usually taken only once per day. There is a slightly increased risk of liver problems with diclofenac compared to other NSAIDs. Therefore, in 2009, the Food and Drug Administration (FDA) recommended that liver tests be performed 4 to 6 weeks after taking *any* product containing diclofenac.

Diclofenac/Misoprostol Combination (Arthrotec)

Tablet size: 50, 75 mg

Arthrotec is a combination pill that contains the NSAID diclofenac as well as a stomach-protecting medication. Arthrotec is usually taken twice per day. Because the tablet contains the stomach protector misoprostol, there is less chance of stomach problems.

Diclofenac Topical (Pennsaid, Voltaren Gel, Flector)

Voltaren Gel: 1%
Pennsaid solution: 1.5%
Flector patch: 1.3%

In 2009, Voltaren Gel became the first NSAID that could be applied directly to the skin (topically) over the joint to treat inflammation. Later Pennsaid topical solution and Flector patches were introduced. Topical treatment of RA is usually prescribed for people with only one or two joints affected with pain or inflammation. This form of NSAID treatment, to date, has been approved by the FDA for use only for osteoarthritis (Voltaren Gel, Pennsaid) or for joint pain caused by an acute injury, such as a sprain (Flector). Because only a small portion of these medications is absorbed into the bloodstream, topical treatment may be an option for individuals with RA who cannot take oral NSAIDS because of complicating illnesses, such as stomach, kidney, or heart conditions, and have only one or two particularly troubling joints. However, people who cannot take oral NSAIDS because of medical issues should always discuss the potential use of topical NSAIDS with their physician, since even a small amount of absorbed medication may present serious problems for some.

Diflunisal (Dolobid brand discontinued)

Tablet size: 500 mg

Diflunisal is taken twice daily. The brand-named diflunisal, called Dolobid, was discontinued in the United States because multiple generic versions quickly became available. Diflunisal differs from most other NSAIDs in being a close relative of the salicylate family, which includes aspirin. It is also one of the more effective NSAIDs for relieving pain.

Etodolac (Lodine brand discontinued)

Tablet size: 400, 500 mg
Extended-release tablet size: 400, 500, 600 mg
Capsule size: 200, 300 mg

Etodolac is generally taken two to four times per day. The brand-named etodolac, called Lodine, was discontinued in the United States; this medication is available in generic form. Extended-release tablets are taken one or two times per day. Etodolac is generally well tolerated.

Fenoprofen (Nalfon)

Tablet size: 600 mg
Capsule size: 200 mg

Fenoprofen is generally taken three or four times daily. There is a possibility of slightly increased risk of kidney problems with fenoprofen compared with other NSAIDs.

Flurbiprofen (Ansaid)

Tablet size: 50, 100 mg

Flurbiprofen is taken two or three times daily. It is an excellent pain reliever and causes comparatively fewer headaches than other NSAIDs.

Ibuprofen

Over-the-counter brand name examples: Advil, Motrin IB
Tablet size: 200 mg
Prescription brand name examples: prescription available in generic only
Tablet size: 400, 600, 800 mg
Liquid form available without prescription

Ibuprofen is generally taken three or four times daily. It is available without a prescription. Ibuprofen is generally well tolerated and is a proven pain reliever. For treatment of RA, the dosage of ibuprofen is greater than that recommended on the manufacturer's package insert. *Do not take large doses of ibuprofen without a physician's guidance.* In addition, to avoid increased toxicity, ibuprofen should not be taken with other NSAIDs.

Ibuprofen/Famotidine (Duexis)

Tablet size: 800 mg/26.6 mg

Duexis is a combination NSAID and stomach protectant that can be used in people who are at risk for stomach ulcers or irritation. It is generally taken three times per day. It contains high-dose ibuprofen and famotidine. Both ibuprofen and famotidine are available without prescription, but the over-the-counter products deliver lower doses.

Indomethacin (Indocin)

Capsule size: 25, 50 mg
Sustained-release capsule: 75 mg
Liquid and suppository forms are available.

Regular indomethacin is generally taken two or three times daily. The sustained-release capsule is taken once or twice per day. Indomethacin results in comparatively more headaches and stomach distress than other NSAIDs. It is generally considered to be one of the most potent NSAIDs in terms of anti-inflammatory effect.

Ketoprofen (Orudis, Oruvail brand discontinued)

Capsule size: 50, 75 mg
Extended-release capsule size: 200 mg

Ketoprofen is generally taken two or three times daily. Extended-release capsules are taken once per day. Brand-named Orudis and Oruvail (extended-release version) are no longer being manufactured; generic versions are available. Ketoprofen appears to be an excellent pain reliever for many people. Do not take this medication with other NSAIDs, even an over-the-counter NSAID.

Magnesium Choline Trisalicylate (Trilisate brand discontinued)

Tablet size: 500, 750, 1000 mg
Liquid form available

This medication is taken two or three times daily. Although the brand-named Trilisate is no longer manufactured, many doctors refer to this medication by the brand name, for simplicity. Magnesium choline trisalicylate differs from most other NSAIDs in being a close relative of the salicylate family, which includes aspirin. However, it is different from aspirin and other NSAIDs in some very important ways. It is one of the safer NSAIDs, because it results in a very low incidence of stomach irritation and ulceration. It also has little or no effect on the kidneys and platelets. The trade-off for this wonderful safety profile is that it may not be as effective for pain relief as other NSAIDs. Like aspirin, it can cause more ear ringing and temporary hearing loss than other NSAIDs. Salicylate levels in the blood are monitored to produce the most effective therapy possible.

Meclofenamate (Meclomen brand discontinued)

Capsule size: 50, 100 mg

Meclofenamate is generally taken three or four times daily. It is available in generic form only. It is a very good pain reliever. Complaints of abdominal cramping and diarrhea, particularly when it is used in high doses, limit its longer-term use in some people.

Meloxicam (Mobic)

Tablet size: 7.5, 15 mg
Liquid form available

Meloxicam became available in the United States in the year 2000. It had been used successfully in other countries for several years before then. Although not technically classified as a **COX-2 inhibitor,** it has many of the same characteristics. Compared to other traditional NSAIDs, it appears to have a less irritating effect on the stomach.

Nabumetone (Relafen brand discontinued)

Tablet size: 500, 750 mg

Nabumetone can be taken once or twice a day. Released in 1992, this NSAID may cause fewer stomach problems than many other traditional NSAIDs.

Naproxen (Naprosyn)

Prescription brand name examples: Naprosyn, Naprosyn EC (enteric coated)
Tablet size: 250, 375, 500 mg
Enteric-coated tablet size: 375, 500 mg
Liquid form available

See description below.

Naproxen Sodium (Aleve, Anaprox, Naprelan)

Over-the-counter brand name example: Aleve
Tablet size: 220 mg
Prescription brand name examples: Anaprox, Anaprox DS, Naprelan
   (extended release)
Tablet size: 275, 550 mg
Extended-release tablet size: 375, 500, 750 mg

Naproxen and naproxen sodium are convenient NSAIDs that are taken twice a day. The availability of an over-the-counter product has made this medication very popular. Both provide excellent pain relief. This medication should *not* be taken with other NSAIDs.

Naproxen/Esomeprazole (Vimovo)

Tablet size: 375, 500 mg

Vimovo is a combination NSAID and stomach protectant that is taken twice per day. The pill is made up of enteric-coated naproxen combined with esomeprazole, which is a member of the family of stomach protectants called proton pump inhibitors or, more commonly, PPIs. Medications in the PPI family have been shown to reduce the incidence of stomach ulcers in people who are on long-term NSAID therapy.

Oxaprozin (Daypro)

Tablet size: 600 mg

Oxaprozin is an NSAID that can be given once daily. The usual dosage is two tablets per day. Some individuals choose to divide the doses.

Piroxicam (Feldene)

Capsule size: 10, 20 mg

Piroxicam's major virtue is its once daily dosage. Excellent compliance with this dosing schedule is usually possible. Because this medication stays in the body longer than other NSAIDs, blood tests may need to be monitored closely in certain individuals (see cautionary notes below).

Salsalate (Disalcid brand discontinued)

Tablet size: 500, 750 mg

Salsalate is taken three or four times daily. It is available in generic forms only. It differs from other NSAIDs in that it is classified in the salicylate family of medications, which includes aspirin. However, it differs from aspirin and from other NSAIDs in many respects. It is one of the safer NSAIDs, carrying a very low incidence of stomach irritation and ulceration. In addition, it has little or no effect on the kidneys and platelets. Unfortunately, this safe and effective anti-inflammatory drug may not relieve pain as well as other NSAIDs. Like aspirin and magnesium choline trisalicylate, it can cause comparatively more ear ringing and reversible hearing loss than other NSAIDs. Salicylate levels in the blood are monitored to produce the most effective therapy possible.

Sulindac (Clinoril)

Tablet size: 150, 200 mg

Sulindac has a simple twice daily dosage. It tends to be well tolerated. There appears to be a *slight* decrease in the risk for kidney problems with this medication as compared with some other NSAIDs. There may be a slight risk that gallbladder and pancreas problems will arise from its use.

Tolmetin (Tolectin brand discontinued)

Tablet size: 200, 600 mg
Capsule size: 400 mg

Tolmetin is usually taken three or four times daily. It is available in generic form only. Its use sometimes results in a false reading of protein in the urine. This can be misleading, because one rare but real side effect of tolmetin and the other NSAIDs is protein in the urine.

Side Effects of Traditional NSAIDs

The negative side effects of NSAIDs are summarized in Table 3. The most common side effect of NSAIDs is stomach upset. Stomach symptoms are generally relieved by taking the medication with a meal or by adjusting the dosage.

Patients who have been taking NSAIDs for a long time can develop serious stomach problems (gastritis or stomach ulcer). Bleeding ulcers are an infrequent side effect of NSAID therapy. If gastritis, stomach ulcer, or bleeding ulcer develop, however, you will need to discontinue taking the NSAID and take medication that treats your stomach problem. At the end of this chapter we will discuss stomach medications that can be used to help reduce the risk of ulcers caused by NSAIDS. After that we will describe and list COX-2 inhibitors. This subset of NSAIDs may be an option for people who have experienced stomach problems or are considered at high risk for stomach problems.

A less common side effect of NSAID therapy is kidney problems. This consequence is rare in healthy individuals, but it can be more likely in people who have known risk factors for developing kidney trouble. Risk factors include

TABLE 3. Side Effects of NSAIDs

SIDE EFFECTS	INCIDENCE	SIDE EFFECT THERAPY
Nuisance		
Heartburn, nausea, and stomach pain	Common	Take with food or try a different NSAID
Cramping or diarrhea	Common	Take with food or reduce dosage
Rash	3–9%	Discontinue NSAID
Fluid retention, weight gain, ankle swelling	Common	Decrease salt intake
Headache, drowsiness, dizziness, difficulty concentrating	Common	Discontinue NSAID or try a different NSAID
Increased bleeding from cuts or tendency to bruise easily	Common	Usually no treatment
Ear ringing or mild change in hearing	Common	Discontinue NSAID or reduce dosage
Serious		
Abnormal liver tests	3%	Discontinue NSAID or reduce dosage if markedly abnormal since hepatitis is a rare consequence of NSAID use
Gastritis or stomach ulcers	Occasional	Discontinue NSAID and take stomach medication
Bleeding ulcers	Infrequent	Obtain prompt medical evaluation, discontinue NSAID, and take stomach medication
Kidney problems	Infrequent	Discontinue NSAID
Blood problems	Rare	Discontinue NSAID
Cardiovascular problems	(See text)	(See text)

diabetes, uncontrolled high blood pressure, being older than sixty, a history of kidney disease, significant liver disease, heart disease, and hardening of the arteries. Most kidney problems caused by NSAIDs resolve when the medication is discontinued.

People who have the above risk factors for kidney side effects may also be at risk for cardiovascular side effects (meaning, literally, heart and blood vessel problems). These issues include high blood pressure as well as increased risk of heart attack and stroke. (You will read more about this below under COX-2 inhibitors.) The potential risk that NSAIDs will cause or worsen cardiovascular problems is much more difficult to quantify than one might expect. Studies to look at cardiovascular risk would have to be long term, since the side effects may take years to manifest themselves in most individuals. This is very similar to the challenges of measuring cardiovascular risk from conditions such as high cholesterol, elevated blood pressure, diabetes, and smoking. Since the vast majority of NSAIDS are now generic, it is not likely that drug manufacturers (frequently the funders of drug research) will sponsor lengthy clinical trials to answer these questions. Because the exact risk is unknown, the FDA has required that all NSAIDs list cardiovascular side effects as a possibility. Thus, you will see this on pharmacy handouts, even though the exact risk is unclear. As with all treatments, the risks and benefits of NSAID therapy should be discussed with your doctor, looking at your individual medical and other needs.

Cautionary Notes

Before starting NSAID therapy, discuss the following with your physician:

- A history of allergy to aspirin or other anti-inflammatory medication. Symptoms of allergy include rash, hives, wheezing, and swollen lips or eyelids.
- Previous history of asthma, nasal polyps, stomach ulcer, bleeding problems, colitis, high blood pressure, or kidney, liver, or heart problems.
- Any medications you are taking, particularly medications for blood thinning, diabetes, gout, high blood pressure, pain, or seizures.

While taking NSAIDs:

- Contact your physician promptly if you notice dark or tar-colored bowel movements, persistent indigestion or nausea, stomach pain that is relieved by eating.

- Never take more than one NSAID at a time. If your doctor prescribes a new NSAID, he or she will almost certainly take you off the other; if the doctor fails to discuss this with you, you should ask about it. *Do not take over-the-counter anti-inflammatory medications, such as ibuprofen, naproxen, or aspirin, while you are taking another NSAID.* If your physician approves, *acetaminophen* (such as Tylenol) may be taken while you are taking an NSAID.

- Unless you are instructed otherwise, you should take the NSAID at mealtime, to reduce indigestion and stomach irritation.

- Inform your dentist, surgeon, and anyone else performing health care procedures on you that you are taking an NSAID. Because NSAIDs can increase the tendency to bleed, these practitioners may need to alter their procedures to account for this risk.

- Wait two to four weeks before judging the effectiveness of the NSAID.

- Avoid drinking alcohol and smoking, because these practices increase your risk of developing an ulcer.

- Your doctor may periodically request blood tests for blood cell counts, kidney and liver tests, and tests for electrolyte (sodium and potassium) levels, as well as examine your stool for blood.

Pregnancy and breastfeeding. Not all NSAIDs have been studied adequately as to their effects on pregnancy, but it is generally recommended that they be discontinued during pregnancy. Most NSAIDs are excreted to some degree in breast milk; hence, their use is usually discouraged during nursing. The manufacturer's package insert can be reviewed by you and your physician for information about the use of a specific NSAID during pregnancy and nursing. Discuss with your obstetrician and your pediatrician *all* medications you are taking or considering taking.

COX-2 INHIBITORS

In December 1998 the FDA approved the first cyclo-oxygenase-2 inhibitor, the brand name Celebrex. In May 1999, a second COX-2 inhibitor, Vioxx, was released in the United States, and in 2001 a third, Bextra. Milder on the stomach, these anti-inflammatory drugs were welcome additions to the pharmaceutical choices for people who have difficulty tolerating traditional NSAIDs.

TABLE 4. COX-2 Inhibitors

DRUG	BRAND NAME	GENERIC AVAILABLE
Celecoxib	Celebrex	no[a]
Rofecoxib	Vioxx[b]	no
Enterocoxib[c]	Arcoxia	no
Valdecoxib	Bextra[b]	no

[a] Expected soon.
[b] No longer on the market.
[c] Only in clinical studies in the United States at the time of this writing; available in many other countries.

Cyclo-oxygenase-2, or COX-2, is an enzyme in the body known to stimulate inflammation by producing prostaglandins. Some prostaglandins can cause pain and swelling. Both COX-2 inhibitors and traditional NSAIDs block the COX-2 enzyme and limit the production of inflammatory prostaglandins, thereby decreasing inflammation. As it happens, traditional NSAIDs also block COX-1, a "good" enzyme that protects the stomach lining by producing protective prostaglandins. Blocking the production of the good variety of prostaglandins can result in stomach irritation and possibly ulcers, as well as a higher risk of bleeding problems. Researchers at the University of Rochester discovered that they could create medications that could block the production of inflammatory prostaglandins (by blocking the COX-2 enzyme) without interfering with the function of the protective prostaglandins (produced by the COX-1 enzyme). The result was a *presumably* safer class of NSAIDs, which were named COX-2 inhibitors. The availability of the COX-2 inhibitors has made it possible for many people who couldn't tolerate traditional NSAIDs to relieve their pain and swelling with less risk of stomach ulceration and bleeding.

However, after the first three COX-2 inhibitors were on the market for a time, it became clear that there were unintended consequences of blocking COX-2 only. By 2004, medical researchers were finding evidence that these medications could increase the risk of cardiovascular problems, namely heart attacks and strokes. This observation led to the withdrawal from the U.S. market of Vioxx (in 2004) and Bextra (2005). Celebrex was allowed to remain on the market with cardiovascular warnings on its label and plans for further research to assess its cardiovascular risk. A fourth COX-2 inhibitor, called Arcoxia, is still in extended clinical trials in the United States but is available in more than 70 countries worldwide. Questions about COX-2 inhibitors' cardiovascular risk have prompted a harder look at our existing traditional NSAIDs, the result being the presumption that all NSAIDs may potentially increase risk of high blood pressure, heart conditions, and strokes.

Unlike traditional NSAIDs, COX-2 inhibitors can be cautiously prescribed for people who are already taking blood thinners, such as Coumadin (warfarin). The doctor will want to monitor your blood tests closely to look for changes in a test called INR or Protime. The dose of your blood thinner may have to be adjusted while you are on both medications. Your physician may also choose to place you on low-dose aspirin while you are on a COX-2 inhibitor. This would depend on your individual risk for side effects, such as a history of bleeding ulcer. Many people will require low-dose aspirin if their personal history makes them at risk for heart attack or stroke. Further discussion of side effects follows these descriptions of the four brand name COX-2 inhibitors mentioned above.

Celecoxib (Celebrex)

Capsule size: 100, 200 mg

Celecoxib can be taken once or twice daily. Some find that taking the medication in the evening helps diminish morning stiffness. This anti-inflammatory agent is very effective and well tolerated. If you have an allergy to sulfa drugs, you may not be able to take Celebrex. Be sure to discuss *all* medication allergies with your physician before starting any new medication.

Enterocoxib (Arcoxia)

Although enterocoxib was initially expected to be available in the United States in 2003, its release was stalled by concerns regarding the safety of COX-2 inhibitors in general. It is expected to remain in long-term clinical studies in the United States until at least 2014. At the time of this writing, Arcoxia is approved for use in more than 70 other countries.

Rofecoxib (Vioxx)

Rofecoxib was voluntarily removed from the world market by its manufacturer, Merck, in 2004 because of concerns about increased risk of heart attacks and strokes.

Valdecoxib (Bextra)

Bextra was removed from the U.S., Canadian, and European Union markets in 2005 because of concerns about increased risk of heart attacks and strokes.

Side Effects of COX-2 Inhibitors

The negative side effects of COX-2 inhibitors and their frequency and treatments are listed in Table 5. The most common side effects of the COX-2 inhibitors are abdominal pain, nausea, indigestion, and diarrhea. Stomach ulceration and bleeding are less likely than with traditional NSAIDs. As you have read above, use of COX-2 inhibitors may increase the risk of cardiovascular side effects, including heart attack and stroke. At the time of this writing, in the United States, only Celebrex is available. In 2006, a study was initiated at the Cleveland Clinic to study 20,000 patients considered at high risk for cardiovascular disease. The study is comparing Celebrex to naproxen and ibuprofen. It is expected that this study will be completed in 2014. Arcoxia is also undergoing long-term safety studies. Studies on these two drugs should help us further define potential risks to cardiovascular health from COX-2 inhibitors.

Cautionary Notes

Before starting a COX-2 inhibitor, discuss the following with your physician:

- History of uncontrolled high blood pressure, ankle swelling, or fluid retention.
- History of sulfa allergy (particularly if considering celecoxib).
- History of allergy to aspirin or other anti-inflammatory medications (symptoms include rash, hives, wheezing, swollen lips or eyelids).
- History of asthma, nasal polyps, stomach ulcer, colitis, or kidney or liver problems.
- History of heart attack, stroke, or blood clots.
- Any medications you are taking, particularly medications for blood thinning, gout, high blood pressure, pain, or seizures.

While taking a COX-2 inhibitor:

- Contact your physician promptly if you notice dark or tar-colored bowel movements, persistent indigestion or nausea, or stomach pain that is relieved by eating.
- Never take more than one COX-2 inhibitor or NSAID at a time. If your doctor prescribes a COX-2 inhibitor, he or she will take you off other NSAIDs; if he or she fails to discuss this with you, you should ask. *Do not take COX-2*

inhibitors with over-the-counter anti-inflammatory medications such as ibu-profen or naproxen. Read labels. Ask your doctor about low-dose aspirin if you are on aspirin for other reasons. If your physician approves, acetamin-ophen (such as Tylenol) may be taken while you are on a COX-2 inhibitor.

- Inform your dentist, surgeon, and anyone else performing health care pro-cedures that you are taking a COX-2 inhibitor.

TABLE 5. Side Effects of COX-2 Inhibitors

SIDE EFFECTS	INCIDENCE	SIDE EFFECT THERAPY
Nuisance		
Heartburn, nausea, and stomach pain	Infrequent	Take with food or try different COX-2 inhibitor
Cramping or diarrhea	Occasional	Take with food
Rash	Infrequent	Discontinue medication
Fluid retention, weight gain, ankle swelling	Common	Reduce dose or decrease salt intake
Headache, drowsiness, dizziness, difficulty concentrating	Occasional	Discontinue medication
Ear ringing or mild change in hearing	Occasional	Discontinue medication or reduce dosage
Serious		
High blood pressure	Occasional	Discontinue medication or reduce dosage
Abnormal liver tests	Infrequent	Discontinue medication if severe
Gastritis or stomach ulcers	Infrequent	Discontinue medication and take stomach medication
Bleeding ulcers	Rare	Obtain prompt medical evaluation; discontinue medication and take stomach medication
Kidney problems	Infrequent	Discontinue medication
Cardiovascular problems	(See text)	Discuss latest research with your doctor

- Avoid drinking alcohol and smoking, which increase your risk of developing an ulcer.
- Your doctor may periodically request blood tests for blood cell counts, kidney and liver tests, and tests for electrolyte (sodium and potassium) levels, as well as examine your stool for blood.

Pregnancy and breastfeeding. COX-2 inhibitors have not been studied adequately as to their effects on pregnancy. It is generally recommended that they be discontinued during pregnancy. COX-2 inhibitors are excreted to some degree in breast milk, so their use is usually discouraged during nursing. The manufacturer's package insert can be reviewed by you and your physician for information about the use of a COX-2 inhibitor during pregnancy and nursing. Discuss all medications with your obstetrician and your pediatrician.

STOMACH MEDICATIONS FREQUENTLY USED WITH NSAIDS

Because aspirin and NSAIDs can cause stomach problems such as gastritis and ulcers, it is sometimes necessary to take medications to treat these conditions. Stomach problems often can be relieved by changing how often, when, and how much of the medication you take. You might switch from a traditional NSAID to a COX-2 inhibitor. Also, there are many medications available for relieving stomach problems. Some stomach medications are listed in Table 6. Lastly, some NSAIDs are available in the form of combination pills that contain both an NSAID and a stomach protectant (see Arthrotec, Duexis, and Vimovo, listed above).

TABLE 6. Stomach Medications

PURPOSE OF DRUG	DRUG NAME	BRAND NAME
Prescription		
Prevents stomach ulcers; protects the stomach	Misoprostol[a]	Cytotec
Decreases acid production	Cimetidine[a]	Tagamet
	Famotidine[a]	Pepcid
	Nizatidine[a]	Axid
	Ranitidine[a]	Zantac
	Omeprazole[a]	Prilosec
	Omeprazole/sodium bicarbonate	Zegerid
	Lansoprazole[a]	Prevacid
	Pantoprazole[a]	Protonix
	Esomeprazole	Nexium
	Rabeprazole	Aciphex
	Dexlansoprazole	Kapidex
		Dexilant
Coats the stomach	Sucralfate[a]	Carafate
Over-the-counter		
Neutralizes acids	Antacid	Mylanta
		Maalox
		Rolaids
		Tums
Decreases acid production	Cimetidine[a,b]	Tagamet[b]
	Famotidine[a,b]	Pepcid AC[b]
	Nizatidine[a,b]	Axid[b]
	Omeprazole[a,b]	Prilosec OTC[b]
	Lansoprazole[a,b]	Prevacid 24 hr[b]
	Omeprazole/sodium bicarbonate	Zegerid OTC[b]

[a] Available in generic.
[b] Generic and over-the-counter brand name product lower dosage than prescribed version of same drug.

Disease-Modifying Antirheumatic Drugs (DMARDs)

The purpose of disease-modifying antirheumatic drugs (**DMARDs**) is to alter the course of rheumatoid arthritis (RA)—to control the arthritis process and prevent damage. DMARDs are also commonly referred to as *second-line* agents, because traditionally they were used only after NSAIDs or other anti-inflammatory medications had failed.

All drugs that are classified as DMARDs are believed to be effective in slowing down the process of RA. In some cases they may even induce a complete remission of the condition (which explains why they are sometimes referred to as *remittive* drugs). Their ability to affect the course of RA distinguishes this group of drugs from NSAIDs, which effectively treat symptoms, such as pain and swelling, but do not change the course of the disease. Although DMARDs do not provide fast pain relief, improved comfort is often a long-term benefit of using them to control the arthritis process.

Twenty-one medications are considered by most rheumatologists to fit into the DMARD family. We generally divide them into two broad categories: biologic and nonbiologic. The eleven nonbiologic DMARDs are usually referred to simply as DMARDs. Seven of these—injectable gold, gold pills, hydroxychloroquine, penicillamine, sulfasalazine, leflunamide, and minocycline—are categorized only as DMARDs. We do not fully understand how most of them work. The other four nonbiologic DMARDs are also categorized as *immunosuppressants*. This group includes methotrexate, azathioprine, cyclophosphamide, and cyclosporine. We *think* we know how they work: immunosuppressants appear to change the course of RA by suppressing, or decreasing the activity of, the immune system.

In RA, parts of the immune system are overactive, so a drug that decreases that hyperactivity of the immune system is useful in controlling the disease. But to maintain health, a person must have a properly functioning immune system, since the immune system is designed to fight infectious disease. For this reason, immunosuppressants must be prescribed with care. The immune system cannot be allowed to become suppressed to the point that it is unable to fight infection. Safe and effective treatment of RA with immunosuppressants requires close supervision by a physician experienced in their use, preferably a **rheumatologist.**

In this chapter, we will be discussing the nonbiologic DMARDs; the nine biologic DMARDs (Enbrel, Remicade, Humira, Kineret, Simponi, Cimzia, Orencia, Actemra, and Rituxan), called biologics, are discussed in detail in Chapter 14. Lastly, there is one new DMARD that has a class of its own: Xeljanz. Because it is very similar to the biologics in many ways, it will be discussed in the next chapter.

NONIMMUNOSUPPRESSANT DMARDS

Injectable Gold: Gold Sodium Thiomalate (Myochrysine); Aurothioglucose (Solganal)

Generic available: no form of injectable gold available in the
    United States *at this time*
Usual dose: weekly to monthly injections
Effective within: six weeks to six months

Gold was first used as a medicine in the early 1900s, to treat people with tuberculosis and other infections. Believing that RA was caused by tuberculosis, Dr. Jacques Forestier began injecting gold into RA patients in the late 1920s, with a degree of success. He published his small study of 48 patients in 1932, suggesting that gold might "be regarded as the best chemical for the treatment of rheumatoid arthritis." During the 1930s and early 1940s, doctors prescribed very high doses of gold and achieved excellent results, although with excessive side effects. Eventually the disadvantages were considered to outweigh the benefits, and gold therapy went through a phase of disfavor.

In the late 1940s, a resurgence in the use of gold therapy began after carefully designed studies proved that lower doses could be effective. Since then, gold injections have been administered to thousands of people, many of whom have enjoyed positive results with few side effects. With the advent of methotrexate and the new biologic medications in the 1990s, the use of intramuscular gold decreased considerably. By 2004, one form of gold, Solganal, had become unavailable in the United States. In 2011, the last manufacturer ceased making Myochrysine, the other form of injectable gold. There are still countries that manufacture injectable gold, but availability internationally is decreasing due to raw material shortages. Oral gold is still available (discussed below).

Although injectable gold is not currently available in the United States, that status could change. The two previously prescribed forms of injectable gold were approximately half gold by weight (and half inactive ingredients). The injections are administered into the buttock muscles. The dose is increased slowly over weeks and months, to limit side effects. Once improvement is noted, the interval between injections can be lengthened, although injections are generally not spaced further apart than one month. This frequency is usually necessary to sustain a remission.

Side effects of injectable gold. About one in every three persons receiving injectable gold will experience side effects from it (see Table 7), skin rash and mouth sores being the most common problems. Approximately 15 percent of people treated will discontinue gold treatment within the first six months because of its toxicity.

The kidneys are sometimes affected by gold therapy, although fewer than 1 percent of people receiving the treatments develop *serious* kidney problems. The most common renal problem is the appearance of protein in the urine. The vast majority of kidney problems reverse themselves when gold injections are discontinued.

Gold-induced blood problems are also rare. In 1 to 3 percent of patients, a low platelet count develops. This is almost always treatable and reversible. In fewer than 0.5 percent of people, serious bone marrow problems occur. Since bone marrow produces red and white blood cells as well as platelets, this complication must be detected as early as possible and gold therapy discontinued. People receiving gold injections must have their blood monitored closely and frequently. Early detection of a blood problem permits prompt treatment and usually reverses the problem.

One occasional side effect, nitritoid reaction, is alarming but usually not dangerous. When it occurs, it happens within ten minutes after the injection

TABLE 7. Side Effects of Injectable Gold

SIDE EFFECTS	INCIDENCE	SIDE EFFECT THERAPY
Nuisance		
Rash or itching	15–25%	Discontinue medication or reduce dosage; apply corticosteroid cream; take antihistamines
Mouth sores	5–10%	Discontinue medication if sores are severe or intolerable
Metallic taste		No treatment
Hair thinning (mild)		No treatment
Serious		
Blood toxicities	1–5%	Discontinue medication
Protein in urine	10–20% (significant in only 1–3%)	Discontinue medication if significant amounts of protein are present
Lung toxicity	Rare	Discontinue medication
Neuropathy	Rare	Discontinue medication
Colitis	Rare	Discontinue medication
Liver problems	Rare	Discontinue medication
Nitritoid reaction	5%	Discontinue medication or use aurothiogluclose (Solganal) instead of gold sodium thiomalate (Myochrysine)

has been given. Flushing, fainting, dizziness, and sweating are its symptoms. Although these symptoms can be frightening, they generally have no serious consequences. Fewer than 5 percent of people taking gold sodium thiomalate (Myochrysine) have this reaction. If this occurs, the gold preparation can be changed to aurothioglucose (Solganal), if available.

Before starting injectable gold therapy, discuss the following with your physician:

- A history of blood disorders, kidney or liver disease, uncontrolled high blood pressure, bleeding problems, or allergic reactions to any drugs.

While receiving injectable gold:

- Contact your physician promptly if you notice a new rash or itching, mouth sores, increased bruising, a tendency to bleed easily, fever, cough, shortness of breath, or a change in skin or urine color.
- Avoid unprotected or prolonged exposure to the sun.
- Your doctor will frequently order complete blood counts and urine studies.

Pregnancy and breastfeeding. Gold should probably be stopped several months before conception if possible. Gold is excreted in breast milk, and the potential exists for serious adverse effects in the nursing infant. Mothers should discontinue either nursing or gold injections.

Oral Gold: Auranofin (Ridaura)

Generic available: no
Capsule size: 3 mg
Usual dose: one pill twice daily
Effective within: six weeks to six months

The introduction of auranofin in the 1980s allowed people with RA to take gold by mouth. This method of treatment can be effective in slowing the progression of RA, particularly if begun in the early stages of the disease. Unlike injectable gold, oral gold is only 29 percent gold by weight. Many physicians believe that auranofin is not as effective as injectable gold.

Side effects of oral gold. Auranofin therapy causes fewer *serious* side effects than does injectable gold (see Table 8). The most common side effects are stomach cramping, diarrhea, nausea, and changes in appetite. Most of these problems can be made tolerable by starting with a low dose, taking the medication with meals and consuming products containing bulk and large amounts of fiber, such as Metamucil.

Before starting auranofin therapy, discuss the following with your physician:

- Previous history of blood disorders, kidney or liver disease, uncontrolled high blood pressure, bleeding problems, or allergic reactions to any drugs.

While receiving auranofin:

- Contact your physician promptly if you notice a rash or itching, mouth sores, increased bruising, an increased tendency to bleed, fever, cough, shortness of breath, or a change in skin or urine color.

- Avoid unprotected or prolonged exposure to the sun.

- Complete blood counts and urine studies need to be done frequently during therapy.

Pregnancy and breastfeeding. Discontinue gold therapy during pregnancy. Gold is excreted in breast milk, and the potential exists for serious adverse effects in the nursing infant. Mothers should discontinue either nursing or auranofin therapy.

TABLE 8. Side Effects of Oral Gold

SIDE EFFECTS	INCIDENCE	SIDE EFFECT THERAPY
Nuisance		
Rash	24%	Discontinue medication or
Itching	17%	reduce dosage; apply corticosteroid cream
Hives	1–3%	Discontinue medication
Mouth sores	13%	Discontinue medication if sores are severe or intolerable
Diarrhea, abdominal cramps, decreased appetite, heartburn, flatulence	40–50%	Take medication with meals, take fiber laxatives, or increase dose slowly
Metallic taste	Rare	No treatment known
Hair loss (minor)	2.4%	No treatment known
Serious		
Blood problems	1–2%	Discontinue medication
Kidney problems	Less than 5%	Discontinue medication
Lung problems	Rare	Discontinue medication
Liver test abnormalities	Rare	Discontinue medication

Hydroxychloroquine (Plaquenil)

Generic available: yes
Tablet size: 200 mg
Usual dose: one or two pills daily
Effective within: six weeks to six months

The healing qualities of quinine have been recognized for centuries. Quinine and its derivatives have been used to treat skin ailments, fever, and, notably, malaria. Commonly used antimalarial drugs are hydroxychloroquine, chloroquine, and quinacrine. Quinacrine was the first antimalarial medication used to treat RA. The FDA approved hydroxychloroquine for use in 1955, so we have many years of experience with this medication. Chloroquine and hydroxychloroquine are both used today in treating RA. Hydroxychloroquine is used most commonly because it causes fewer side effects and is more available.

Side effects of hydroxychloroquine. Hydroxychloroquine may be the safest of all the DMARDs. Estimates are that only 5 percent of patients discontinue using the medication because of its side effects. The most commonly reported side effects of hydroxychloroquine are nausea, decreased appetite, diarrhea, and rash (see Table 9). Most of these problems can be eliminated with dose changes and by taking the medication at mealtime. With long-term use, some patients may notice areas of darkened skin color. This is particularly common in areas that have been bruised badly. Hydroxychloroquine appears to bind to pigments in the skin, including melanin, creating darkening. This discoloration is not harmful and will fade over time with discontinuation of the medication.

The principal concern with all antimalarial drugs is the risk of eye problems (*retinopathy*). With long-term use, these medications can cause changes in the eye's retina. When hydroxychloroquine is taken in the customary dose for RA, however, the risk of this is very small, particularly in the first 5 years of usage. According to the largest study to date, the risk of damage to the retina increases from less than 0.3 percent at 5 years to more than 2 percent at 15 years of usage (Wolfe and Marmor, 2010). When eye examinations are performed by an **ophthalmologist** as recommended and the medication is discontinued immediately on the ophthalmologist's advice, the risk of permanent eye damage is low. Chloroquine use involves a slightly higher risk of permanent eye damage. People with pre-existing retina problems appear to be at greater risk for problems. Your eye doctor will advise you on how often your eyes should be examined.

TABLE 9. Side Effects of Hydroxychloroquine

SIDE EFFECTS	INCIDENCE	SIDE EFFECT THERAPY
Nuisance		
Nausea, decreased appetite, diarrhea, bloating	11–20%	Take medication with meals or divide dosage
Rash	Occasional	Reduce dosage and apply corticosteroid cream
Skin pigment changes	10–25%	Discontinue medication if significant
Nervousness, headache, dizziness	Infrequent	Discontinue medication or reduce dosage
Serious		
Blood abnormalities	Rare	Discontinue medication
Eye problems Retinal damage Corneal deposits	(See text) 18–46%	Discontinue medication Continue medication
Muscular weakness	Rare	Discontinue medication

There are also newer objective tests that can be performed, including *spectral domain ocular coherence tomography, fundus autoflourescence*, and *multifocal electroretinography*. These new technologies make it possible to detect very early changes in the retina before you have any noticeable changes in your vision.

Your ophthalmologist may also mention that he or she has detected deposits on the cornea. This appears to be a reversible side effect that does not warrant a change in therapy.

When hydroxychloroquine is first taken, your vision may be temporarily blurred. This does not mean that there is a problem with your retina; the blurring will clear within a week.

Before starting hydroxychloroquine therapy, discuss the following with your physician:

- A history of psoriasis, liver disease, porphyria, or eye problems.
- Any medications that you are presently taking, particularly the heart medication digoxin.

- If you have been diagnosed as having glucose-6-phosphate dehydrogenase (G-6-PD) deficiency. This condition appears in approximately 10 percent of people of African descent and in some people of Mediterranean background. A blood test for G-6-PD deficiency can be performed before you start treatment with hydroxychloroquine.

- A baseline examination (an examination performed before treatment begins) by an ophthalmologist is recommended to look for pre-existing retina problems.

While taking hydroxychloroquine:

- Contact your physician promptly if you notice a change in vision, a rash, muscle weakness, fever, or easy bleeding or bruising.

- Avoid unprotected or prolonged exposure to the sun.

- You should be checked by your ophthalmologist according to the screening schedule that he or she advises.

Pregnancy and breastfeeding. Because the eyes of the fetus can (though rarely) be affected by hydroxychloroquine, it is recommended that use of this medication be avoided during pregnancy. Hydroxychloroquine is excreted in breast milk, and therefore mothers should discontinue either nursing or use of the medication.

Penicillamine (Cuprimine, Depen)

Generic available: no
Cuprimine capsule size: 250 mg
Depen (scored) tablet size: 250 mg
Usual dose: two to four pills daily
Effective within: two to nine months

Penicillamine has been used since the 1960s to treat people with RA, and it is quite effective. It takes a long time to become effective, because its dose has to be increased very slowly to minimize side effects. This DMARD is very rarely used today, however, because there are now safer and more effective medications.

The chemical structure of penicillamine is similar to that of penicillin. Nevertheless, there seems to be no increased incidence of allergic reactions to this drug in individuals who are allergic to penicillin.

Side effects of penicillamine. Penicillamine therapy produces numerous side effects, which limits its use (see Table 10). Withdrawal rates of up to 40 percent in the first year have been reported. Some of the serious side effects are similar to those of injectable gold. A chief concern is the development of blood abnormalities, the most common being a decrease in platelets, a condition that is usually reversible (approximately 4 percent of people taking penicillamine develop this condition). The white blood cell count decreases in approximately 2 percent of individuals using this drug. Low white blood cell counts are also usually reversible, but the risk of infection is increased while the count is low.

Kidney problems can develop with penicillamine treatment. Almost all of these problems can be reversed if they are detected early. Penicillamine therapy also can, rarely, result in the development of autoimmune conditions such as myasthenia gravis, pemphigus, Goodpasture's syndrome, or systemic lupus erythematosus. All of these conditions are serious but can be treated successfully.

TABLE 10. Side Effects of Penicillamine

SIDE EFFECTS	INCIDENCE	SIDE EFFECT THERAPY
Nuisance		
Rash	12–25%	Discontinue medication or reduce dosage; take antihistamines
Upset stomach, nausea, vomiting, anorexia, diarrhea	12–20%	Reduce dosage
Change in taste	4–33%	Discontinue medication or reduce dosage
Breast enlargement	Rare	Continue medication
Mouth sores	10%	Reduce dosage
Serious		
Blood toxicities	5–10%	Discontinue medication
Protein in urine	6–20%	Discontinue medication or reduce dosage
Autoimmune syndromes	2%	Discontinue medication
Liver test abnormalities	Rare	Discontinue medication
Lung problems	Rare	Discontinue medication
Muscle weakness	1–2%	Discontinue medication

Before starting penicillamine therapy, discuss the following with your physician:

- A diagnosis of lupus.

- A history of lung conditions, skin conditions, or kidney or liver disease.

While taking penicillamine:

- Contact your physician promptly if you notice a new rash or itching, mouth sores, increased bruising, easy bleeding, fever, sore throat, cough, shortness of breath, or a change in urine or skin color.

- Take medication on an empty stomach (at least one hour before or two hours after a meal).

- Complete blood counts and urine studies need to be performed frequently during therapy.

Pregnancy and breastfeeding. Since penicillamine can cause birth defects, this medication is not to be taken during pregnancy. Nursing mothers should not take this medication.

Sulfasalazine (Azulfidine)

Generic available: yes
Tablet size: 500 mg
Enteric-coated tablets: 500 mg
Liquid form available
Usual dose: two or three pills twice daily
Effective within: two to six months

Sulfasalazine is commonly prescribed to treat colitis, although when it was developed in the 1930s by Professor Nanna Svartz in Stockholm it was designed for the treatment of RA. Sulfa drugs were just being developed at that time, and RA was considered to be an infectious condition caused by *streptococci* bacteria in milk (Svartz, 1948). Sulfasalazine contained both an antibiotic (sulfa) and an anti-inflammatory component (salicylate). It was used to treat RA throughout the 1940s, with proven effectiveness, but eventually fell into disuse largely because the new miracle drug, cortisone, had become available.

Since the late 1980s, there has been a resurgence of interest in and use of sulfasalazine for RA. This drug did not receive formal FDA approval for use in RA until 1996. Studies have determined that sulfasalazine can be used effectively alone or in combination with other DMARDs, such as methotrexate. Many rheumatologists prescribe sulfasalazine for RA because of its effectiveness and low incidence of serious side effects.

Side effects of sulfasalazine. Individuals taking this medication complain more frequently of stomach problems than of any other side effect (see Table 11). Although sulfasalazine is most effective when taken on an empty stomach, taking it with meals is acceptable and helps prevent stomach discomfort. Enteric-coated tablets also help in this regard. Beginning treatment with low doses and increasing the dose slowly also improves stomach acceptance.

Decreased sperm counts and changes in the sperm can occur, temporarily decreasing fertility. Sperm counts return to normal approximately two months after sulfasalazine use has been discontinued.

Serious side effects are quite rare and usually appear early in the course of treatment. Most worrisome are severe sulfa allergic reactions, hepatitis, fever, and a decrease in the number of white blood cells, red blood cells, and platelets. The majority of people recover from these side effects when the medication is discontinued and proper treatment is given.

Before starting sulfasalazine therapy, discuss the following with your physician:

- Allergy to sulfa or other antibiotics; allergy to aspirin or history of nasal polyps or bronchial asthma.
- A history of kidney or liver problems.
- Any medications you are taking to treat diabetes, blood pressure, seizures, or heart ailments or to thin the blood.

While taking sulfasalazine:

- Avoid or protect yourself against sun exposure.
- Inform your physician immediately if you develop a rash, blood in your urine, fever, bruising or easy bleeding, sore throat, cough, or shortness of breath.
- Your physician will intermittently order complete blood counts, liver function tests, and urine tests to monitor and control the side effects.

Pregnancy and breastfeeding. Avoid use of this medication during pregnancy. Although birth defects have not been reported, caution suggests the use of birth control methods until sulfasalazine has been discontinued for two months.

TABLE 11. Side Effects of Sulfasalazine

SIDE EFFECTS	INCIDENCE	SIDE EFFECT THERAPY
Nuisance		
Nausea, vomiting, upset stomach	Greater than 20%	Take medication with meals; take enteric-coated tablets
Headache, irritability, dizziness	Less than 5%	Discontinue medication or reduce dosage
Rash	1–5%	Discontinue medication
Reduced sperm count		Discontinue medication
Serious		
Blood problems	0.5–4.0%	Discontinue medication
Liver toxicity	Rare	Discontinue medication
Allergic reaction	Common if sulfa allergic	Discontinue medication

Leflunamide (Arava)

Generic available: yes

Tablet size: 10, 20 mg

Usual dose: 20 mg tablet daily; daily dose can be decreased to 10 mg if side effects appear

Effective within: one to three months

Leflunamide (as Arava) became available for use in 1998. Unlike many of its predecessors, leflunamide was developed specifically to treat rheumatoid arthritis. Like other DMARDs, leflunamide helps to reduce joint swelling as well as slow the progression of joint damage. It appears to work differently from other available medications in that it affects a particular stage in the process of RA. It is an immune system modifier that interferes with the proliferation (multiplication) of activated lymphocytes. (See sections on inflammation in Chapter 1.)

Studies suggest that leflunamide is an effective DMARD, comparable to methotrexate and sulfasalazine in effectiveness. Leflunamide is approved by the FDA for inhibiting structural damage to the joints as evidenced by x-ray studies. Studies have also demonstrated that leflunamide reduced tenderness and swelling in joints, and patients reported reduced pain levels and less difficulty performing activities of daily living, such as walking and dressing.

Side effects of leflunamide. The most commonly reported side effects associated with leflunamide are diarrhea and other gastrointestinal symptoms, such as bloating, nausea, and abdominal pain (see Table 12). These problems are usually mild and short lived. Some patients experience more serious symptoms, requiring a reduction of dosage or discontinuation of medication. Other side effects include skin rash, reversible hair loss, and elevations of liver enzymes. Cases of severe liver problems have been reported but are uncommon. (These cases have mostly occurred within the first six months of treatment. Many of these patients had other serious conditions or were on other medications that could be toxic to the liver.)

Leflunamide should be used with caution if you are taking other medications that can affect the liver. People with a history of heavy alcohol use, hepatitis, or other severe liver problems should avoid its use. It is recommended that liver function tests be checked monthly during the first six months of usage, and every six to eight weeks thereafter.

Before starting leflunamide therapy, discuss the following with your physician:

- The form of contraception you are using to avoid pregnancy.
- Any medications you are currently taking, but in particular rifampin or cholestyramine.
- Any history of kidney or liver problems.
- Present or past history of excessive alcohol use.
- Any history of serious immune deficiency or uncontrolled infections.

While taking leflunamide:

- Call your doctor if the onset of menstruation is delayed or you suspect pregnancy.
- Contact your physician if you notice yellowing of your skin or eyes or if there is a change in the color of your urine or stool.
- Avoid drinking alcohol.
- Inform your doctor if you develop signs of infection such as fever, chills, cough, burning with urination, or sore throat.
- Contact your physician if you develop a rash, shortness of breath, blood in your urine, or easy bruising.

TABLE 12. Side Effects of Leflunamide

SIDE EFFECTS	INCIDENCE	SIDE EFFECT THERAPY
Nuisance		
Diarrhea	17–27%	Usually goes away; if not, discontinue medication or reduce dosage
Nausea, vomiting, abdominal pain, decreased appetite	3–9%	Take medication with meals; discontinue medication or reduce dosage
Headache, dizziness, numbness	2–7%	Discontinue medication or reduce dosage
Hair loss	9–10%	Discontinue medication or reduce dosage
Rash	4–10%	Discontinue medication or reduce dosage
Serious		
Serious infection	Rare	Treat infection; discontinue medication until infection better
Liver problems	(See text)	Reduce dosage and eliminate alcohol; possibly discontinue medication
Severe allergic reaction	Rare	Discontinue medication and consider drug elimination procedure with cholestyramine

- You may experience diarrhea; contact your doctor if the diarrhea is severe or does not diminish after the first two weeks of treatment.
- Your physician will initially order frequent laboratory tests to rule out potential side effects; in particular, complete blood counts and liver function tests should be monitored. After initial testing, your doctor will set up a schedule for routine blood tests.
- If you miss a dose, do not double your dose the next day; just take routine dose.

Pregnancy, breastfeeding, and fatherhood. Animal testing indicates that leflunamide may result in birth defects if taken by a pregnant woman. Please be certain that you are not pregnant before starting this medication. Your physician may request a pregnancy test for you, to be certain. Reliable birth control measures are imperative while a woman is taking leflunamide. If you wish to become pregnant within two years of taking leflunamide, a drug elimination procedure will be required to remove the drug from your body. This is accomplished with the use of a medication called cholestyramine. This medication is given for 11 days, and then the blood is tested to confirm that leflunamide has been successfully eliminated. The test will then be repeated in another 14 days to be 100 percent certain of complete removal. Without cholestyramine, it takes *up to two years* for the body to remove leflunamide.

If you suspect you are pregnant, stop leflunamide immediately and contact your doctor for a pregnancy test. If you are pregnant, a drug elimination procedure is recommended with the use of cholestyramine. Further counseling from your obstetrician is then recommended. Leflunamide should not be used by nursing mothers.

Although studies on men are limited, men are encouraged to stop treatment with leflunamide if considering a child. A drug elimination procedure with cholestyramine is suggested before attempting insemination.

Minocycline (Minocin)

Generic available: yes
Capsule size: 50, 100 mg
Usual dose: 100 mg twice daily
Effective within: two to four months

Minocycline is an antibiotic in the tetracycline family. Its story as it relates to RA is a very interesting one. For more than fifty years, researchers have been trying to prove that there is an infectious cause or "trigger" for RA. One physician, Thomas McPherson Brown, ardently believed this to be true. Just before World War II, this young researcher isolated a microorganism, mycoplasma, from the joint fluid of a woman with RA. This finding could not be confirmed by other researchers, and so it was discounted by the scientific world. Despite this, Dr. Brown started treating patients with tetracycline-type antibiotics and had good results. He published a report on 98 of his patients in 1985; because his study was not a "double-blind" study, his results were not considered scientifically valid. Dr. Brown wrote a widely circulated book called *The Road Back* describing his unique perspective as an early pioneer in this area (Brown's book is incorporated into Scammell, 1998).

In the past decade, several scientific studies have shown that minocycline *is* a safe and effective treatment for RA. The largest of these trials, called the MIRA trial (for "minocycline in rheumatoid arthritis") was published in 1995 (Tilley et al., 1995). After this report, many physicians began prescribing minocycline for RA. Researchers are not certain whether the antibiotic effect of minocycline is what renders it effective for RA or if some other mechanism of action comes into play. The tetracycline family of antibiotics appears to have other effects on the immune system and on inflammatory proteins that may play a role in RA. There are strong proponents of the "microorganism theory" and the "immunomodulatory theory" for its effectiveness. Minocycline has not been approved by the FDA for use in RA and likely will never be. The studies needed for FDA approval are very costly, and since this medication is available in a generic form, there is no source of funding to perform the necessary testing required for approval (drug manufacturers usually pay for such studies). The drug has been approved for long-term treatment of acne. Its use to treat RA is technically experimental, but because of its widespread use, effectiveness, and safety, this medication has become a commonly prescribed DMARD, particularly in patients with mild, early RA.

Side effects of minocycline. Minocycline has very few side effects compared to other DMARDs (see Table 13). The most common complaint is dizziness. In most cases this is mild, but it can be significant enough to make some patients discontinue use. Other potential side effects are rash and stomach problems. Infrequently, some patients describe changes in skin pigmentation. A bluish discoloration can occur on the skin and inside the mouth. Although the rash is not harmful, most individuals choose to discontinue the medication if it occurs. At times, this bluish discoloration can be seen in the cartilage during surgery. Like other antibiotics, minocycline can cause overgrowth of fungi or yeast in some patients. This is more likely to occur if someone has had a previous history of yeast or *Candida* infections. Increased sensitivity to the sun is a possibility, so persons taking minocycline need to be cautious about intense sun exposure. Rarely, this medication has been associated with the development of lupus-like symptoms.

Before starting minocycline therapy, discuss the following with your physician:

- Any side effects that you have had with antibiotics, particularly the tetracycline family of antibiotics.

- Use of birth control pills, because minocycline may make oral contraceptives less effective.

- Use of warfarin or Coumadin; close observation and dosage adjustment may be required.

- History of serious kidney or liver disease.

- History of yeast infections.

While taking minocycline:

- Contact your physician with any new or unusual symptoms.

TABLE 13. Side Effects of Minocycline

SIDE EFFECTS	INCIDENCE	SIDE EFFECT THERAPY
Nuisance		
Rash	Infrequent	Discontinue medication
Photosensitivity	Occasional	Avoid intense sun; use sun protection
Pigmentation of skin and mucous membranes	Infrequent	Discontinue medication if significant
Lightheadedness, dizziness or vertigo	Occasional	Contact your physician; often self-limiting; may need to discontinue medication
Nausea, diarrhea, decreased appetite	Infrequent	Discontinue if significant
Yeast or *Candida* infections	Infrequent	Treat yeast infection; may need to discontinue if severe or recurrent infection
Serious		
Severe dizziness and headache	Rare	Discontinue medication
Abnormal liver tests; hepatitis	Rare	Discontinue medication
Severe allergic reaction	Rare	Discontinue medication
Decreased hearing	Rare	Discontinue medication
Blood abnormalities	Rare	Discontinue medication
Lupus-like condition	Rare	Discontinue medication

- Avoid taking this medication at the same time as antacids, calcium, magnesium, or iron, since they may interfere with absorption of minocycline.

- Be careful to avoid high-intensity sun exposure and tanning beds; use sun blockers and protective clothing.

- If you experience dizziness while on minocycline, avoid driving vehicles or using hazardous machinery; contact your physician if dizziness is severe.

- Temporarily stop minocycline if you are on another antibiotic for an infection, since the antibiotics may compete with each other.

Pregnancy and breastfeeding. Minocycline can cause fetal harm when taken by a pregnant woman. The use of minocycline during fetal tooth development (latter half of pregnancy) may cause permanent discoloration of the teeth. Minocycline is excreted in breast milk. Nursing infants would be at risk for permanent tooth discoloration.

IMMUNOSUPPRESSANTS

Methotrexate (Rheumatrex, Trexall, Otrexup)

Generic available: yes for 2.5 mg tablet
Tablet size: 2.5 mg (most common); Trexall: 5, 7.5, 10, 15 mg
Autoinjector size (Otrexup): 10, 15, 20, 25 mg
Usual dose: two to eight (2.5 mg) pills per week all on one day,
    or one weekly injection
Effective within: four to eight weeks

Methotrexate was used initially in the 1940s to treat people with leukemia and is still frequently taken in very high doses as an anticancer drug. It later became widely used as a treatment for severe psoriasis and a form of arthritis associated with that skin condition. Since the early 1980s, its use in the treatment of RA has skyrocketed, and it is still the most commonly prescribed oral DMARD.

The continued popularity of methotrexate for RA treatment has many explanations. First, it becomes effective more rapidly than the traditional DMARDs: improvement is sometimes noted within four weeks of the first use. Second, it is very effective. Third, it is very convenient in that it can be taken once a week. Fourth, it is often used successfully in combination with the biologic DMARDs.

Side effects of methotrexate. Like the other immunosuppressants, methotrexate can produce side effects (see Table 14). The most commonly reported ones involve stomach problems and mouth sores. Nausea, vomiting, and diarrhea can usually be minimized by dividing up the weekly dose; that is, taking the weekly dose of pills one pill every several hours (if your dose is three pills per week, for example, you would take one pill every eight hours on the day of your treatment). The dose should not be divided throughout the week, however; it needs to be taken over the course of a single day. Your doctor will help you with a schedule that is tolerable for you. Other ways to avoid stomach problems include taking the medication with food, adjusting the dose, and taking antinausea medications. Some people tolerate methotrexate better when it is taken by shot than by pill. Injections can be administered weekly in your doctor's office. However, most patients choose to self-administer shots of methotrexate at home, if they can master the proper and safe technique. Home injections are usually given **subcutaneously** ("sub Q"), that is, just under the skin. Autoinjectors are now available as well.

The side effect of methotrexate that most frequently causes concern involves the liver. In people taking methotrexate, blood tests that measure liver enzymes are frequently elevated slightly, but this is rarely an indication of a serious liver problem. With long-term use, however, inflammation and scarring of the liver can take place. Although cirrhosis of the liver is a distinctly rare side effect, some people with psoriatic arthritis have developed cirrhosis of the liver from methotrexate. Scarring and cirrhosis appear to be much less common in rheumatoid arthritis patients. The risk of liver problems can be minimized greatly if the person avoids alcohol and keeps his or her weight down. After several years of methotrexate use, a liver biopsy may be indicated, particularly if liver function test abnormalities appear and persist.

Blood counts (white and red blood cells and platelets) can be lowered by methotrexate use. At the dose used to treat RA, this side effect is unusual. When it occurs, it is almost always reversible by discontinuing the use or reducing the dose of the drug. Reduced platelet counts increase bleeding risks in some people. When the white blood cell count is markedly lowered, serious infections can occur; much more rarely, unusual, "atypical," infections develop even though white blood counts may be at *normal* levels. These infections can develop because of methotrexate's effect on the immune system.

Another rare but serious side effect is lung inflammation, or pneumonitis. This inflammation is generally reversible with discontinuation of methotrexate

TABLE 14. Side Effects of Methotrexate

SIDE EFFECTS	INCIDENCE	SIDE EFFECT THERAPY
Nuisance		
Rash	1–11%	Discontinue medication or reduce dosage
Stomach problems		
Nausea	10–23%	Take medication with meals,
Vomiting	4%	adjust dosage, or take nausea medication
Diarrhea	8%	Take medication with meals
Mouth sores	3–10%	Reduce dosage or take folate or folinic acid
Headache	9%	Reduce dosage
Hair loss or thinning	1–5%	Reduce dosage
Dizziness	2%	Reduce dosage
Increase in nodules	Unknown	Possible benefit from hydroxychloroquine
Serious		
Liver problems	15%	Reduce dosage, eliminate alcohol, and reduce weight; possibly discontinue medication
Blood problems	1–10%	Reduce dosage or discontinue medication
Lung inflammation	2–5.5%	Discontinue medication and take corticosteroids
Stomach ulcers	Rare	Discontinue medication and take stomach medication
Infection	3.8%	Treat infection and discontinue medication

and treatment with **corticosteroids.** Pneumonitis can, on rare occasions, be life threatening. Smoking appears to increase the risk.

Studies suggest that taking daily folic acid (or folate) supplements decreases the side effects of methotrexate. Some physicians also prescribe folinic acid before each methotrexate dose if side effects are significant.

Before starting methotrexate therapy, discuss the following with your physician:

- A history of liver problems (especially hepatitis), stomach ulcer, alcohol use, kidney or lung problems, blood problems, human immunodeficiency virus (HIV) infection, or a positive tuberculin skin test or tuberculosis.

- Any medications you are currently taking, but particularly sulfa drugs, other antibiotics (particularly those containing trimethaprim), NSAIDs, diuretics (water pills), probenecid (gout medication), and medications to treat seizures or diabetes.

While taking methotrexate:

- Contact your physician promptly if you have mouth sores, nausea or vomiting, black or tar-colored stools, fever or chills, sore throat, unusual bleeding or bruising, a change in skin or urine color, cough or shortness of breath, or a marked increase in fatigue.

- Inform your doctor if you contract an infection; methotrexate is often temporarily discontinued to help a patient's immune system fight an infection.

- Inform your physician, surgeon, or dentist that you are taking methotrexate *well before* he or she performs any medical procedure.

- Ask your physician before you receive any "live" vaccines; flu and pneumonia vaccinations are generally recommended.

- *Never* take this medication more than one day a week.

- Alcohol ingestion is prohibited.

- Take *every* precaution to avoid pregnancy (see below).

- Frequent liver function tests and blood tests to obtain complete blood counts are required. Blood tests for kidney function and urine studies may be requested periodically by your physician.

Pregnancy and breastfeeding. Methotrexate is an extremely dangerous medication for the fetus. It has been known to cause fetal death and birth defects. Women should avoid getting pregnant for *at least* one full menstrual cycle after stopping methotrexate. Men should wait *at least* three months after discontinuing methotrexate treatment before trying to father children. Do not breastfeed while taking methotrexate.

Azathioprine (Imuran, Azasan)

Generic available: yes (for 50 mg)
Tablet size: 50, 75, 100 mg
Usual dose: variable
Effective within: six weeks to six months

Azathioprine was initially introduced as a form of cancer chemotherapy and is still being used for that purpose. It is also used to prevent rejection in organ transplant recipients. It was the first immunosuppressant to be approved by the FDA for treatment of rheumatoid arthritis and has been shown to be effective. Many physicians prefer to reserve this therapy for patients who have not responded to treatment with other DMARDs. Azathioprine is a notable component in many combination drug therapies.

Side effects of azathioprine. The negative side effects of azathioprine are listed in Table 15. The side effect of most concern is blood abnormalities, especially a lowered white blood cell count (Table 15). Infection can result and can become severe when insufficient numbers of white blood cells are present to destroy infection-causing bacteria. As with other immunosuppressants, there is also an increased risk of unusual infections, even without a change in the white blood cell count. Less common blood abnormalities include decreased numbers of platelets or of red blood cells (resulting in **anemia**). With low numbers of platelets, bruising or bleeding may occur more easily. Blood abnormalities almost always improve when azathioprine is discontinued. Life-threatening situations are rare. Any person taking azathioprine *must* be monitored vigilantly by a physician who is an expert in immunosuppressant therapy.

Another side effect that has received a great deal of attention is the risk of developing cancer after prolonged use of azathioprine. This issue is debated in rheumatology circles. Findings from studies of large numbers of RA patients taking azathioprine in the United Kingdom are reassuring. Those studies suggest that the additional risk of cancer in people taking azathioprine as compared with others with RA, exists but is actually quite small.

Before starting azathioprine therapy, discuss the following with your physician:

- A history of blood problems, liver or kidney disease, HIV infection, or a positive tuberculin skin test or tuberculosis.

- All medications that you are taking, but in particular allopurinol (gout medicine) and angiotensin converting enzyme (ACE) inhibitors (a blood pressure medicine).

While you are taking azathioprine:

- Contact your physician promptly if you have fever or chills, sore throat, cough, unusual bruising or bleeding, a marked increase in fatigue, nausea or stomach pain, or a change in urine or skin color.

- Inform your doctor if you have an infection; azathioprine is often discontinued on a temporary basis to help the patient's immune system combat an infection.

- Ask your doctor before you receive any "live" vaccines; flu and pneumonia vaccinations are generally recommended.

- Take your medication with meals.

TABLE 15. Side Effects of Azathioprine

SIDE EFFECTS	INCIDENCE	SIDE EFFECT THERAPY
Nuisance		
Nausea, vomiting, diarrhea	12–16%	Take medication with meals or divide dosage
Rash	2%	Discontinue medication or reduce dosage
Mouth sores	Rare	Reduce dosage
Hair loss	Rare	Reduce dosage or discontinue medication
Serious		
Infection	1–3%	Take antibiotics and discontinue medication
Liver problems	Rare	Discontinue medication
Blood problems	28%	Reduce dosage or discontinue medication
Cancer risks	(See text)	(See text)
Pancreatitis	Rare	Discontinue medication

- *Never* take a dose higher than the doctor has prescribed.
- Try to avoid close contact with anyone who has a bacterial or viral infection.
- Frequent blood tests for blood cell counts and to check liver function are required.

Pregnancy and breastfeeding. Because problems can develop in the fetal immune system when the mother takes azathioprine, this medication should not be used during pregnancy, nor should it be taken if the mother is nursing.

Cyclophosphamide (Cytoxan)

Generic available: yes
Tablet size: 25, 50 mg
Intravenous administration possible
Dose: variable
Effective within: two weeks to three months

Cyclophosphamide is by far the most potent and dangerous of the oral immunosuppressive drugs used in the treatment of RA. Like azathioprine, it was first used as a form of cancer chemotherapy. Its effectiveness in the treatment of rheumatoid arthritis is undisputed, but its potentially severe side effects preclude its use in the treatment of mild or moderate RA. Cyclophosphamide is generally reserved for the treatment of unusually severe cases or those with life-threatening complications, such as **vasculitis, Felty's syndrome,** and other rare complications with organ involvement (see Chapter 4 for more about such complications). In these very serious situations, the benefits of cyclophosphamide outweigh the risks.

Side effects of cyclophosphamide. Cyclophosphamide has essentially the same potential side effects as azathioprine (see above and Table 16). Because cyclophosphamide has a more potent effect on the bone marrow and immune system than azathioprine does, the occurrence and severity of these side effects are higher in people taking cyclophosphamide, although the precise risk is difficult to ascertain. We do know that a low white blood cell count occurs so frequently during cyclophosphamide therapy that it is considered an *expected effect* rather than a side effect. The risk of severe blood abnormalities and infection increases in proportion to the dose and length of time over which cyclophosphamide is taken.

TABLE 16. Side Effects of Cyclophosphamide

SIDE EFFECTS	INCIDENCE	SIDE EFFECT THERAPY
Nuisance		
Nausea, vomiting, decreased appetite	Common	Take nausea medication
Rash	Less than 5%	Discontinue medication or reduce dosage
Hair loss	Common[a]	Reduce dosage if possible
Serious		
Blood problems	(See text)[a]	Discontinue medication or reduce dosage
Bladder problems	17%	Discontinue medication and drink ample fluid to facilitate frequent urination
Infection	(See text)[a]	Treat infection and discontinue medication if possible
Cancer risks	(See text)[a]	Treat cancer
Liver problems	Rare	Discontinue medication
Lung problems	Rare	Discontinue medication
Infertility	Common[a]	No treatment known

[a] Frequency depends on dose and length of time medication is taken.

Unlike azathioprine, cyclophosphamide can cause *cystitis*, bladder inflammation. Uncomfortable urination and the appearance of blood in the urine are symptoms of cystitis.

Hair loss can occur, particularly at very high doses. The amount of hair loss is highly variable, but in almost all patients the hair regrows after the treatment is discontinued.

An important concern in cyclophosphamide therapy is the long-term increased risk of bladder cancer or blood cancers (leukemias and lymphomas). It is estimated that with long-term daily cyclophosphamide use the risk of developing these cancers nearly doubles. Because cyclophosphamide is prescribed almost exclusively for severe, unremitting RA or for life-threatening complications, this potential risk of cancer in the future is usually regarded, by patients and physicians, as a tolerable risk.

Before starting cyclophosphamide therapy, discuss the following with your physician:

- A history of blood problems, kidney or liver conditions, HIV infection, previous x-ray therapy or chemotherapy, or a positive tuberculin skin test or tuberculosis.

- Any medications you are taking, but in particular sleeping medications (barbiturates), diuretics (water pills), or gout medications (such as allopurinol).

While taking cyclophosphamide:

- Contact your physician promptly if you have fever or chills, sore throat, cough, unusual bleeding or bruising, a change in urine color, burning or pain with urination, a change in skin color, or a marked increase in fatigue.

- Contact your physician at any sign of infection; cyclophosphamide is often discontinued on a temporary basis to help a patient's immune system combat an infection.

- Ask your doctor before you receive any "live" vaccines; flu and pneumonia vaccinations are generally recommended.

- Monitor your urination while you are taking cyclophosphamide. Make certain that the frequency of urination has not decreased. Drink large amounts of water each day to flush out your bladder.

- Never take this medication at bedtime.

- Avoid close contact with anyone who has a viral or bacterial infection.

Pregnancy and breastfeeding. Both men and women must use contraception while taking cyclophosphamide. *Birth defects are a distinct possibility should a pregnancy occur during this therapy.* Decreased fertility and sterility are potential side effects of this medication. Nursing is not recommended.

Cyclosporine (Neoral, Gengraf)

Generic available: yes
Capsule size: 25, 100 mg
Liquid form: oral solution 100 mg/ml
Usual dose: varies with weight; usually taken twice per day
Effective within: four to eight weeks

When a single DMARD is not effective, your physician may choose to begin combination therapy, using more than one medication, and that is how cyclosporine is most often prescribed in the United States. Cyclosporine plus methotrexate has been recommended for patients with severe active RA that is not responding to methotrexate alone. This combination treatment for RA was approved by the FDA in the late 1990s.

Cyclosporine is a powerful immunosuppressant that has been approved for use in the United States since the early 1980s for people who have undergone organ transplantation. It helps keep the immune system from rejecting the newly transplanted organ.

Because of its effect on the immune system, cyclosporine has also been shown to benefit patients with RA. Although sometimes prescribed alone for RA, cyclosporine is most commonly prescribed with methotrexate. The FDA has not approved its use singly as a DMARD. In research studies, patients with severe rheumatoid arthritis who had partially responded to methotrexate alone had meaningful improvement with the combination of methotrexate and cyclosporine. These patients experienced a reduction of tenderness and swelling in their joints. Also, pain and degree of disability were reduced. Because of potential side effects, the lowest effective dose should be used. If adverse effects do occur, the dose should be further reduced. Cyclosporine should be discontinued if there is no additional benefit after 16 weeks or if dose reduction does not eliminate side effects.

Side effects of cyclosporine. Side effects that may occur with the use of cyclosporine include high blood pressure and kidney problems (see Table 17). The physician will likely check blood pressure and order kidney function tests frequently when a patient is starting with this medication. In clinical research trials, cyclosporine had to be discontinued in 5.3 percent of patients because of high blood pressure and in 7 percent of patients because of abnormal kidney tests (elevated creatinine). These serious side effects usually resolve after discontinuing the medication. Other potential problems include headache, stomach problems, and abnormal hair growth. As with other immunosuppressants, patients must be watched closely for possible infections. If you are on methotrexate as well, monthly blood counts and liver tests are recommended in order to detect potential side effects early (see section on methotrexate). Only physicians experienced in management of immunosuppressive therapy for RA should prescribe cyclosporine and methotrexate in combination.

TABLE 17. Side Effects of Cyclosporine

SIDE EFFECTS	INCIDENCE	SIDE EFFECT THERAPY
Nuisance		
Tremor	7–13%	Reduce dosage or discontinue medication
Headache	17–25%	Reduce dosage or discontinue medication
Dizziness	6–8%	Reduce dosage or discontinue medication
Burning or tingling sensations	7–11%	Reduce dosage or discontinue medication
Rash	7–12%	Reduce dosage or discontinue medication
Increased body hair	15–19%	Reduce dosage or discontinue medication
Nausea, diarrhea, upset stomach	15–24%	Reduce dosage or discontinue medication
Leg cramps	2–12%	Reduce dosage or discontinue medication
Reduced kidney function (by >30%)	39–48%	Reduce dosage or discontinue medication
Serious		
High blood pressure	8–26%	Reduce dosage or discontinue medication
Fluid retention	5–14%	Reduce dosage or discontinue medication
Reduced kidney function (by >50%)	18–24%	Reduce dosage or discontinue medication
Upper respiratory complications	3–14%	Reduce dosage or discontinue medication
Cancer (lymphoma)	Rare	Discontinue medication

Before starting cyclosporine therapy, discuss the following with your physician:

- Any history of kidney problems or high blood pressure.
- All current medications, because drug interactions are common.
- Any history of immune deficiency or severe infections.
- Any history of tuberculosis or a positive tuberculin skin test.

While taking cyclosporine:

- Contact your doctor immediately with any signs of fever, chills, sinus pain, severe headache, cough, shortness of breath, pain or burning with urination, bleeding gums, or severe bruising.

- Contact your physician if you have an infection; he or she may want to discontinue the cyclosporine temporarily to help your immune system fight infection.

- You will need frequent monitoring of blood pressure, complete blood count, kidney function tests, and liver enzyme checks. Blood lipids, magnesium, potassium, and cyclosporine concentration may also require monitoring.

- Do *not* get any "live" vaccines; ask your doctor about any vaccines; flu and pneumonia vaccination are generally recommended.

- Alert your prescribing physician about *all* new medications (even over-the-counter ones) but, in particular, antibiotics, anti-inflammatory, stomach, blood pressure, heart, or seizure medications.

Pregnancy and breastfeeding. There are no adequate studies of cyclosporine in pregnant women. Discontinuation of cyclosporine in non-life-threatening conditions is recommended. Cyclosporine is excreted in breast milk and should be avoided during breastfeeding.

Biotherapies: Biologics, Kinase Inhibitors, and a Biologic Medical Device

UNDERSTANDING CYTOKINES AND INFLAMMATION

Before reading this chapter, you may want to reread Chapter 1, which explains the disease process in rheumatoid arthritis and defines some RA terminology. Scientists are getting closer to understanding the very complex nature of rheumatoid arthritis. Researchers are discovering critical changes that occur in the immune system in people with RA. As these key elements are discovered, each piece of the puzzle gives us a new opportunity to target treatment. We use the word *target* because that is exactly what this next class of medications does.

Starting in the late 1990s, a new form of treatment was developed that revolutionized the treatment of RA. Each member of this category of medication focuses on a very small part of the complicated cascade of events that create and perpetuate RA. These medications are biologic agents, more commonly called *biologics*; later in this chapter, we will review the biologics that are currently available. Understanding this complex area is not easy, even for physicians. The following information is meant to give the reader a basic understanding of how current biologics function. We will also be reviewing the newest group of oral medications, called the **kinase inhibitors.** Although the kinase inhibitors are *not* biologics by definition, they are very similar to biologics in many ways. Because of these similarities, they are presented in this chapter rather than with the other oral disease-modifying antirheumatic drugs (**DMARDs**).

Biologics are bioengineered proteins designed to interfere with the cascade of events that leads to inflammation and damage. (See Figure 4 for a schematic of the RA cascade.) Before you can understand how the biologics work, it is important to understand some of the fundamental changes in the immune system that occur with rheumatoid inflammation, which is a malfunction of a normal process.

The normal immune system relies upon various types of immune cells and the communication that occurs between them. Chemical messengers called **cytokines** enable the communication between immune cells. Cytokines communicate their message by attaching to *receptors* on the cells intended to receive the message. When the messenger (cytokine) connects to the receiving cell's receptor, the message is delivered. When a cytokine's message is "promote inflammation," the attachment of that "pro-inflammatory" cytokine to its receptor "turns on" the receiving immune system cell (see Figure 18). Once activated, the receiving cell releases chemicals that lead to inflammation; allowed to continue too long, the inflammation will cause damage. RA inflammation is caused by a complex array of many cell-to-cell communications among immune cell types relying on several different cytokines. When the inflammation message is started, it spreads like a ripple to multiple kinds of immune cells, each delivering different cytokine messages to the next immune cell. This chain of communications results in inflammation in several areas of the body. Interrupting this domino-like pathway to inflammation is the goal of the biologics.

Since the creation of the biologics, our RA treatment strategies fall into two broad categories:

1. Cytokine-based therapies

   • Treatment aimed at preventing the pro-inflammatory cytokine from delivering its inflammatory message

   • Cytokines whose inflammatory message gets disrupted by currently available biologics include TNF (tumor necrosis factor), IL-1 (Interleukin-1), and IL-6 (Interleukin-6)

2. Immune cell–based therapies

   • Treatment directed at subduing the activity of overactive immune cells

   • Cells whose immunologic activity is altered by currently available biologics include T cells and B cells

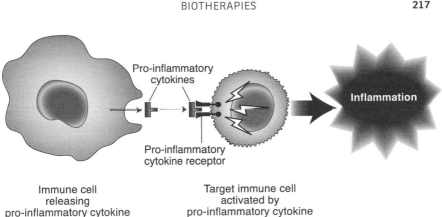

Pro-inflammatory
cytokines

Inflammation

Pro-inflammatory
cytokine receptor

Immune cell
releasing
pro-inflammatory cytokine

Target immune cell
activated by
pro-inflammatory cytokine

FIGURE 18. Pro-inflammatory cytokines

Using the Body's Secrets to Tame Inflammation: Balancing the Cytokines

There are many cytokines in the rheumatoid cascade that have been targeted for clinical research. Three of these cytokines have been proven to have a major role in the inflammation pathway in RA and have currently available biologics directed against them. These cytokines are tumor necrosis factor (TNF), interleukin-1 (IL-1), and interleukin-6 (IL-6). To balance these pro-inflammatory cytokines in normal inflammation there are naturally occurring proteins made by the body that decrease inflammation by overpowering the pro-inflammatory messengers. The pro-inflammatory cytokines are not in themselves bad; they appear to have an important role in helping the immune system function properly. While pro-inflammatory cytokines like TNF, IL-1, and IL-6 seem to have important *beneficial* functions in the body under normal circumstances, in RA their concentrations are abnormally high. *Completely* eliminating these pro-inflammatory cytokines is not the goal of treatment; putting them back in balance is.

Naturally occurring anti-inflammatory proteins represent the body's built-in mechanism for balancing increased numbers of pro-inflammatory cytokines. One type of these proteins works by preventing the pro-inflammatory cytokine from hooking up to its receptor and delivering its message to the receiving immune cell. These blocking agents are called *receptor antagonists*. These naturally occurring *cytokine receptor blockers* work by plugging up the receptor so it cannot receive the inflammation message delivered by the pro-inflammatory cytokine (see Figure 19). Some biologics work by mimicking this type of anti-inflammatory protein. One such medication is the biologic anakinra (Kineret). Kineret is a man-made receptor antagonist that disables the IL-1 cytokine by preventing IL-1 from delivering its inflammation message.

The body also makes protective *free-floating receptors* that are *not* bound to cells. They can intercept the pro-inflammatory cytokines and knock them out of commission. These are called *soluble receptors*. These protective proteins intuitively increase in the body when there is a need to control inflammation. In essence, these naturally occurring *cytokine blockers* snatch up the cytokine, so it doesn't get to the target cell's receptor to deliver its inflammation message (see Figure 20). An example of how we mimic this type of protein is a medica-

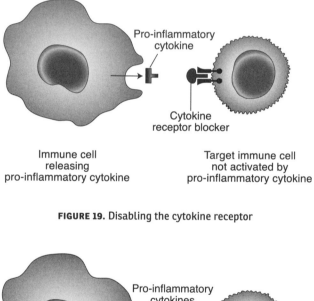

Pro-inflammatory
cytokine

Cytokine
receptor blocker

Immune cell
releasing
pro-inflammatory cytokine

Target immune cell
not activated by
pro-inflammatory cytokine

FIGURE 19. Disabling the cytokine receptor

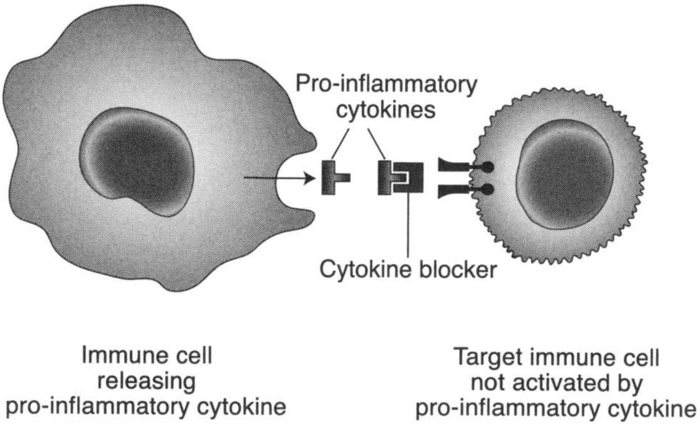

Pro-inflammatory
cytokines

Cytokine blocker

Immune cell
releasing
pro-inflammatory cytokine

Target immune cell
not activated by
pro-inflammatory cytokine

FIGURE 20. Disabling the cytokine

tion called etanercept (Enbrel). Enbrel is a biogenetically engineered soluble receptor that captures TNF before it can connect to its receptor and deliver its inflammation message. Enbrel is sometimes called a "decoy" protein because it fools the pro-inflammatory cytokine into connecting to it, leaving the cytokine unable to go on to the real receptor on the receiving immune cell.

In addition to copying the body's built-in defenders against inflammation, unique biologic agents are being designed that perform similar processes. One prominent example of this is the assembling of man-made antibodies called *monoclonal antibodies*. Although not found naturally in the body, these "designer" molecules are created to attach to and disable a chosen target. Many of the RA biologic medicines are bioengineered monoclonal antibodies designed to render pro-inflammatory cytokines inoperative. These unique antibodies are very specific and are designed to disable either a specific cytokine (as in Figure 20) or its cytokine receptor (as in Figure 19). Monoclonal antibodies that disable a cytokine include the TNF blockers: infliximab (Remicade), adalimumab (Humira), golimumab (Simponi), and certolizumab pegol (Cimzia). Monoclonal antibodies designed to disable a cytokine receptor include the IL-6 blocker tocilizumab (Actemra). These agents are listed in Table 18 and are described individually below.

TABLE 18. Treatments to Reduce or Block Pro-inflammatory Cytokines

PRO-INFLAMMATORY CYTOKINE	TYPE OF BLOCKER	AVAILABILITY
Tumor necrosis factor (TNF)	TNF soluble receptor	Enbrel (etanercept)—1998
	Monoclonal antibody against TNF	Remicade (infliximab)—1999 Humira (adalimumab)—2003 Simponi (golimumab)—2009 Simponi Aria (golimumab)—2013
	Antibody fragment against TNF	Cimzia (certolizumab pegol)— 2008/2009[a]
Interleukin-1 (IL-1)	IL-1 receptor antagonist	Kineret (anakinra)—2001
Interleukin-6 (IL-6)	Monoclonal antibody against IL-6 receptor	Actemra (tocilizumab)—2010/2013[b]

[a] Approved first for Crohn's disease, then RA.
[b] Approved first for infusion, then self-injection.

Thus, our *current* strategies for balancing inflammation via cytokine manipulation fall into two basic categories. The first strategy is to knock the inflammatory cytokine itself out of commission. The second is to disable the receptor on the immune cells so that it cannot bind to the cytokine and receive its inflammatory message.

Redirecting the Message Makers: Calming the B Cell and T Cell

The biologic strategies discussed so far are aimed at disruption of the delivery of the cytokine inflammation message from one immune cell to the next. A different biologic strategy is directed at immune cells involved in creating the inflammation message in the first place. There are many immune cells involved in the inflammatory process, but two are particularly important in RA: the B cell and the T cell. Both of these immune cells fall into the category of cells called **lymphocytes.** Each of these cells has a pivotal role in creating and directing the production of inflammatory messages. Treatments in this strategy are intended to "calm down" these cells but *not* to eliminate their function completely. This form of treatment is called immune cell "modulation," and the medications are called T cell and B cell *modulators.* They are listed in Table 19, and specific details about them are given below.

THE BIOLOGICS: PRACTICAL CONSIDERATIONS

The introduction of the biologics in the late 1990s forever changed the way we look at treating rheumatoid arthritis. The immense effectiveness of these agents has made it possible to expect extraordinary results in even the toughest cases of RA. In the years since their introduction, we have seen a considerable reduction in surgeries, hospitalizations, disabling consequences, and premature death related to uncontrolled RA. These therapies have raised the bar for our treatment expectations. With the biologics, a vast majority of people with RA can expect to live very full and functional lives.

With any treatment, there are always risks and other considerations. Given the complexity of these drugs, their use comes with more technical particulars and general precautions than do traditional medications. Notably, most **DMARDs** are taken by mouth; because biologics are proteins, they need to be given either by intravenous (IV) infusion or **subcutaneous** injection (more de-

TABLE 19. Treatments That Modulate Immune Cells

IMMUNE CELLS	TYPE OF MODULATOR	AVAILABILITY
T cell	T cell selective co-stimulation modulator	Orencia—2005/2011[a]
B cell	Monoclonal antibody against B cell	Rituxan—2006
Immune cells	JAK kinase inhibitor[b]	Xeljanz—2012

[a] Approved first for infusion, then self injection.
[b] Not in the biologic family; see text.

tails about these two methods of administration below). In the realm of molecules, proteins are considered to be very large, and as such they cannot be absorbed intact by our digestive systems. If taken by mouth, the protein-based biologic would be broken down by stomach enzymes and not be effective.

Subcutaneous Injections: Can I Give Myself the Shot?

Many of the biologics are given by self-injection. When a medication is given as an injection just beneath the skin, it is called a subcutaneous or "sub-Q" injection. Many people are initially frightened to give themselves an injection. Almost everyone, however, learns, under the guidance of their physician or nurse, to self-inject biologics without too much difficulty. It is important to receive training by a health care provider on the right way to prepare for and give injections, so don't attempt it on your own, and don't decline instruction assuming you can figure it out on your own. Some biologics are available with auto-injectors, which are invaluable in helping needle-shy individuals self-inject, since you never have to see the needle. The area of injection is "rotated" from site to site (thigh, abdomen, and arm) so that no one area gets too tender.

Injection-site reactions can include pain, redness, and swelling of the skin. Most of these reactions are temporary and decrease over time with most biologics. Applying a cold pack to the site immediately after injection can decrease reactions. Discuss injection-site itching with your doctor, since this could be an early sign of an allergic reaction. Do not inject into any area that is sore, bruised, red, itchy, scaly, or hard. Try to avoid scars, stretch marks, and visible veins. If shots are painful, try different injection locations, such as the stomach. Make certain that the alcohol you apply to the skin to prepare the injection site has dried before injecting, to prevent stinging. Removing the syringe or auto-injector from the refrigerator 30 to 60 minutes before injection allows the medicine to reach room temperature, which reduces discomfort. Do not attempt to speed up the warming process in any way or leave the medication out longer than an hour. Usually, with some adjustment in technique, injections are well tolerated. For sensitive people, placing a cold pack on the skin before injections is very helpful.

It is best to have a friend or another person in the household also learn to give the injections. Then, if the arthritis in your hands has made them too sore for precise work, this care partner can help you. He or she can also inject areas that you cannot reach, if that is needed. Of course, your physician and his or her staff will always be there if problems with self-administration develop.

Being proteins, biologics need to be refrigerated at 36° to 46° F (these medications must not freeze). If something has kept your medication from staying cool for an extended period of time, call the manufacturer to determine if it is still safe to use. If you are traveling, an insulated bag or cooler will be required to keep the biologic at the correct temperature. Many pharmacies sell such insulated carriers for this purpose. You should be allowed to carry your medication with you on an airplane in an insulated bag or case. I tell my patients to ask that the medications *not* go through the x-ray scanner, although no tests have been done to determine if x-raying is harmful to the medication. To be safe, I provide my patients with a note to say that they are on a medication that is injectable and needs to avoid x-ray exposure. This note usually avoids unnecessary hold ups. Do not put your medication in your checked luggage; carry it on with you. For safety, needles, syringes, and auto-injectors (called "sharps") must be disposed of in a puncture-resistant container out of the reach of children. Do *not* throw used syringes or auto-injectors into regular trash or recycle bins. Ask your doctor or nurse how you should dispose of the container in your community. In addition, many of the manufacturers of subcutaneous biologics offer programs for "sharps" disposal.

Intravenous Infusions: What to Expect

Some biologics are given by intravenous (IV) infusion. Some physicians give IV biologics in their office. Others prefer that you receive the medication at an infusion center or hospital. Infusion involves placing a needle into one of your veins, usually in the arm, and taping it in place so it doesn't move around. The medication is then fed into the vein slowly through sterile tubing. During the infusion a nurse will monitor you. This is often a good time to read a book, listen to music, or get some well-deserved relaxation. Most infusions are uneventful. However, you will be monitored closely for "infusion reactions." Most reactions are mild and include symptoms like flushing or chills. Often, the problem is solved by slowing down the infusion rate, that is, letting less medication per minute enter the vein. Sometimes, pretreatment with other medications will be necessary to decrease infusion reactions. Fortunately, severe infusion reactions are rare; they can include hives, difficulty breathing, chest pain, low or high blood pressure, swelling of the face or hands, or a severe allergic reaction called anaphylaxis. Infusion centers are very capable of taking care of patients in the event of one of these unusual reactions. It is most important to tell the infusion nurse of any new symptoms that you are experiencing during or after your infusion.

Cost Issues

The biologics are all very expensive, which can present a serious obstacle for many people. Your insurance company may require a "prior authorization," "precertification," or "letter of medical necessity" from your prescribing physician. Biologics that are given by sub-Q injections are generally subject to your medical insurance prescription policy and considered a "pharmacy benefit." Biologics given by IV are generally treated differently than other prescriptions by most insurance plans. They are often considered a "major medical" benefit rather than a "pharmacy benefit." For instance, under some Medicare plans, intravenous infusions are covered under Medicare B whereas subcutaneous injections are covered under Medicare D. This can often mean considerable differences in the co-pays, deductibles, and "out-of-pocket maximum" for these treatments, depending on how the medication is given. If biologics are being considered, call your insurance company to inquire about specific requirements before you start the medication. I also tell my patients to ask this very specific question: "What will be the maximum yearly out-of-pocket expense for this type medication?" Then compare the yearly maximum costs for an IV-administered biologic with the yearly maximum costs for a subcutaneously administered biologic.

Many of the manufacturers of biologics have co-pay assistance programs. These can make a major difference in affording biologic treatment. Unfortunately, because of federal guidelines, the pharmaceutical or biotechnology companies are not allowed to offer these programs to people with Medicare or any other federally funded insurance plan. In these circumstances, there are private, independent foundations that work with the companies to offer help. However, funding from these foundations can be limited. Contact information for financial help with individual medications is listed at the end of this chapter. Also listed are several resources that may be able to direct you to other potential sources of financial assistance.

In the near future, we may see *some* cost break in the biologic drugs. Many companies are studying a new group of biologics called **biosimilars.** They are like *generic* drugs in that they will be less expensive versions of brand-name biologic drugs. Unlike small-molecule oral drugs, branded biologics are incredibly complex, large protein molecules that cannot be duplicated exactly. Since these copy products are similar but not *identical* in their structure to the branded biologics, they are termed biosimilars. Many biosimilars are being tested in clinical studies at this time. These medications will still be very expensive, but there are predictions that they will cost 10–25 percent less than branded biologics.

Which Biologic Should I Take?

Just as every person is different, every biologic medication brings with it a different set of benefits and risks. This is one of the times when a trusted relationship with your rheumatologist comes into play. Your doctor will talk to you about the options available to you given your medical history, the circumstances in your community, and, alas, the requirements of your insurance company. Reading this chapter in its entirety will familiarize you with the potential options and enable you to ask your doctor pertinent questions. You may need to read the chapter several times to understand all its complex information. There is so much information to take in and think about.

Risk of Infection: The Most Serious of Biologic Side Effects

Biologics have dramatically changed the outlook for people with RA in a very positive way. As you read about these medications, you will likely feel a little afraid. You may even think that taking a biologic is not worth the risk. Please know that for the vast majority of people, the use of biologic medications offers life-altering improvement with a small risk of serious side effects. We also know that the introduction of these drugs has actually *reduced* the most serious risks associated with RA: the risk of hospitalizations, disability, joint replacement surgery, and premature death.

There is one area of risk, however, that deserves special attention, and that is the risk of infection. By lowering the body's infection-fighting capacity, these drugs make it easier to catch an infection and, more importantly, harder to fight it off. Being vigilant for the warning signs of infection makes a very big difference in the risk of serious problems. If you are taking a biologic and get an open sore or develop symptoms like fever, chills, cough, burning with urination, or any other evidence of infection, stop the biologic immediately and call your doctor. Stopping the biologic temporarily and treating the infection promptly will ward off most serious consequences of infection. Always lean in the direction of over-cautiousness regarding infection. Don't be shy about reminding your other doctors that you are on medications that affect your immune system. Your rheumatologist will be very aware of your risks and will not need this reminder, but other physicians involved with your care may not be as well versed in the nature of these medications, given the rapidly expanding number of new treatments that are being used for RA. So, a respectful reminder will always be appreciated.

BIOLOGIC AGENTS AGAINST TUMOR NECROSIS FACTOR: THE TNF BLOCKERS

As mentioned above, cytokines, such as tumor necrosis factor, can increase inflammation. Although a small amount of TNF is necessary for the immune system to function normally, this cytokine is found in very high amounts in rheumatoid joints. High levels of TNF are believed to contribute to the pain, swelling, stiffness, and fatigue of rheumatoid arthritis. Currently available TNF-blocking drugs mimic the function of the naturally occurring soluble TNF receptors (as seen in Figure 20). Like their natural protein counterparts, they bind to TNF so that the TNF cannot connect to cells and communicate its message to cause inflammation. These man-made agents work *with* the natural proteins to disarm the extra TNF that is produced in RA.

The introduction of TNF blockers into our arsenal against RA has made an enormous impact on the lives of thousands of people with RA. The TNF blockers can dramatically reduce the pain, stiffness, and swelling that many people with RA experience. This group of biologics has been shown to improve quality of life and physical function while reducing the damage that can occur with untreated RA. We have had almost two decades of experience with this form of biologic agent, and having this many years of successful use is encouraging in regard to long-term safety concerns. Currently, there are five anti-TNF drugs on the market used to treat RA. Some of these TNF blockers are used to treat other conditions as well, such as psoriasis, psoriatic arthritis, ankylosing spondylitis, and Crohn's disease.

The following anti-TNF biologics are used for patients with rheumatoid arthritis. The individual TNF blockers are described first, then important information that is common to all of the anti-TNF biologics is reviewed.

Etanercept (Enbrel)

Generic available: no
Usual dose: 25 mg, by self-administered injection twice weekly or 50 mg injection once weekly
Delivery options: Enbrel is available in:
   Single-use prefilled syringe
   Single-use prefilled SureClick auto-injector
   Multiple-use vial
Effective within: two weeks to three months

Released in 1998, Enbrel was the first biologic available for the treatment of rheumatoid arthritis. Its introduction has forever changed the way we treat RA, giving patients and doctors an exciting and powerful way to manage the damaging effects of RA.

Enbrel is a biogenetically engineered protein called a soluble receptor fusion protein; it is designed to resemble the naturally occurring soluble receptors that bind TNF. Enbrel is unique in this way, because all of the other TNF blockers use monoclonal antibody technology. Like all of the other TNF blockers, Enbrel was designed to attach to and disable TNF. Enbrel has to be injected by needle through the skin by subcutaneous (sub-Q) injection, as described above. The injection can be given using an auto-injector, the Enbrel SureClick. Injections can also be given using a prefilled syringe. It is also available in a vial that needs to be reconstituted into a solution. A health professional will teach you how to reconstitute the concentrated solution provided by the pharmacy.

In medical studies, Enbrel has been shown to decrease joint pain, swelling, and stiffness in patients with RA. In addition to a reduction of arthritis symptoms, patients also report improvement in day-to-day functioning and vitality.

Enbrel is used to treat adults with moderately to severely active RA. Enbrel has been proven in clinical studies to inhibit the progression of structural damage that can occur with RA. Long-term studies reveal that most patients have continued benefit with an acceptable risk of side effects.

Enbrel can be used alone, as a *monotherapy*, or, if you are already on methotrexate and have had an inadequate result, Enbrel can be added as part of a *combination therapy.*

Side effects of Enbrel. Fortunately, Enbrel has few side effects for the vast majority of people (see Table 20). The most common side effect is redness, itching, pain, or swelling at the injection site. These injection-site reactions occur in just over one-third of people. They generally occur at the beginning of treatment, are usually mild, and resolve without specific treatment. Other than site reactions, side effects reported most during medical studies include upper respiratory infections (like a cold), other infections, diarrhea, rash, and itchy skin. Although uncommon, serious side effects can occur. Please refer to the section "Important Safety Information regarding TNF Blockers" later in this chapter.

Pregnancy and breastfeeding. Studies in other animals have not revealed harm to the fetus. There have been no formal studies done with pregnant women. Because safety in animal studies cannot assure safety in humans, this drug should

TABLE 20. Side Effects of Enbrel

SIDE EFFECTS	INCIDENCE	SIDE EFFECT THERAPY
Nuisance		
Injection-site reactions	37–43%	Review injection technique; observe closely
Rash	3–13%	Discontinue if severe; treat rash
Itching	2–5%	Treat symptoms
Diarrhea	8–16%	Treat symptoms
Fever	2–3%	Watch closely for infection
Serious		
Infection	Increased risk	Discontinue medication

Adverse effects that were reported in 2% or more of patients in clinical trials.

not be used during pregnancy unless it is absolutely necessary. The makers of Enbrel have a registry for pregnant women who take Enbrel. The purpose of this registry is to check the health of the pregnant mother and her child. Talk to your doctor if you are pregnant and contact the registry at 1-877-311-8972. It is not known if Enbrel is excreted in human milk. Because of the potential for serious harm to the infant, the mother will need to decide whether to refrain from nursing or remain off Enbrel until the child is weaned.

Geriatric use. Enbrel has been successfully used to treat people over 65 years of age. Because older adults, in general, are at higher risk for infection, watching closely for this side effect is particularly important. (For most RA drugs, the safety and effectiveness in geriatric patients specifically has not been studied.)

Infliximab (Remicade)

Generic available: no
Usual dose: varies based on weight; intravenous infusions at weeks 0, 2,
    and 6, then every six to eight weeks
Delivery options: by intravenous infusion only
Effective within: two weeks to three months

Infliximab became available to treat RA in November 1999. It reduces the quantities of TNF in the body. Infliximab, so far available only as the brand-name drug Remicade, is a biogenetically engineered **antibody** that was specifically designed to attach to the TNF molecule and *permanently* inactivate it. Remicade was developed using *monoclonal antibody* technology.

Remicade is administered intravenously by a health care professional in a two-hour outpatient infusion. There are three initial doses, and then treatments are usually given every eight weeks. In people with very active arthritis, the interval between doses can be decreased to six weeks. Medical studies have shown that when used with methotrexate, Remicade effectively decreases the signs and symptoms of RA. It has also been proven to inhibit the progression of joint damage in patients with moderate or severe active RA who have had an inadequate response to methotrexate alone. In most cases, Remicade is used in combination with methotrexate.

Side effects of Remicade. Remicade is generally well tolerated (see Table 21). Because it is given intravenously, Remicade can sometimes be associated with "infusion reactions." Most reactions are mild, such as itching and stinging at the site where the IV line enters the skin. Much less commonly, these reactions can include rash, fever, achiness, chills, hives, chest pain, difficulty breathing, or low blood pressure. If reactions are severe, the medication must be discontinued. Many physicians "pretreat" the patient with diphenhydramine (Benadryl) and acetaminophen (Tylenol), which in many cases reduces these reactions significantly. If you are treated with Benadryl, which is sedating, you will need to discuss with your physician whether you should drive after an infusion or not. In medical studies, less than 2 percent of people needed to discontinue Remicade due to infusion reactions.

TABLE 21. Side Effects of Remicade

SIDE EFFECTS	INCIDENCE	SIDE EFFECT THERAPY
Nuisance		
Infusion reactions	~20%	Pretreatment with Tylenol or Benadryl
Nausea	21%	Treat nausea
Abdominal pain	12%	Seek physician's advice
Diarrhea	12%	Treat symptoms; seek physician's advice
Dyspepsia	10%	Treat stomach pain
Headache	18%	Treat headache
Fatigue	9%	Get extra rest
Rash	10%	Seek physician's advice
Achy joints	8%	Treat pain
Itching	7%	Pretreatment with Tylenol or Benadryl
Serious		
Infusion reactions requiring discontinuation	<2%	Discontinue medication
High blood pressure	7%	Seek physician's advice
Infections	Increased risk	Halt treatment; seek medical care
Lupus-like syndrome	Rare	Discontinue medication

Adverse effects occurring after receiving 4 or more infusions.

Treatment with Remicade may result in the development of *autoantibodies*, antibodies that are directed against one's own body. Usually, these autoantibodies cause no harm. Rarely, though, people with autoantibodies develop a lupus-like syndrome, and treatment should be discontinued. The most common side effects of Remicade reported during medical studies were upper respiratory infections (including sinus infection and bronchitis), nausea, headache, stomach pain, and diarrhea. Although uncommon, other serious side effects can occur. Please refer to the section "Important Safety Information regarding TNF Blockers" later in this chapter.

Pregnancy and breastfeeding. Because of its specificity to humans, Remicade cannot be studied in pregnant animals. It is not known if it can cause harm to a fetus. Remicade should be given to pregnant women only if it is clearly needed. It is not known whether Remicade is excreted in breast milk. Because other antibodies can be found in breast milk and because of the potential for harm to nursing infants, a decision should be made to stop the medication or refrain from nursing.

Geriatric use. In medical studies, there was no difference in safety between younger and older adults' responses to Remicade. Because older adults are at higher risk for infection, watching closely for this side effect is particularly important.

Adalimumab (Humira)

Generic available: no
Usual dose: 40 mg, self-administered injections every two weeks
Delivery options: Humira is available in:
    Single-dose prefilled pen (Humira Pen)
    Single-dose prefilled syringe
Effective within: two to twelve weeks

Adalimumab became available in the United States in 2003, as Humira. Like Remicade, Humira is a *monoclonal antibody* against the TNF cytokine. Unlike Remicade, which is made partly with mouse proteins, Humira is a fully human protein, which may lessen its side effects. Also it is given by self-administered injection and not by intravenous infusion. Injections are required every two weeks. Humira is available in a syringe or a prefilled pen (the Humira Pen) which is often preferred by needle-shy individuals.

In medical studies, Humira has been shown to be highly effective as a monotherapy or as a part of combination therapy with other DMARDs, such as methotrexate. It has been proven effective in decreasing the symptoms of RA, such as pain, swelling, and stiffness.

Side effects of Humira. Like its subcutaneous predecessor Enbrel, Humira is generally well tolerated (see Table 22). The most common side effect is redness, itching, pain, or swelling at the injection site. These injection-site reactions occur in about 8% of people. They generally occur at the beginning of treatment, are usually mild, and resolve without specific treatment. In addition to injection-site reactions, the most common side effects reported in medical studies include upper respiratory infection (including sinus infection), headache, rash, and nausea. Although uncommon, serious side effects can occur. Please refer to the section "Important Safety Information regarding Taking TNF Blockers" later in this chapter.

Pregnancy and breastfeeding. It is not known if Humira will harm an unborn baby. Humira should be used during a pregnancy only if needed. Abbott Laboratories, the maker of Humira, has a registry for pregnant women who take

TABLE 22. Side Effects of Humira

SIDE EFFECTS	INCIDENCE	SIDE EFFECT THERAPY
Nuisance		
Headache	12%	Treat headache
Rash	12%	Seek physician's advice
Nausea	9%	Treat nausea
Injection-site reaction	>8%	Review injection technique; ice area before injection
Back pain	6%	Treat back pain
Serious		
Infection	Increased risk	Halt treatment; seek medical care
High blood pressure	5%	Seek physician's advice

Adverse effects reported in 5% or more of patients in pooled clinical trials.

Humira. Talk to your doctor if you become pregnant, and contact the registry at 1-877-311-8972. You should not breastfeed while under treatment with Humira.

Geriatric use. In clinical studies, there was a higher rate of serious infections and malignancy reported in patients over the age of 65 than those under the age of 65. Because of this higher incidence, caution is advised when treating older individuals.

Golimumab (Simponi, Simponi Aria)

Generic available: no
Subcutaneous dose: 50 mg by self-administered subcutaneous injection
    once per month
Intravenous dose: variable dose based on weight by intravenous infusions
    at weeks 0 and 4, then every 8 weeks
Delivery options:
    Subcutaneous: Simponi comes in a:
        Single-dose SmartJect auto-injector
        Single-dose prefilled syringe
    Intravenous: Simponi Aria is available for intravenous infusion
Effective within: two to three months

Golimumab was released in 2009 as the subcutaneously administered biologic Simponi. In 2013, Simponi Aria became available for intravenous administration. In both forms, Simponi uses *monoclonal antibody* technology to disable TNF. Like Humira it is a "fully human" monoclonal antibody. Simponi is given only once per month, by subcutaneous (sub-Q) injection just beneath the skin. It can be given with a prefilled syringe or with the SmartJect auto-injector. Simponi Aria is given by a health care provider through a needle placed in a vein. When given by intravenous infusion, the first two doses are given one month apart, and then every eight weeks thereafter. The infusion is usually given in an arm and takes approximately 30 minutes. When used in combination with methotrexate, both Simponi and Simponi Aria have been proven to reduce the pain, swelling, and stiffness associated with RA.

Side effects of Simponi/Simponi Aria. Like other TNF blockers, golimumab is generally well tolerated (see Tables 23 and 24). For self-administered injections, a potential side effect is redness, itching, pain, or swelling at the injection site. Simponi was designed using a different buffer than other subcutaneously

TABLE 23. Side Effects of Simponi Used with DMARDs

SIDE EFFECTS	INCIDENCE	SIDE EFFECT THERAPY
Nuisance		
Injection site reactions	6%	Review injection technique; ice area before injection
Dizziness	2%	Discuss with physician
Tingling	2%	Discuss with physician
Serious		
Infections	Increased risk	Halt medication; seek medical care
Abnormal liver tests	3–4%	Discontinue medication if severe; seek physician's advice
High blood pressure	3%	Seek physician's advice

Adverse effects reported in 2% or more of patients in clinical trials.

TABLE 24. Side Effects of Simponi Aria with Methotrexate

SIDE EFFECTS	INCIDENCE	SIDE EFFECT THERAPY
Nuisance		
Infusion fever	2%	Inform infusion nurse; halt infusion
Rash	3%	Discuss with physician
Serious		
Infections	Increased risk	Halt medication; seek medical care
High blood pressure	3%	Seek physician's advice; treat
Leukopenia	1%	Discuss with doctor

Adverse effects reported in 1% or more of patients in clinical trials.

administered TNF blockers, which may explain why injections of Simponi appear to be less uncomfortable and to result in injection-site reactions in only 6 percent of people. When they happen, such reactions generally occur at the beginning of treatment, are usually mild, and resolve without specific treatment. In addition to injection-site reactions, the most common side effects reported in clinical research trials included upper respiratory infections, runny nose, abnormal liver tests, and high blood pressure.

For Simponi Aria, the most commonly reported side effects were upper respiratory infections (runny nose, sore throat, or laryngitis), viral infections such as the flu, bronchitis, high blood pressure, and rash. Reactions that occur during the infusion should be immediately reported to the nurse (see the section on intravenous infusions earlier in this chapter).

Although uncommon, serious side effects can occur. Please refer to the section "Important Safety Information regarding TNF Blockers" later in this chapter.

Pregnancy and breastfeeding. There are no adequate studies of Simponi use during pregnancy, so it is best to avoid its use while pregnant unless absolutely necessary. It is not known whether Simponi is excreted in breast milk or if it can be absorbed by the baby if ingested. The decision should be made to either breastfeed or take Simponi, but not both.

Geriatric use. In medical studies, there was no significant difference in serious adverse effects between those older and younger than 65. However, because infections are more common in older individuals, particular caution should be exercised with geriatric patients on Simponi.

Certolizumab pegol (Cimzia)

Generic available: no
Usual dose: 400 mg at weeks 0, 2, and 4; then either 200 mg every two weeks
    or 400 mg every month
Delivery options: Cimzia is available in:
    Prefilled syringe (for home administration)
    Lyophilized powder for reconstitution (for administration in a doctor's
        office)
Effective within: one to twelve weeks

Cimzia is a member of the TNF blocker family that was first approved for Crohn's disease and later for rheumatoid arthritis. Although it is considered a monoclonal antibody against TNF, like Humira, Remicade, and Simponi, it has some important differences. Unlike the other monoclonal antibodies that are manufactured as complete antibodies, this technology uses only a fraction of an entire antibody. That fraction of the antibody is called the *Fab' fragment.* This bioengineered antibody fragment attaches to TNF, knocking it out of commission just as the full monoclonal antibody biologics do. However, because of its smaller size and other factors, the fragment needs to be attached to a chemical called polyethylene glycol or PEG. This process is called *PEGylation*. By becoming PEGylated, the antibody fragment can remain in the body longer, thus requiring less frequent injections.

Cimzia can be taken alone as a monotherapy or be may be taken with other RA medications, like methotrexate. Cimzia has been proven effective in decreasing the pain, swelling, and other symptoms associated with RA, and it improves day-to-day functioning. It has also been shown to reduce the structural damage to joints.

Side effects of Cimzia: The most common side effects of Cimzia reported in medical research trials include rash, upper respiratory infection (flu, cold), urinary tract infections, headache, fatigue, and nausea (see Table 25). Burning and stinging at the injection site was very low, less than 2 percent, during clinical trials, which is less than some of the other biologics. Serious allergic reactions have been reported. Although uncommon, other serious side effects can occur. Please refer to the section "Important Safety Information regarding TNF Blockers" later in this chapter.

TABLE 25. Side Effects of Cimzia in Combination with Methotrexate

SIDE EFFECTS	INCIDENCE	SIDE EFFECT THERAPY
Nuisance		
Headache	5%	Treat headache
Nasopharyngitis	5%	Seek physician's advice
Back pain	4%	Treat back pain
Rash	3%	Halt medication; seek physician's advice
Fatigue	3%	Get extra rest
Serious		
Infection	Increased risk	Halt medication; seek medical care
High blood pressure	5%	Seek physician's advice

Adverse effects reported in 3% or more of patients in clinical trials.

Pregnancy and breastfeeding. Limited human studies have shown that there is low transfer of Cimzia across the placenta. However, Cimzia may be eliminated more slowly from the body of an infant than from an adult. This drug should not be used during pregnancy unless clearly needed. There is a pregnancy exposure registry that monitors pregnancy outcomes in women exposed to Cimzia during pregnancy. To enroll, call 1-877-311-8972.

It is not known if Cimzia is excreted in breast milk. Therefore, a decision should be made to either refrain from breastfeeding or remain off Cimzia.

Geriatric use. Cimzia studies do not include enough individuals over the age of 65 to determine if there is a difference in response to the drug or difference in side effects by age. Since older individuals in general are more likely to get infections, particular care is suggested when there is a question of infection in an older person being treated with Cimzia.

Important Safety Information regarding TNF Blockers

The most serious problem with the TNF blockers is the increased risk of infection. This includes risk of acquiring new infections and worsening of infections while on treatment. Most infections can be treated and get better with the appropriate therapy given promptly. However, TNF blockers lower the body's ability to fight infections. Also, many patients on TNF blockers are also on methotrexate or corticosteroids which also decrease the immune system's ability to react against infection. There have been reports of serious infections caused by bacteria, fungi, or viruses that have spread throughout the body. Some of these infections have been fatal. Some of the infections contracted by people on TNF blockers are considered "opportunistic infections." This means that normally the body would fight them off, but they have the "opportunity" to become infections because the immune system is weakened. These infections include tuberculosis (TB) and histoplasmosis as well as some more rare infections. Your doctor will test you for TB before starting a TNF blocker and will monitor you for signs of TB during treatment. Tell your doctor if you have been in close contact with anyone you know has TB. Tell your doctor if you have been in a region (such as the Ohio and Mississippi River Valleys and the Southwest) where certain fungal infections like histoplasmosis or coccidioidomycosis are common.

TNF blockers can rarely cause other serious side effects, including the following: active hepatitis B, if you have had it and it had become dormant; nervous system problems, such as multiple sclerosis, seizures, and inflammation of the nerves of the eyes; blood problems, such as low white blood cells and decreased platelets; new or worsening heart failure; new or worsening psoriasis; allergic reactions; autoimmune reactions, including a lupus-like syndrome and auto-immune hepatitis.

Product labels for the different TNF blockers reveal that there have been some cases of unusual cancers reported in children and teenage patients who started using tumor necrosis factor blockers before 18 years of age. Also, for children, teenagers, and adults taking TNF blockers, the chances of getting lymphoma or other cancers may increase. However, patients with RA, in general, may be more likely to get lymphoma. Hence, there is considerable controversy about how much of that particular risk can be attributed to the TNF blockers; long-term studies are under way. If you use TNF blockers, your chance of getting two forms of skin cancer may increase (basal cell cancer and squamous cell cancer). These two forms of skin cancer are not life threatening if treated.

Before starting a TNF blocker, discuss the following with your physician:

- Any history of diabetes, HIV, or weakened immune system.
- If you have open cuts or sores, signs of infection, predisposition to infection, or history of serious infections.
- If you have TB, been in close contact with someone who has had TB, or were born in or traveled to countries where there is more risk of getting TB.
- The need for a TB skin test and/or TB blood test and a chest x-ray to see if there is evidence of previous tuberculosis.
- If you live in, have lived in, or have traveled to certain parts of the country (such as the Ohio and Mississippi River Valleys or the Southwest) where there is a greater risk for certain kinds of fungal infections, such as histoplasmosis, coccidioidomycosis, or blastomycosis.
- If you have or have had hepatitis B.
- If you have or have had congestive heart failure.
- If you have a latex allergy, since some needle covers may contain latex.
- If you have had a disease that affects your nervous system, such as multiple sclerosis (MS).
- If you are planning to have surgery.

- If you are pregnant or planning to become pregnant or breastfeed.
- If possible, all vaccines should be brought up to date prior to starting TNF blockers, particularly any live vaccines (such as the shingles vaccine).

While receiving a TNF blocker:

- Do not take another biologic agent; previous biologics should be cleared from your body before starting a new biologic agent. Discuss with your doctor how long to wait when changing from one biologic to another.
- Contact your physician if you think that you are developing any kind of infection. Your TNF blocker will be temporarily discontinued in most situations.
- If you are on a subcutaneously administered TNF blocker and you experience severe skin redness, itching, pain, swelling, or any worrisome symptoms at an injection site, notify your doctor. Never inject into a tender, red, or hard area on the skin.
- If you are on an intravenously administered TNF blocker and have any new symptoms during the infusion, notify the nurse. In particular, immediately make the nurse aware of chills, chest tightness, shortness of breath, flushing, hives, itching, or dizziness.
- If you develop any signs of fever, bruising, bleeding, or paleness, call your physician.
- Numbness, tingling, muscle weakness, or vision changes should be reported to your doctor.
- If you develop increased achiness, pain with breathing, mouth sores, sensitivity to the sun, or a new rash, tell your health care provider.
- Never inject a biologic that has not been properly refrigerated.
- Do not get any "live" vaccines while you are receiving a TNF blocker. Flu shots are a form of "killed" or inactivated vaccine and should be given in most circumstances. Pneumonia vaccinations are generally recommended.
- Contact your prescribing doctor if you are planning a surgery; many physicians choose to discontinue TNF blockers temporarily around the time of an operation to reduce the risk of infection.

BIOLOGIC AGENTS AGAINST INTERLEUKIN-1:
THE IL-1 BLOCKERS

Interleukin-1, like TNF, is a cytokine that causes inflammation. Higher levels of IL-1 have also been shown to correlate with the degree of joint damage that can occur with RA. While all currently available TNF blockers bind to the cytokine TNF, disabling it before it can attach to immune cells, our only available IL-1 blocker, Kineret, functions differently. It disables the IL-1 receptors on the cell, keeping the IL-1 cytokine from being able to attach and deliver its inflammatory message. It is a man-made version of the naturally occurring protein called interleukin-1 receptor antagonist (IL-1Ra). (See general information earlier in the chapter and Figures 19 and 20.) The one IL-1 blocker approved for use in the United States at this time, Kineret, is described below.

Anakinra (Kineret)

Generic available: no
Usual dose: 100 mg by self-administered subcutaneous injection once per day
Delivery options: Kineret is available as a prefilled syringe
Effective within: four to thirteen weeks

In November 2001 Kineret became the third biologic to be released for use in the treatment of rheumatoid arthritis. Kineret is approved by the FDA for patients with moderate to severe active RA who have failed to respond to at least one DMARD. Medical studies reveal that Kineret decreases the signs and symptoms of RA, including pain and swelling. There is evidence that this medication may prove to be very valuable in preventing injury to the cartilage and bones that surround joints affected by RA. Kineret can be used alone or in combination with methotrexate or other DMARDs. It is advised that Kineret not be used with biologics that block TNF. This is due to concern that if both IL-1 and TNF are blocked at the same time, risk of infection will be dangerously increased by so much interference with natural immune system responses.

Side effects of Kineret. The most frequently reported side effect of Kineret is injection-site reactions (see Table 26). Most such reactions involve minor redness, bruising, swelling, or pain where the needle penetrates the skin. These symptoms typically last for 14 to 28 days. Injection-site reactions were described in 71 percent of patients in the early studies. Injection-site swelling can be decreased by applying a cold pack on the site immediately after injection. For particularly sensitive individuals, placing a cold pack on the skin before injections is very helpful.

As with other biologics, the side effect that causes greatest concern is the risk of infection. In studies, Kineret has been associated with an increased incidence of serious infections. Your doctor should discontinue treatment with Kineret if you develop a serious infection and should not start Kineret if you have an active infection. Decreases in white blood cell counts have been seen in 8 percent of patients on Kineret. Seriously low white blood cell count (neutropenia) was seen in only 0.3 percent of people receiving monotherapy with Kineret. Because of this potential side effect, complete blood counts (CBCs) should be performed as a baseline and monthly for three months after treatment begins, then quarterly for the first year.

Before starting Kineret therapy, discuss the following with your physician:

- Any history of poorly controlled diabetes, presence of open wounds or signs of infection, predisposition to infection, history of tuberculosis or other serious infections.
- Any history of low white blood cell count.

TABLE 26. Side Effects of Kineret

SIDE EFFECTS	INCIDENCE	SIDE EFFECT THERAPY
Nuisance		
Injection-site reaction	71%	(See text)
Headache	12%	Treat headache
Nausea	8%	Treat nausea
Diarrhea	7%	Treat diarrhea
Abdominal pain	5%	Treat symptoms; seek physician's advice
Flu-like symptoms	6%	Treat symptoms
Serious		
Infection	Increased risk	Discontinue medication; seek medical care

- Any history of hypersensitivity to *E. coli*–derived proteins.
- If you have latex allergy, since the needle cover contains latex.

While receiving Kineret:

- Contact your physician if you think that you are developing any kind of infection. Kineret will be temporarily discontinued in most situations.
- If you experience severe redness, itching, pain, swelling, or any concerning symptoms at an injection site, notify your doctor.
- Never inject into a tender, red, or hard area on the skin.
- Never inject Kineret that has not been properly refrigerated.
- Do not get any "live" vaccines. Flu shots are a form of "killed" or inactivated vaccine and should be given in most circumstances. Pneumonia vaccinations are generally recommended.

Pregnancy and breastfeeding. Reproductive studies performed on animals have not revealed problems. There are, however, no adequate studies in pregnant women. Because animal reproduction studies are not always predictive of human response, Kineret should be avoided during pregnancy. It is not known whether Kineret is secreted in breast milk. Because many drugs are secreted in human milk, caution should be exercised if Kineret is administered to nursing mothers.

Geriatric use. There have been no reported differences in safety or effectiveness among different age groups, but an increased sensitivity in geriatric patients cannot be ruled out. Because there is an increased risk of infections in older persons, caution must be exercised when taking this drug.

BIOLOGIC AGENTS AGAINST INTERLEUKIN-6: THE IL-6 BLOCKERS

Like TNF and IL-1, interleukin-6 is a pro-inflammatory cytokine. During testing of people with RA, elevated amounts of this cytokine were found in the blood and synovial fluid. Furthermore, the degree of elevation of IL-6 appeared to correlate with the extent of pain, swelling, stiffness, and other signs of RA activity.

There is also evidence that IL-6 has a very prominent role in the development of systemic inflammation or inflammation that affects the entire body and causes such symptoms as fatigue and blood test abnormalities, such as anemia. Hence, it made very good sense to target this pro-inflammatory cytokine. At the time of this writing there is only one approved IL-6 blocker, but there are several more in clinical trials.

The pro-inflammatory cytokine IL-6 delivers its message of inflammation upon its successful attachment to the receptor on the receiving immune cell. Our only currently available IL-6 blocker, Actemra, functions by disabling that cytokine receptor (as shown in Figure 19). Actemra is a bioengineered *monoclonal antibody* that attaches to the receptor and interferes with its ability to bind with the oncoming IL-6. With the connection of IL-6 to its destination receptor blocked, the message of inflammation is not transmitted.

Tocilizumab (Actemra)

Generic available: no

Intravenous dose: dose adjusted based on weight; given by infusion
    every four weeks

Subcutaneous dose: 162 mg by self-administered subcutaneous injection
    once per week or once every two weeks dependent on weight and
    other factors

Delivery options:
    Intravenous: Actemra is available for intravenous infusion
    Subcutaneous: Actemra is available as a prefilled syringe

Effective within: two to twelve weeks

Approved for use in 2010, Actemra is the first IL-6 inhibitor to come to market. First approved as an IV infusion drug, it became available for self-injection in 2013. Actemra can be given as an IV infusion into the vein, either in a doctor's office or in a hospital or infusion center. The infusions take approximately one hour and are given every four weeks. The self-injection dose is initially determined by weight. Patients who weigh less than 220 pounds will start with one subcutaneous injection every two weeks. Those over 220 pounds will administer their injection weekly. For patients starting with injections every two weeks, the dose can be changed to weekly if adequate results are not achieved.

Actemra has been approved by the FDA for use in patients with RA who have active signs of inflammation despite being treated with at least one DMARD. It can be given alone as a monotherapy or in combination with methotrexate or other nonbiologic DMARDs used to treat RA. Actemra cannot be used in combination with other biologic drugs. Medical studies have shown that Actemra can improve RA pain, swelling, and stiffness, as well as other symptoms of arthritis. Research has also shown that it slows or prevents the joint damage associated with RA. Actemra appears to be particularly effective in the correction of anemia, which is a common problem in people with RA.

Side effects of Actemra. Table 27 summarizes the side effects of Actemra, their frequency, and how to respond to them. As with other biologics when given by IV, there is a risk of infusion reactions. These reactions can include fever, chills, or rashes. Slowing the rate of infusion can often relieve mild reactions such as flushing and chills. Very rarely, there is a risk of serious allergic reaction, which would require stopping medication immediately and treating the reaction. When given by subcutaneous injection, there is a risk of injection-site reactions. Most such reactions involve minor redness, bruising, swelling, or pain where the needle penetrates the skin. Injection-site reactions were described in 4–10 percent of patients in clinical studies. Injection-site swelling can be decreased by applying a cold pack on the site immediately after injection. For particularly sensitive individuals, placing a cold pack on the skin before injections is very helpful.

Like other biologics, Actemra can lower the ability of the immune system to combat infection. Therefore, the most concerning potential side effect is the increased risk of infection. The most reported infections are common ones such as upper respiratory infections, including the common cold and sinus infections. However, more serious bacterial infections and unusual or atypical infections also present a concern. These infections can be life-threatening, so early detection and treatment are important. Although tuberculosis has not been seen frequently with Actemra, screening for prior exposure to TB is recommended before starting treatment. Your doctor will decide which screening tests are necessary given your previous treatment history and testing. Although the unusual infections are very rare, your doctor will also watch you closely for uncommon ones such as those caused by fungi and atypical bacteria and viruses. Many people carry the hepatitis B virus in their blood without knowing it. This virus can become active while taking Actemra or any other of the biologics, given their effect on the immune system. If it hasn't already been done, your doctor may require testing for previous exposure to hepatitis B.

TABLE 27. Side Effects of Actemra

SIDE EFFECTS	INCIDENCE	SIDE EFFECT THERAPY
Nuisance		
Nasopharyngitis	4–7%	Seek physician's advice
Headache	5–7%	Treat headache
Dizziness	2–3%	Discuss with physician
Rash	2–4%	Seek physician's advice
Mouth ulceration	1–2%	Treat mouth sores; discuss with physician
Abdominal pain	2–3%	Discuss with physician
Gastritis	1–2%	Treat gastritis
Serious		
Hypertension	4–6%	Seek physician's advice
Abnormal liver tests	3–6%	Pause or discontinue medication; discuss with physician
Serious infections	Increased risk	Discontinue medication; seek medical care

Actemra has some potential side effects that are not seen with other biologics. For instance, some patients taking Actemra have developed an increase in blood cholesterol. Commonly reported side effects included headache and high blood pressure. 3–6 percent of people taking Actemra have been shown to have increased liver enzyme values. Treatment with Actemra is not recommended in people with known liver impairment. Other laboratory abnormalities that have been reported include a decrease in the white blood cells and/or platelets. White blood cells are important in fighting infection, and platelets help blood to clot. Your doctor will suggest blood tests periodically to monitor for these abnormalities. A very rare complication that was seen with Actemra use during the early clinical studies was the occurrence of stomach or bowel perforations (tears in the wall of the intestine). This appeared to occur most often in people who were also taking NSAIDS, corticosteroids, or methotrexate.

As with other biologics, there is a very small but potential risk of other serious conditions. The impact of treatment with Actemra on the development of malignancies is unknown. However, like other biologics that suppress the immune system, use of Actemra may result in an increased risk of malignancy. Patients on Actemra should also be monitored closely for conditions that affect the nervous system, such as multiple sclerosis, although the rate of increased risk for these diseases is unknown.

Pregnancy and breastfeeding. There are no adequate studies in pregnant women taking Actemra. Therefore, its use should be considered only if the potential benefit justifies the potential risk to the fetus. Genentech, the maker of Actemra, has a registry for pregnant women who have taken Actemra. The purpose of this registry is to gather information about the health of mothers and newborns in the presence of the medication, to protect women who may become pregnant during treatment, and their babies. If you become pregnant while taking Actemra, please call the registry at 1-877-311-8972 to enroll. It is not known if Actemra is excreted in breast milk. If you are considering breastfeeding, you and your health care provider should decide if you will take Actemra or breast-feed. You should not do both.

Geriatric use. In clinical studies, the frequency of serious infections was higher among patients over the age of 65. Because infections are more common in the elderly population in general, caution should be used while taking Actemra to avoid infection and to recognize and treat all infections promptly.

Before starting Actemra, discuss the following with your physician:
- Any history of diverticulitis, stomach ulcers, or other bowel problems.
- Any history of diabetes, HIV infection, or history of weakened immune system.
- Open cuts or sores, signs of infection, predisposition to infection, or history of serious infections.
- If you have TB, have been in close contact with someone who has had TB, or were born in or have traveled to countries where there is more risk of getting TB.
- The need for a TB skin test and/or TB blood test and a chest x-ray to see if there is evidence of previous tuberculosis.

- If you live in, have lived in, or have traveled to certain parts of the country (such as, the Ohio and Mississippi River Valleys, or the Southwest) where there is a greater risk for certain kinds of fungal infections, such as histoplasmosis, coccidioidomycosis, or blastomycosis.
- If you have or have had hepatitis B; testing to confirm the absence of hepatitis B is recommended.
- If you have or have had any condition that has caused abnormal liver tests or are taking medications that can affect your liver function.
- If you have had a history of low white blood cell levels or low platelet levels.
- If you have had a disease that affects your nervous system such as multiple sclerosis.
- If you are planning to have surgery.
- If you are pregnant or planning to become pregnant or to breastfeed.

While receiving Actemra:

- Do not take another biologic agent; previous biologics should be cleared from your body before starting a new biologic agent. Ask your doctor how long to wait when changing from one biologic to another.
- Contact your physician if you think that you are developing any kind of infection. Your medication will be temporarily discontinued in most situations.
- If you have any new symptoms during the infusion, notify the nurse. In particular, immediately make the nurse aware of chills, chest tightness, shortness of breath, flushing, hives, itching, or dizziness.
- If you develop any signs of fever, bruising, bleeding, or paleness, call your physician.
- Numbness, tingling, muscle weakness, or vision changes should be reported to your doctor.
- If you develop increased achiness, pain with breathing, mouth sores, sensitivity to the sun, or a new rash, tell your health care provider.
- Do not get any "live" vaccines. Flu shots are a form of "killed" or inactivated vaccine and should be given in most circumstances. Pneumonia vaccinations are generally recommended.

- Contact your prescribing doctor if you are planning a surgery; many physicians choose to discontinue Actemra temporarily around the time of the operation to reduce the risk of infection.
- Your doctor will be ordering periodic blood tests to monitor your cholesterol, liver enzymes, and blood counts.

BIOLOGIC AGENTS THAT AFFECT THE T CELL: THE T CELL MODULATORS

The T cell lymphocyte is an important cell in our body's immune defense system. It also plays a major role in the development of inflammation with RA. Above we discussed the pro-inflammatory cytokines, including TNF, IL-1, and IL-6, and how they are protein messengers that are sent from one immune cell to another triggering inflammation. The other biologic medications we have discussed have been directed against these pro-inflammatory cytokines. The T cell is one of the immune cells involved in *starting* that chain of cytokine messages sent down the inflammation cascade from immune cell to immune cell. The T cell becomes "turned on" very early in the chain of events that lead to inflammation (as illustrated in Figure 4). Hence, T cell activation is often called an "upstream" event. The production of cytokines, including TNF, IL-1, and IL-6, is considered a "downstream" event. In order for the T cell to become involved in inflammation, it has to be activated or stimulated. So, interfering with the activation of T cells can result in a reduction in the downstream production of many of the pro-inflammatory cytokines. With fewer pro-inflammatory cytokines, there is less inflammation and less damage. The biologics that accomplish this interference are called T cell modulators; they do not completely block the activation of T cells. It is very important to have some continued T cell activation, since this immune cell is critical to helping us fight infections. More about the precise function of these agents is given below, in the description of the only T cell modulator so far approved, Orencia.

Abatacept (Orencia)

Generic available: no

Intravenous dose: dependent on weight; weeks 0, 2, and 4, followed by a
monthly dose

Subcutaneous dose: 125 mg per week self-injected; dosage the same,
     regardless of weight
Delivery options:
     Intravenous: Orencia is available for intravenous infusion
     Subcutaneous: single-dose, prefilled glass syringe
Effective within: four weeks to six months

Orencia came to market in 2005. First introduced as an IV infusion drug, it became available for self-injection in 2011. As noted above, the T cell is an immune cell involved early in the process of the inflammation cascade of RA. To participate in the inflammatory process, the T cell has to be "activated" or "stimulated." You will recall from Chapter 1 that an *antigen-presenting cell* (APC) presents an *antigen* (foreign substance) to the T cell to activate it (as shown in Figure 4). The activation of T cells is, in itself, a complex process that requires two signals from another immune cell. Because there are two signals needed, the T cell is activated in a process called "co-stimulation" (see Figure 21A). It is this process that Orencia disrupts (Figure 21B). Hence, Orencia is formally considered a "T cell selective co-stimulation modulator," since it interferes with the second signal required to fully activate the T cell. Don't be concerned if this seems a lot to take in. It may be useful to you to be familiar with the science behind the terminology, since you will see these terms in your reading. What is important is that this is a very different class of medications than the ones that we have previously reviewed.

Orencia can be given as either an IV infusion or by subcutaneous (sub-Q) injection. (These two methods of drug administration are discussed earlier in this chapter.) For the intravenous form, a health care provider administers Orencia through a vein in your arm. It takes approximately 30 minutes to receive the full infusion. After your initial dose, you receive Orencia two weeks later, then two weeks after that, and then every four weeks thereafter. The dosage is adjusted according to your weight. The subcutaneous form is given weekly by self-injection, just below the skin using a prefilled syringe. The dosage is the same for everyone regardless of weight.

Orencia has been shown in clinical studies to reduce joint pain and swelling and other symptoms of RA. It has also been shown to inhibit the progression of joint damage and to improve physical function. It can be used as a monotherapy or in conjunction with other nonbiologic DMARDS, such as methotrexate.

Side effects of Orencia. The most common side effects reported in medical studies were headaches, upper respiratory infections, nasopharyngitis (sore throat),

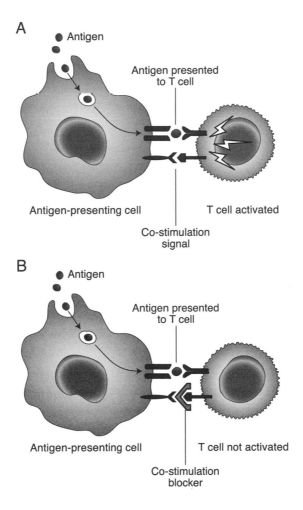

A

● Antigen

Antigen presented
to T cell

Antigen-presenting cell

T cell activated

Co-stimulation
signal

B

● Antigen

Antigen presented
to T cell

Antigen-presenting cell

T cell not activated

Co-stimulation
blocker

FIGURE 21. T cell modulation

and nausea (see Table 28). For those receiving IV infusions, the risk of reactions occurring during infusion was about 9 percent. Most of these infusion reactions were mild and resolved uneventfully with the discontinuation of treatment and/or adjusting the speed of infusion. Most common infusion complaints included dizziness, headaches, and high blood pressure. Serious infusion reactions occurred in less than 1 percent of people. For those taking subcutaneous injections, the risk of injection site reactions was about 2.6 percent. The most common issue was redness or itching, and no one in the studies needed to stop the injections because of these. Serious allergic reactions can occur in less than

1 percent of people treated with Orencia. Tell your doctor immediately if you develop hives, swollen face or tongue, or difficulty breathing.

As with other biologics, the most important side effect is the risk of developing a serious infection. The most commonly reported infections were upper respiratory infections, nasopharyngitis (nasal congestion/sore throat/runny nose), sinusitis, urinary tract infection, influenza, and bronchitis. Serious infections were reported in 3 percent of treated patients and included infections such as pneumonia, kidney infections, cellulitis (skin infection), and diverticulitis. If you are a carrier of hepatitis B infection, there is a risk that the virus can become active while you are taking Orencia. Your doctor may do a blood test for hepatitis B before starting any biologic. Although you should not receive "live" vaccinations while on Orencia, other vaccines, like the one for pneumonia and the yearly flu vaccine, are recommended. Orencia may lessen the effectiveness of some vaccines, so you will still need to use care around sick friends and family members. If vaccination with a live vaccine is deemed necessary, you need to be off Orencia for three months before you can receive the live vaccine.

TABLE 28. Side Effects of Orencia

SIDE EFFECTS	INCIDENCE	SIDE EFFECT THERAPY
Nuisance		
Headache	18%	Treat headache
Nasopharyngitis	12%	Seek physician's advice
Dizziness	9%	Discuss with physician
Cough	8%	Treat cough; seek physician's advice
Back pain	7%	Treat back pain
Dyspepsia	6%	Treat symptoms; seek medical advice
Rash	4%	Seek physician's advice
Serious		
Hypertension	7%	Seek medical care
Infection	Increased risk	Halt medication; seek medical care

Adverse effects reported in 3% or more of patients in clinical trials.

People with emphysema or COPD (chronic obstructive pulmonary disease) can have more problems with cough, shortness of breath, worsening of COPD, and pneumonia while taking Orencia. Caution is advised in prescribing this drug for people with known lung disease. As with other biologics, there may be unknown risks that haven't been revealed in the brief life of these new drugs. In clinical trials, the overall risk of malignancies was similar between those treated with Orencia compared to those on a **placebo.** However, more cases of lung cancer were reported in those treated with Orencia (0.2% versus 0%). Lymphomas were reported at a higher rate compared to the general population. However, in patients with very active RA, there is a known increased risk of developing lymphoma, even without use of a biologic drug. Hence, it is not known if Orencia increases your risk of developing a malignancy.

If you are taking *intravenous* Orencia and have diabetes or another reason to check your blood sugar, be aware that Orencia can *falsely* increase your blood sugar readings on the day of treatment. This is because the IV form contains maltose, which can affect some glucose test strips. There are test methods available that do not react to maltose. Ask your doctor if you are not sure about yours. This problem does not occur with the subcutaneous version of Orencia, which does not contain maltose.

Pregnancy and breastfeeding. There are no adequate studies on the use of Orencia in pregnant women. Therefore, it should not be used by a pregnant woman unless the potential benefit to the mother outweighs the unknown risk to the fetus. To monitor the outcomes of pregnant women and babies exposed to Orencia, a pregnancy registry has been established. Pregnant women receiving Orencia are encouraged to enroll in this registry by calling 1-877-311-8972. It is not known if Orencia is excreted in breast milk or absorbed by the nursing infant. Therefore, a decision should be made whether to refrain from nursing or to discontinue the drug.

Geriatric use. Although medical studies did not show a statistical difference in overall effectiveness and safety between those over and under age 65, the numbers of geriatric patients were too small to be sure. The frequency of serious infections and malignancies reported among Orencia-treated patients over the age of 65 was higher. Because serious infections and cancers are more common in the elderly population in general, caution is advised when prescribing Orencia for older persons.

Before starting Orencia, discuss the following with your physician:

- Any history of diabetes, HIV, or history of weakened immune system.
- Open cuts or sores, signs of infection, predisposition to infection, or history of serious infections.
- If you have TB, have been in close contact with someone who has had TB, or were born in or have traveled to countries where there is more risk of getting TB.
- The need for a TB skin test and/or TB blood test and a chest x-ray to see if there is evidence of previous tuberculosis.
- If you have or have had hepatitis B.
- If you have or have had emphysema, COPD, or any serious lung disorder.
- If you are planning to have surgery.
- If you are pregnant or planning to become pregnant or to breastfeed.
- If possible, all vaccines should brought up to date prior to starting Orencia, particularly any "live" vaccines (such as the shingles vaccine).

While receiving Orencia:

- Do not take another biologic agent; previous biologics should be cleared from your body before starting a new biologic agent. Ask your doctor how long to wait when changing from one biologic to another.
- Contact your physician if you think that you are developing any kind of infection. Your Orencia will be temporarily discontinued in most situations.
- If you are on subcutaneous administered Orencia and you experience severe skin redness, itching, pain, swelling, or any worrisome symptoms at an injection site, notify your doctor. Never inject into a tender, red, or hard area on the skin.
- If you are on an IV-administered Orencia and have any new symptoms during the infusion, notify the nurse. In particular, immediately make the nurse aware of chills, chest tightness, shortness of breath, flushing, hives, itching, or dizziness.
- If you develop any signs of fever, bruising, bleeding, or paleness, call your physician.
- If you have emphysema or other lung conditions, and notice an increase

in shortness of breath, cough, or wheezing, make your doctor aware immediately.

- Never inject a biologic that has not been properly refrigerated.

- Do not get any "live" vaccines. Flu shots are a form of "killed" or inactivated vaccine and should be given in most circumstances. Pneumonia vaccinations are generally recommended. Live vaccines should not be given within three months of stopping Orencia because it may blunt the effectiveness of some immunizations.

- Contact your prescribing doctor if you are planning a surgery; many physicians choose to discontinue Orencia temporarily around the time of the operation to reduce the risk of infection.

BIOLOGIC AGENTS THAT AFFECT THE B CELL: THE B CELL MODULATORS

The B cell is a very important part of our immune system. Once activated it is transformed into another form of immune cell called the *plasma cell*. Plasma cells are responsible for producing a wide range of antibodies that fight infection. In people with RA, the B cell becomes misdirected and creates dysfunctional plasma cells that produce antibodies that react against a person's own body. This is called an *autoimmune* response. These antibodies are called *autoantibodies* (meaning antibodies against oneself). For many decades, the misdirected B cell has been known to be key in the development of RA. It is responsible for the production of *rheumatoid factor* (*RF*), an abnormal antibody that is present in 60–70 percent of people with RA. Rheumatoid factor was discovered in the 1940s by researchers Erik Waaler and H. M. Rose. The test for the presence of rheumatoid factor was the first test that allowed us to categorize rheumatoid arthritis as a specific disease, separate from other forms of arthritis. The dysfunctional plasma cells are also responsible for production of the more recently discovered *anti-citrullinated peptide antibodies* (*ACPAs*). Their presence is now routinely tested for in patients with RA. (Read more about RF and ACPA in Chapter 3.)

The misdirected B cell is implicated in RA in other ways, too. For instance, it is one of the immune cells known to produce inflammatory cytokines and to activate the T cell. We have talked a lot about the domino-like series of events that occurs in the immune system and ultimately results in the symptoms of RA (Figure 4). Unlike the T cell changes described above, which represent early or "upstream" abnormalities in the rheumatoid cascade, the changes in the B cell are considered "downstream" changes. B cell activation, with its subsequent production of autoantibodies, is in part responsible for many of the more severe complications of uncontrolled RA. Not only are these antibodies involved in pain, stiffness, and swelling of joints, but they can also cause problems in other parts of the body, including the skin, lungs, and kidneys (see Chapter 4). Fortunately, the introduction of new medications, including the biologics, has made these RA complications blessedly rare in the twenty-first century. In those unusual situations when the DMARDs and the other biologics cannot control RA, we are grateful that we now have B cell therapies and that they have been shown to be effective in the most stubborn cases of RA. Below we present some information on how B cell modulators work, in a description of the only one on the market, Rituxan.

Rituximab (Rituxan)

Generic available: no
Usual dose: two doses, 1000 mg each, given by IV fifteen days apart (some have used 500 mg, although 1000 is the approved dose). The treatment can be repeated as directed by the treating physician.
Delivery options: intravenous infusion
Effective within: six weeks to three months

The B cell gone awry is not an event that is exclusive to RA. In fact, abnormal B cells are responsible for some types of lymphoma and chronic leukemia (forms of blood cancer). Studying one of these malignancies, B cell non-Hodgkin's lymphoma, helped us discover ways to treat RA. Rituxan was initially developed and approved to treat this form of lymphoma. Later, in 2006, it was approved for the treatment of RA in patients who have failed treatment with one or more of the TNF blockers.

On the mature B cell, there is a molecule called the CD20. This molecule is not present on growing or immature B cells or on plasma cells (the cells that B cells become when they are ready to produce antibodies). Rituxan is a *monoclonal antibody* that is targeted against the CD20 molecule and disables the B cell. Rituxan treatment reduces the number of mature B cells, including the misdirected B cells present in RA. This course of action is referred to as "B cell depletion" (see Figure 22). After the medication is out of the system, the blood becomes repopulated with new B cells that, we hope, will produce more normal antibodies and fewer abnormal or harmful antibodies.

Rituxan is given in combination therapy with methotrexate. It is reserved for people who have not responded to other biologic therapy, in particular, the TNF blocker family of biologics. Rituxan is given as an intravenous infusion into a vein. The infusion takes between two and four hours to complete for most people. Prior to the infusion of Rituxan, the patient is given a pretreatment with an IV form of corticosteroid (discussed in Chapter 15) called methylprednisolone. The patient is also given acetaminophen (Tylenol) and an antihistamine (such as Benadryl) before the infusion. These medications reduce some of the

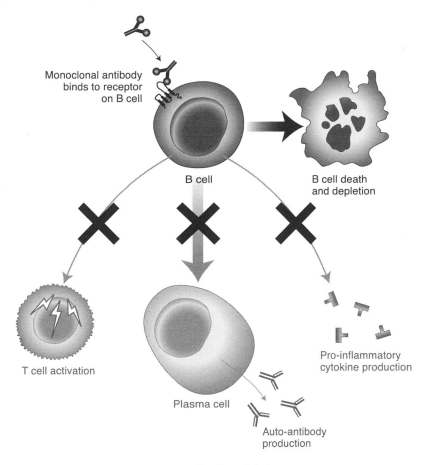

Monoclonal antibody binds to receptor on B cell

B cell

B cell death and depletion

T cell activation

Plasma cell

Auto-antibody production

Pro-inflammatory cytokine production

FIGURE 22. B cell modulation

side effects of the infusions, such as fever and chills. Re-treatment can occur at six months, but whether to do so varies widely among patients and depends upon each individual's response to the treatment and other factors. In clinical studies, Rituxan has been found to reduce the symptoms of RA when other treatments have failed. It has been shown to slow the progression of structural damage caused by RA.

Side effects of Rituxan. Side effects are listed in Table 29. In medical studies, 32 percent of people experienced a side effect during the infusion or within the first 24 hours following it. These reactions occurred in 11 percent after the second infusion. Acute infusion reactions—those occurring within two hours of the infusion—(such as fever, chills, shakes, itching, rash or hives, face swelling, sneezing, sore throat, cough, wheezing, high or low blood pressure) happened in 27 percent of first infusions and 9 percent of second infusions. Other side effects included body aches, headache, nausea, sweating, nervousness, muscle stiffness, tiredness, and tingling. Many of these side effects can be reduced by receiving IV corticosteroids before the infusion, along with acetaminophen (such as Tylenol) and diphenhydramine (such as Benadryl). Often, adjusting the dose or rate of infusion helps as well. Being on high blood pressure medications may increase the risk of low blood pressure during the infusion, so adjustments may need to be made. Fortunately, serious acute infusion reactions were experienced by fewer than 1 percent of patients. Severe, life-threatening infusion reactions, which include shock, heart rhythm abnormalities, and anaphylaxis (a severe allergic reaction) are fortunately rare.

Rituxan can lower your ability to fight infection. If you have had hepatitis B or are a carrier of hepatitis B, Rituxan could cause the virus to become active. As with other biologics, the risk of infection remains of greatest concern; 39 percent of treated patients in medical studies contracted an infection. The majority of these illnesses were upper respiratory infections (common cold or sinus infection) and urinary tract infections. Serious infections, including pneumonia, cellulitis (skin infection), and sepsis (bacteria in the blood), were reported in 2 percent of patients. After the treatment, some patients can have a prolonged period when levels of good antibodies in their blood remain low. This can increase the risk of infection. It is very important to consider all infections as potentially serious when taking this or any other biologic drug. Rarely, Rituxan can decrease the white blood cell count, as well as other blood cell counts, so the doctor may choose to do a blood test during the treatment.

TABLE 29. Side Effects of Rituxan with Methotrexate

SIDE EFFECTS	INCIDENCE	SIDE EFFECT THERAPY
Nuisance		
Acute infusion reaction	9–27%	(See text)
Nausea	8%	Treat nausea
Joint aches	6%	Treat joint aches
Fever	5%	See physician to rule out infection
Itching	5%	Seek medical care
Chills	3%	See physician to rule out infection
Dyspepsia	3%	Treat symptoms
Runny nose	3%	Watch closely for infection; treat symptoms
Tingling	2%	Discuss with physician
Hives	2%	Report to physician
Abdominal pain	2%	Discuss with physician
Sore throat	2%	See physician to rule out infection
Anxiety	2%	Discuss with physician
Migraine	2%	Treat headache
Asthenia	2%	Treat symptoms
Serious		
High blood pressure	8%	Seek medical attention
Infection	Increased risk	Halt medication; seek medical attention

Adverse effects reported in 2% or more of patients in clinical trials.

Pregnancy and breastfeeding. There are no adequate studies of Rituxan in pregnant women. Low numbers of B cells have been reported in infants exposed to Rituxan while in the mother's uterus. It is not known if Rituxan is secreted in human milk. The unknown risks to the infant from oral ingestion of Rituxan should be weighed against the known benefits of breastfeeding.

Geriatric use. In clinical studies, only 14 percent of patients were over the age of 65. The overall risk of side effects in this older group was similar to that in the younger patients. However, the risk of serious side effects, including heart issues, malignancies, and serious infections, was higher in the older patients. Therefore, extreme caution is advised when treating older individuals.

Before starting Rituxan, discuss the following with your physician:

- Any history of diabetes, HIV, or history of weakened immune system.

- Open cuts or sores, signs of infection, or predisposition to infection.

- If you have or have had a history of serious infections, including hepatitis B, hepatitis C, herpes simplex virus, shingles, parvovirus, cytomegalovirus, and West Nile virus.

- If you have TB, have been in close contact with someone who has had TB, or were born in or have traveled to countries where there is more risk of getting TB.

- The need for a TB skin test and/or TB blood test and a chest x-ray to see if there is evidence of previous tuberculosis.

- If you live in, have lived in, or have traveled to certain parts of the country (such as, the Ohio and Mississippi River Valleys or the Southwest) where there is a greater risk for certain kinds of fungal infections, such as histoplasmosis, coccidioidomycosis, or blastomycosis.

- If you have or have had heart problems, including irregular heartbeat or chest pain.

- If you have or have had lung or kidney problems.

- If you have had a disease that affects your nervous system, such as multiple sclerosis.

- If you are planning to have surgery.

- If you are pregnant or planning to become pregnant or to breastfeed during the twelve months after an infusion of Rituxan.

- All vaccines should be discussed with your treating doctor. Your doctor might want to bring your vaccinations up to date prior to treatment with Rituxan, if there are no contraindications. Vaccines that are considered "live vaccines" must not be given after receiving Rituxan, because this treatment can weaken the immune system significantly. Some vaccines are not as effective if given after receiving Rituxan. Therefore, non-live vaccines should be given at least four weeks prior to treatment with Rituxan.

While receiving Rituxan:

- Do not take another biologic agent; previous biologics should be cleared from your body before starting a new biologic agent. Ask your doctor how long to wait when changing from one biologic to another.
- Contact your physician if you think that you are developing any kind of infection. Rituxan should not be given during an infection.
- If you have any symptoms during the infusion, notify the nurse. In particular, immediately make the nurse aware of chills, chest tightness, shortness of breath, flushing, hives, itching, or dizziness.
- If you develop any signs of fever, bruising, bleeding, or paleness, call your physician.
- Numbness, tingling, muscle weakness, or vision changes should be reported to your doctor.
- If you develop increased achiness, pain with breathing, mouth sores, sensitivity to the sun, or a new rash, tell your health care provider.
- Do not get any "live" vaccines. Flu shots are a form of "killed" or inactivated vaccine and should be given in most circumstances.
- Contact your prescribing doctor if you are planning a surgery.
- Your doctor may intermittently do laboratory tests to monitor your blood cells (blood count) and antibodies (immunoglobulin levels) as well as kidney function.

THE ORAL BIOTHERAPIES—A LOOK INSIDE
THE IMMUNE CELL: THE KINASE INHIBITORS

The last 30 years have been devoted to the development and production of the biologics that are given by IV or by subcutaneous injection. Recall that these must be given this way because of the large size of their molecules and their protein-like makeup. Until recently, these large-molecule therapies were the only agents specific enough in their function and powerful enough in their action to have marked effectiveness with RA. There has been a longstanding desire to create an oral biotherapy that has the potency and specificity for RA to rival the biologics. Unlike their large-molecule counterparts, oral agents must have molecules small enough to be absorbed by the human digestive system and remain intact. The challenge of developing a small-molecule drug with similar effectiveness to biologics has been the focus of research for the past decade. In 2012, these efforts came to fruition with the *oral kinase inhibitors*. We have reviewed how immune cells pass messages from one to another by way of messengers, the cytokines, and how the biologics interfere with those messengers while they are still *outside* of these immune cells. The focus of the oral biotherapies is to alter what is happening *inside* the immune cell, the intracellular process that creates inflammation.

When a given cytokine messenger attaches to an immune cell receptor and activates that cell, it does so by jump-starting an intracellular signaling pathway. There are several different signaling pathways that exist within each of these cells, interconnecting in a very complex network. Some of these pathways are specifically involved with inflammation. Once an inflammatory signaling pathway is activated, the cell is instructed to manufacture other cytokines and inflammatory substances that cause further inflammation. So, these very intricate internal signaling mechanisms enable an immune cell to both *accept* an inflammation message and send it along to other cells.

Important in the functioning of one of these signaling pathways is a family of proteins called the kinases. Kinases are enzymes that are directors of these internal signaling pathways. It is toward these proteins that this newest class of medication, the kinase inhibitors, is directed. By interfering with the function of specific kinases, the medication halts the relay of information along the immune cell's signaling pathway, shutting down the delivery of the inflammatory message. Different kinases direct each of the signaling pathways. Chief among them is a family of kinases called the Janus kinases, named for the mythological Roman god Janus, who had two faces looking in opposite directions and presided over all beginnings and transitions. Described below is a drug that inhibits this family of kinases, Xeljanz, the first kinase inhibitor available for the treatment of rheumatoid arthritis.

Tofacitinib (Xeljanz)

Generic available: no

Usual dose: 5 mg twice per day (dose may need to be adjusted if kidney problems, liver problems, or changes in blood count)

Delivery options: oral tablets
Effective within: six weeks to three months

Xeljanz was released in 2012. Although not formally considered a biologic, it shares similar potency and was developed using the science gleaned from the development of the biologics. Unlike the oral DMARDS reviewed in Chapter 13, Xeljanz was developed with a very specific target: to disrupt an overactive intracellular signaling pathway that perpetuates inflammation. In people who have RA, the kinases that direct the intracellular signaling pathways in immune cells are "ramped up," overexcited. Included among these is the Janus kinase (JAK) family. When a pro-inflammatory cytokine connects to its receptor on the outside of an immune cell, it activates the JAK proteins that reside inside the immune cell (see Figure 23). JAK proteins pass the inflammation message to another set of proteins called the STAT proteins. This passage is often called the JAK pathway or the JAK-STAT pathway. STAT proteins then move into the *nucleus* of the immune cell. The nucleus is the manufacturing part of the cell and houses the cell's genes. The STAT directs the genes to start the manufacture of new pro-inflammatory cytokines, which will be released from the immune cell to communicate with other immune cells. Xeljanz works by disrupting the JAK-controlled signaling pathway, thereby interrupting the inflammatory process inside the cell. Because Xeljanz targets Janus family kinases specifically, it is often referred to as a JAK inhibitor, a JAK-STAT inhibitor, or a "jakinib," in addition to the broader term "kinase inhibitor."

Xeljanz has been approved for people with RA who have not improved enough with methotrexate treatment. It can be used as a monotherapy or in combination with methotrexate or other nonbiologic DMARDs. The medication is taken twice daily by mouth. The dose may have to be reduced in individuals with kidney or liver problems. If there are significant problems with these organs, this medication may need to be avoided. Numerous drugs interact negatively with Xeljanz, including ketoconazole, fluconazole, and rifampin, so always review new medications with your prescribing physician.

Side effects of Xeljanz. Table 30 summarizes the side effects of Xeljanz. In clinical trials, the most common side effects noticed in the first three months of use included upper respiratory infections (including common cold and sinus infections), nasopharyngitis (producing nasal congestion, sore throat, runny nose), diarrhea, and headache. Xeljanz inhibits the immune system, and the most common serious side effects are infections. The overall frequency of infection was 20 percent during the clinical trials. The most commonly reported infections were upper respiratory infection, nasopharyngitis, and urinary tract infections. Serious infections were fortunately uncommon. Serious infections include those caused by bacteria, fungi, and viruses, as well as tuberculosis. Some of such infections can be life-threatening, so all infections should be taken seriously. In people who are carriers of the hepatitis B or hepatitis C virus, the virus can be become active during Xeljanz treatment. Some people on Xeljanz have reported increased blood cholesterol levels. Some had slightly increased creatinine (a possible sign of decreased kidney function). Less than 2 percent of patients have changes in liver function tests or in their complete blood count. These changes include decreased numbers of white blood cells (lymphocytes and neutrophils), red blood cells (anemia), or platelets (clot-

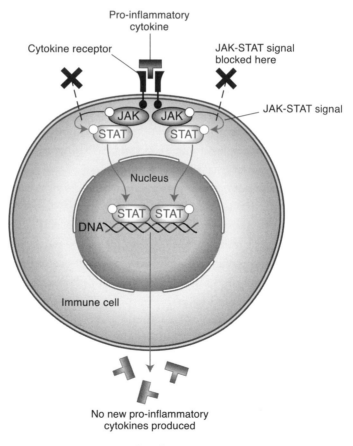

FIGURE 23. Intracellular signaling pathway: JAK inhibitor

ting cells). The doctor may have to decrease the dose or discontinue Xeljanz in these circumstances. Other serious but rare side effects have been reported, including the development of lymphoma and other malignancies. Rarely, small tears (perforations) in the stomach or intestines have been reported, but it is not clear that Xeljanz was the cause of these complications, given that most of these people were also on NSAIDS, corticosteroids, or methotrexate, each of which can also cause this side effect.

TABLE 30. Side Effects of Xeljanz

SIDE EFFECTS	INCIDENCE	SIDE EFFECT THERAPY
Nuisance		
Diarrhea	2.9–4%	Treat diarrhea
Headache	3.4–4.3%	Treat headache
Serious		
Infection	Increased risk	Stop medication; seek medical attention
High blood pressure	1.6–2.3%	Seek physician's advice

Pregnancy and breastfeeding. There are no adequate studies of Xeljanz in pregnant women. Animal studies did reveal possible harm to the fetus at high doses. The makers of Xeljanz have established a pregnancy registry that monitors and reports pregnancy outcomes. Pregnant women exposed to Xeljanz are encouraged to register by calling 1-877-311-8972. Xeljanz is secreted in the milk of lactating rats, so we are assuming that human mothers should not take any chances. Nursing mothers will need to either stop Xeljanz or refrain from nursing.

Geriatric use. In medical studies of Xeljanz, the frequency of serious infections was higher in patients over the age of 65. Since there is higher risk of infection in the elderly in general, caution should be used when older individuals are being treated with Xeljanz.

Before starting Xeljanz, discuss the following with your physician:

- Any history of diabetes, HIV, low white blood cells, or history of a weakened immune system.
- Any open cuts or sores, signs of infection, predisposition to infection, or history of serious infections.

- If you have TB, have been in close contact with someone who has had TB, or were born or have traveled in countries of higher TB risk.

- The need for a TB skin test and/or TB blood test and a chest x-ray to see if there is evidence of previous tuberculosis.

- If you live in, have lived in, or have traveled to certain parts of the country (such as the Ohio and Mississippi River Valleys or the Southwest) where there is a greater risk for certain kinds of fungal infections, such as histoplasmosis, coccidioidomycosis, or blastomycosis.

- If you have or have had hepatitis B, other forms of hepatitis, or any liver problems.

- If you have or have had a history of cancer, high cholesterol, or kidney problems.

- If you have any history of diverticulitis or other inflammation in the bowel or ulcers in the stomach or intestines.

- Review all prescription and nonprescription medicines including herbal preparations and dietary supplements.

- If you are planning to have surgery.

- If you are pregnant or planning to become pregnant or to breastfeed.

While receiving Xeljanz:

- Do not take biologic agents or potent immunosuppressants such as azathioprine and cyclosporin; previous biologics should be cleared from your body before starting Xeljanz. Ask your doctor how long to wait when changing from a biologic to Xeljanz.

- Contact your physician if you think that you are developing any kind of infection. Xeljanz will be temporarily discontinued in most situations.

- Avoid contact with people who have colds or infections; notify your doctor if you have fever, chills, cough, sore throat, change in urination, or muscle aches.

- If you develop a painful rash or blisters, ask your doctor about the possibility of shingles.

- If you develop fever, bruising, bleeding, or paleness, call your physician.

- Contact your health care professional if you have fever, pain in your abdomen, or change in bowel movements.

- Seek immediate medical attention if you have signs of a severe allergic reaction (rash, hives, itching, difficulty breathing, tightness in chest, swelling of the mouth, face, lips, or tongue).

- Lab tests, including complete blood cell counts, liver tests, and cholesterol levels should be ordered intermittently to monitor for potential side effects.

- Be careful to store this medication out of reach of children and animals.

- Contact your doctor if you believe you may be pregnant.

- Do not get any "live" vaccines. Flu shots are a form of "killed" or inactivated vaccine and should be given in most circumstances. Pneumonia vaccinations are generally recommended. Always ask your doctor first.

- Contact your prescribing doctor if you are planning a surgery.

A BIOLOGIC MEDICAL DEVICE FOR PROTEIN A IMMUNOADSORPTION

Protein A immunoadsorption is a therapy for people with severe, longstanding rheumatoid arthritis whose disease has not responded to medications. It is designed to remove from the blood certain antibodies that are believed to be harmful to people with RA. This is accomplished with the Prosorba column, a device that filters the blood, attracting out of it the target antibodies. Although this procedure was not approved for RA until 1999, a similar procedure has been used for people with a blood condition called ITP since 1987.

The Prosorba column consists of a plastic cylinder. The procedure, called apheresis, is much like dialysis. During treatment, the patient will be seated or lying down. A nurse places a needle into a vein in each arm, and the blood drawn from one arm passes through a machine that separates the blood cells from the plasma (the liquid portion of the blood). The plasma is then filtered through a column coated with a sand-like substance, protein A, which attracts harmful antibodies. The purified plasma is recombined with the blood cells and returned to the patient through the other arm. The procedure takes two to three hours and is performed weekly for twelve weeks. It is usually performed in a blood bank, like the Red Cross, or a hospital's apheresis center.

This procedure is reserved for only the most severe cases of RA. Approximately half of those treated have a beneficial response. That response lasts 20 to 84 weeks, with an average effectiveness of 37 weeks.

Side effects of Prosorba column therapy. The most common side effects are flu-like symptoms of chills, fever, nausea, and achiness. Other potential side effects include anemia, low blood pressure, and fatigue. The Prosorba column treatment is not recommended if you are taking a form of blood pressure pill called an ACE inhibitor or if you have heart problems, high blood pressure, or blood clotting problems. Use in pregnant women has not been studied.

Medicare covers Prosorba column therapy in people who meet certain criteria. If you are considering Prosorba column therapy, contact your insurance company to find out whether this treatment is covered and if special authorization procedures are required.

FOR MORE INFORMATION

The makers of Actemra offer an educational program, co-pay assistance, and other support resources. For more information, visit www.actemra.com. For information on patient assistance programs, call 1-866-681-3261 or visit www.GenentechAccessSolutions.com.

The makers of Cimzia offer a toll-free information line and Web site with information on financial assistance, co-pay assistance, educational materials, free needle disposal, and nursing support. Call 1-866-4CIMZIA (1-866-424-6942) or visit cimzia.com/cimplicity.

The makers of Enbrel offer a toll-free patient support telephone line, an educational program, co-pay assistance, sharps mail-back program, helpful resources, and a Web site: visit www.enbrelsupport.com and www.enbrel.com or call 1-888-4ENBREL (1-888-436-2735). Encourage Foundation is a nonprofit patient assistance program sponsored by the makers of Enbrel that provides Enbrel at no cost to qualifying patients with no or limited drug coverage. For more information call 1-800-282-7752 or visit www.encouragefoundation.com.

The makers of Humira offer a toll-free information line and Web site with information on insurance questions, practical information, sharps mail-back service, and access to registered nurses 24/7. Call 1-800-4HUMIRA (1-800-448-6472) or visit www.humira.com. The AbbVie Patient Assistance Foundation provides Humira at no cost to qualified patients who are experiencing financial difficulties and who generally do not have coverage available through private insurance or government-funded programs. Call 1-800-222-6885 or visit www.abbviepaf.org.

The makers of Kineret offer a toll-free patient support telephone line, educational programs, co-pay assistance and a Web site. For general questions about Kineret, call 1-866-773-5274; for co-pay assistance support, call 1-866-547-0644 or visit www.kineretrx.com.

The makers of Orencia offer a toll-free information line and Web site with information on insurance questions, co-pay assistance, educational materials about infusions and injections, needle disposal assistance, and nursing support. Call 1-800-ORENCIA (1-800-673-6242) or visit www.ORENCIA.com. Bristol-Myers Squib Patient Assistance Program is a nonprofit organization that assists eligible patients who need temporary assistance paying for Orencia. For more information, call 1-800-736-0003 or visit www.bmspaf.org/pages/home.aspx.

The makers of Remicade offer a toll-free information line, co-pay assistance, a support program, and other useful information. Call 1-888-222-3771 or visit www.remicade.com/rheumatoid-arthritis.

The makers of Simponi offer a toll-free information line and Web site with support information on cost, auto-injector use, sharp returns, and nursing support. Call 1-877-MY SIMPONI (1-877-697-4676) or visit SimponiOne.com. Visit www.JanssenPrescriptionAssistance.com/simponi if you have questions about affording your medication. Johnson & Johnson Patient Assistance Foundation is a nonprofit foundation that provides Simponi to eligible applicants without insurance and with limited incomes. Call 1-800-652-6227 or visit www.jjpaf.org.

The makers of Xeljanz have a patient support program called Xelsource. They offer a toll-free line with information on samples, insurance questions, funding assistance, educational information, and nursing support. Call 1-855-4XELJANZ (1-855-493-5526). Pfizer Pfriends helps eligible patients get discounts on Xeljanz from participating pharmacies. For more information, call 1-800-706-2400 or visit www.phahelps.com and look for assistance programs: Pfizer Pfriends.

There are several independent foundations that help people pay for medications or direct them to other resources that are available. If you need assistance, try all of them to see if you qualify. Availabilty of funds varies from time to time, so calling back intermittently may be worth the effort. Here are a few of these nonprofit agencies:

NeedyMeds is a nonprofit information resource devoted to helping people find programs to help them afford their medications and other costs related to health care. Their Web site is very up to date and lists options for each individual drug. For more information, call 1-800-503-6897 or visit www.needymeds.org.

The Patient Access Network (PAN) is an independent organization that offers help to people with chronic illness for whom cost limits access to breakthrough medical treatments. The Patient Access Network Foundation provides financial assistance to eligible Medicare patients with RA, funding permitting. Patients can apply for assistance by calling 1-866-316-7263 or applying on-line at www.panfoundation.org.

The Partnership for Prescription Assistance helps qualifying patients without prescription drug coverage get the medicines they need through the program that is right for them. Many applicants will get their medications free or nearly free. Call 1-888-4PPA-NOW (1-888-477-2669) or visit www.pparx.org.

The HealthWell Foundation is a nonprofit organization that provides financial assistance to eligible individuals who cannot afford their medications or health insurance premium. To see if you are eligible for funds call 1-800-675-8416 or go to their Web site, www.healthwellfoundation.org.

The Patient Advocate Foundation (PAF) provides patients with advocacy services to assist in getting the medical care they need. The Co-Pay Relief (CPR) Division of PAF is a donor-funded division that disperses funds when available to qualified patients. Call 1-866-512-3861, Option 1, for live assistance regarding co-pay relief. To see what other resources are available call 1-800-532-5274 or visit www.patientadvocate.org.

The Chronic Disease Fund is a foundation that offers several services including co-payment assistance for people with chronic illnesses. For more information, call 1-877-968-7233 or visit www.cdfund.org/Copay-Assistance.aspx.

Corticosteroids

Corticosteroid medications, better known as *cortisone* or *steroids*, are useful in treating rheumatoid arthritis (RA) and a variety of other conditions. Corticosteroid medications are artificially manufactured to resemble the body's own natural hormones in chemical makeup. Cortisone and hydrocortisone, two such hormones, are produced naturally by the adrenal gland. These hormones have a protective function: when a person suffers any kind of stress, the levels of these hormones increase to help the person cope physically with the particular situation.

One of the helpful abilities of these hormones is to reduce inflammation. When man-made medications resembling the body's natural cortisone are taken in larger amounts than the body normally produces, inflammation is markedly decreased. For this reason, corticosteroid medications can be an important part of the treatment of RA.

ORAL CORTICOSTEROIDS

Corticosteroids were first prescribed for patients with RA in the 1940s, when Dr. Phillip Hench and a colleague of his, biochemist Edward Kendall, discovered the mystery compound later called "cortisone." Cortisone was at first hailed as a "miracle drug" and the "cure" for RA. High-dose cortisone was so potent and dramatically effective in the treatment of RA that Hench and Kendall received the Nobel Prize in 1950 for their work. They shared this award with Tad Reichstein, an organic chemist who simultaneously described the chemical composition of natural cortisone.

It soon became apparent, however, that this powerful medication caused some serious side effects, particularly at the very high doses being prescribed at that time. Because of this, most physicians in the 1960s and 1970s tried to avoid prescribing corticosteroids. They are now again being given to treat RA (see Table 31), but physicians have become more cautious in prescribing the medication. Doctors generally heed the following guidelines when prescribing corticosteroids. The drugs are to be used

- by people whose arthritis cannot be controlled adequately by nonsteroidal anti-inflammatory drugs (NSAIDs), disease-modifying antirheumatic drugs (DMARDs), or biologics or by people who cannot take NSAIDs, DMARDs, or biologics because of unacceptable side effects;

- in the smallest dose that allows the person to function (the medication should be taken in the morning as a single dose); and

- for the shortest course of treatment that is expected to be effective.

If the dose and duration of use of a corticosteroid are limited, the number of side effects will be diminished significantly. Treatment of some of the rare and severe complications of RA (see Chapter 4) does involve taking larger doses of corticosteroids.

It is common practice for doctors to prescribe low-dose corticosteroids on a temporary basis. If NSAIDs prove ineffective or cause intolerable side effects, corticosteroids can be substituted temporarily to control inflammation rapidly while awaiting the effects of a slower-acting DMARD. This is called *bridge therapy*. After the inflammation is controlled, corticosteroids need to be tapered off slowly under a physician's guidance. One should *never* abruptly discontinue corticosteroids without the supervision of a doctor, because medical complications are possible.

TABLE 31. Corticosteroids Available in Pill Form

DRUG	BRAND NAME
Betamethasone	Celestone
Cortisone	Cortone
Dexamethasone	Decadron, Hexadrol
Methylprednisolone	Medrol
Prednisolone	(none)
Prednisone	Deltasone, Orasone
Triamcinolone	Aristocort

Note: All of the above drugs are available in generic form.

A further note of caution is in order here: the relief provided by corticosteroids can lull a person into a false sense of security and the temptation to avoid treatment with DMARDs or biologics. Corticosteroids are extremely potent anti-inflammatory drugs, but they usually do not halt the disease process.

Side Effects of Oral Corticosteroids

The side effects of oral corticosteroids tend to be of two types: those that are immediate and those that occur as a consequence of long-term use (see Table 32). The frequency and intensity of these side effects vary in accordance with dose, length of treatment, and the individual. In general, small daily doses (5 mg of prednisone, for example) cause few side effects, whereas larger doses (more than 20 mg of prednisone daily) are commonly associated with side effects if continued for more than a month. Note that there is a difference between oral corticosteroids and those injected into the joints; the injected form rarely causes any of the side effects listed in Table 32.

Nausea, bloating, and changes in mood are the most common immediate side effects of oral corticosteroid therapy. Long-term use can affect the muscles, bones, eyes, and hormones and make the person susceptible to infection. Many of the side effects resulting from long-term use will subside after corticosteroid treatment is discontinued. If a person develops a serious infection, the infection needs to be treated and the person gradually taken off the corticosteroids if possible.

Cautionary Notes

Before starting oral corticosteroid therapy, discuss the following with your physician:

- A history of diabetes, glaucoma, high blood pressure, heart disease, osteoporosis, thyroid problems, stomach ulcer, or tuberculosis or positive tuberculin skin test.

While taking this medication:

- Contact your physician if you have fever or chills; cough; sore throat; blurred vision; increased frequency, duration, or severity of headaches; eye pain; increased thirst; frequent urination; increased weakness.
- Take with meals, preferably breakfast.
- Avoid alcohol and tobacco products.

TABLE 32. Side Effects of Oral Corticosteroids

SIDE EFFECTS	SIDE EFFECT THERAPY
Immediate	
Changes in mood	
Nervousness	Reduce dosage
Insomnia	Take pill in early morning
Depression	Reduce dosage
Euphoria	No treatment necessary
Nausea	Take with meals or antacid
Changes in appearance	
Weight gain due to increased appetite	Limit fats, sweets, and baked goods; eat more fresh fruits and vegetables
Puffiness	Limit salt intake
Acne	Apply topical antibiotics
Facial hair growth	Electrolysis; laser
Increased bruising	No treatment
Salt and fluid retention	
High blood pressure	Limit salt intake
Ankle swelling	Limit salt intake and elevate legs as often as possible
Long-term	
Osteoporosis (bone thinning)	Exercise; calcium, vitamin D, medications for osteoporosis
Muscle weakness	Slowly stop medication or decrease dosage; exercise
Eye problems	
Cataracts or increased eye pressure	Close observation and treatment by an ophthalmologist
Hormonal problems	
Onset of or worsening of diabetes	Reduce dosage; consult a dietitian; take diabetes medication
Menstrual irregularities	Will return to normal after discontinuation of medication
Further changes in appearance "Moon face," "buffalo hump," stretch marks, easy bruising, fragile skin	Reduce dosage
Decreased blood supply to bones (osteonecrosis), particularly hip and knee	Evaluation by orthopedic surgeon; temporary use of crutches
Susceptibility to infections	Treat infections and slowly reduce medication after infection improves

- *Never stop corticosteroids abruptly.* This can be hazardous if you have been on corticosteroids for an extended period. If you run out of medication, call your doctor immediately. Corticosteroid use must be supervised by a doctor, and discontinuation of it must also be supervised by a doctor.

- If you have a surgical or another medical procedure planned, inform your doctor that you are on corticosteroids. Your doctor may want to *increase* your dose temporarily. This is called *stress dosing*.

- If you have been on corticosteroids for more than one month, wear a medical identification tag that states that you have RA and lists the medications you are taking. This will provide valuable medical information if you are ever in an accident or become so ill that you are unable to speak for yourself.

- If you have severe nausea, vomiting, or diarrhea, you may not be absorbing your medication because it isn't staying in your system long enough. You should alert your physician immediately.

- If you are on long-term corticosteroids, get **bone density testing** to check for osteoporosis, and discuss with your doctor the advisability of treatment to prevent bone loss (see next chapter).

Pregnancy and breastfeeding. Corticosteroid use is considered *relatively* safe during pregnancy.

INTRA-ARTICULAR CORTICOSTEROID INJECTIONS

In RA it is common for one joint to become more swollen than others or to lag behind the others in improvement. An injection of corticosteroids directly into the joint (intra-articular) will decrease the pain, warmth, and swelling in the joint that is giving the person the most trouble. The beneficial effects generally last four to six weeks.

This frequently performed and effective procedure is generally safe and well tolerated. Before the injection is administered, the skin is generally numbed with a local anesthetic. (Be certain to warn your doctor if you have ever had a reaction to a local anesthetic, such as Novocain or Xylocaine.) A needle is then introduced through the skin and into the joint, into which the corticosteroid is injected.

The side effects of the small amount of corticosteroid injected into the joint are minimal. If a given joint is injected no more frequently than every four months, adverse effects from the corticosteroid itself are unlikely.

Injection of corticosteroid into the same joint more frequently than every three to four months, however, may cause joint damage. In fewer than 5 percent of patients the injected corticosteroid can temporarily *increase* inflammation, for a very short period. This is known as a *postinjection flare.* Although uncomfortable, this inflammation will decrease within two to three days. It is impossible to tell in advance of the injection whether a particular individual will experience this side effect.

Occasionally, a dimple in the skin or a mild change in skin color will be noticed at the site of injection. These skin changes almost always lessen with time.

As with any medical procedure, complications related to the procedure itself can arise. During the injection, care must be taken to avoid injuring surrounding tendons or other structures. Sterile technique is required, of course, to prevent the possibility of introducing bacteria or infection into the joint. Experienced physicians who perform this procedure, generally **rheumatologists** and **orthopedic surgeons,** take exceptional care to avoid these complications.

What to Do After a Joint Injection

Apply ice packs to the joint for twenty minutes as soon as possible after the procedure. Rest the joint for at least forty-eight hours after the injection, sparing it from normal use as much a possible. Wear a **splint** if a wrist has been injected; consider using crutches to avoid putting weight on a knee or ankle that has been injected. Avoid carrying heavy objects when a shoulder or elbow has been treated by injection.

For the first week or two after injection, avoid any activity that might stress the joint.

Call your physician if there is increased pain, swelling, or fever after forty-eight hours (increased discomfort and even swelling within the first twelve hours after an injection are common). Repeated applications of ice may help alleviate the discomfort.

16

Osteoporosis Treatments

Many people with RA also have osteoporosis. This is related to several factors. First, RA and osteoporosis are both more common in women than in men, so part of the co-occurrence is statistical coincidence. Second, inflammation can increase the risk of osteoporosis. And third, some medications, particularly corticosteroids, can increase bone loss and thus greatly increase the risk of osteoporosis. Osteoporosis can be diagnosed easily by **bone density testing**, a painless low-radiation x-ray that is suggested for women over 50 anyway.

DIETARY AND LIFE-STYLE TREATMENTS

Eating a diet rich in calcium and vitamin D can help slow osteoporosis. Calcium is a critical building block of bone, and vitamin D helps your body absorb calcium. Calcium-rich foods include dairy products, leafy green vegetables, and shellfish. Vitamin D comes from sunlight but can also be found in fortified dairy products. In the last few years, studies have shown that we require less calcium than we previously believed. Also, consuming too much calcium may lead to other health problems, such as premature heart disease. Table 33 lists the daily amounts of calcium recommended for adults, as determined by the Institute of Medicine (IOM) in 2010 and approved by the National Osteoporosis Foundation (NOF). In calculating how much additional calcium you may need, make sure to subtract from the total daily requirement the calcium that you are already getting in your multivitamin and in your food. Both the NOF and the New York State Osteoporosis Prevention and Education Program offer worksheets to help you calculate your daily calcium intake (see end of this chapter).

The daily requirement of vitamin D is much more controversial. In 2010 the IOM changed the recommended daily allowance (RDA) for vitamin D intake to 600 international units (IU) for adults and 800 IU for adults older than 70.

These recommendations are for otherwise healthy Americans. However, expert opinion varies widely in regard to the best dose of supplemental vitamin D to take. The variation between these experts boils down to differences of opinion as to what level of vitamin D in the bloodstream is considered "necessary" for good health. You will read more about vitamin D in Chapter 18. It appears that higher blood levels of vitamin D may have beneficial effects for rheumatoid arthritis and other health conditions. Please consider the official RDAs as *minimum* recommendations and review the possibility of higher doses of vitamin D with your rheumatologist. Your doctor can also do a blood test to make certain that you are getting enough of this vitamin.

Vitamin D deficiency is common in people with RA. People of color are particularly prone to vitamin D deficiency. Dark-skinned individuals have higher concentrations of the pigment melanin in their skin, and it blocks UVB sunlight and limits the body's ability to make vitamin D. People who are overweight are also prone to deficiency, since vitamin D is fat-soluble and can be hidden inside fat cells and become unavailable for the body's use.

People on corticosteroids, in addition to obtaining generous amounts of calcium in their diet, may require additional calcium and vitamin D supplements as compared to the average adult. If you are on prednisone or another corticosteroid, ask your rheumatologist specifically about calcium and vitamin D supplements.

TABLE 33. National Osteoporosis Foundation
Recommended Daily Intakes of Calcium

GROUP	AMOUNT (MG/DAY)
Men 19–70 years	1,000
Men 71 and older	1,200
Women 19–50 years	1,000
Women 51 and older	1,200

Source: Food and Nutrition Board, Institute of Medicine, National Academy of Sciences, 2010.

Diet and exercise both play a role in keeping or improving bone strength. The best exercises to stimulate bone formation are weight-bearing exercises. These include brisk walking, running, jogging, weight lifting, and team sports. Weight-bearing exercise should be done three to five times per week. Rheumatoid arthritis, however, can limit exercise options. Remember the lessons of joint protection reviewed in Chapter 8. Your physician can help you develop an exercise program that is right for you.

MEDICINAL TREATMENTS

Hormone Replacement Therapy

Hormone replacement therapy (HRT) is drug therapy using various forms of estrogen with or without progesterone. HRT, and the controversy over its benefits and risks, is the subject of many professional and popular books. Here we will speak only to its beneficial effects on the prevention and treatment of osteoporosis. HRT has been shown to prevent bone loss after the menopause in women. Also, many studies suggest that HRT reduces the risk of hip and spine fracture in people who already have osteoporosis. You must be cautious about taking estrogen if you have a history of phlebitis or blood clots or if you have a strong family history of breast cancer.

Selective Estrogen Receptor Modulators

Estrogen-like medications called selective estrogen receptor modulators (SERMS) are used to prevent and treat osteoporosis in women who are past the menopause. Raloxifene (Evista) was the first medication of this type to be available in the United States. Raloxifene has been shown to reduce spine fractures. Unlike hormone replacement treatment, raloxifene does not stimulate the breast or uterus. In clinical trials, raloxifene did not increase the risk of breast cancer. An infrequent side effect is blood clots in the veins, particularly in people who are immobile for long periods.

Bisphosphonates

Bisphosphonates are a class of medication used to prevent and treat osteoporosis, including steroid-induced bone loss. As a group they are among the most potent medications to treat osteoporosis. These medications are very poorly absorbed, however, and therefore must be taken first thing in the morning on an empty stomach with a large glass of water. After taking a bisphosphonate, the person must stand or sit upright for the next 30–60 minutes *before* eating breakfast.

The three oral bisphosphonates approved for use in the United States are alendronate (Fosamax), risedronate (Actonel and Atelvia), and ibandronate (Boniva). Two bisphosphonates are available for intravenous use, ibandronate (Boniva) and zoledronic acid (Reclast). Both oral and IV forms of these medications have been shown to reduce the risk of fractures. Oral alendronate, risedronate, and ibandronate are available in generic versions.

Calcitonin
Calcitonin is a man-made version of a hormone that is found in nature. This hormone is not in the estrogen family. Calcitonin helps to regulate normal calcium levels and reduces bone loss. Miacalcin and Fortical are brands of salmon calcitonin that are taken by nasal spray. Calcitonin has been shown to reduce the risk of spine fractures.

Parathyroid Hormone (Forteo)
Most forms of osteoporosis treatment work by preventing bone loss. To date, there is only one treatment available that builds new bone and helps to replace depleted bone stores. Teriparatide (brand named Forteo) was the first injectable treatment for osteoporosis to be introduced in the United States (2002). Forteo is a synthetic form of parathyroid hormone (PTH), a nonestrogen hormone that is found in nature. Forteo has to be taken by daily injection, because, like the other biologics, it is a protein and gets digested by stomach enzymes if taken orally. It can only be given for two years in a lifetime so it is generally reserved for those with the most severe cases of osteoporosis. Other synthetic forms of this hormone are undergoing clinical studies at this time, including forms that are given by nasal inhaler and by pill.

Denosumab (Prolia)
In 2010, the Food and Drug Administration (FDA) approved Prolia (denosumab), another biologic to be used for osteoporosis. Like the biologics used for RA, Prolia is a protein that has to be given by **subcutaneous** injection. It uses **monoclonal antibody** technology, which we have described for several of the RA biologics. It is given every six months in a doctor's office. This powerful treatment is generally reserved for those who have failed other treatments or cannot tolerate them. Prolia has been shown to decrease the risk of spine and hip fractures. Because this drug has been associated with an increased risk of infections, patients are often advised *not* to take this medication with other drugs that suppress the immune system. That caution applies to many of the

medications that we use for RA. So, as with any other medication, make sure that your rheumatologist is aware of any new medications that you are considering.

Odanacatib

At the time of this edition, a new treatment, odanacatib, is in late stage studies for the treatment of osteoporosis. It is in a new class of medications called the *cathepsin K inhibitors*. This medication will be taken once per week in tablet form. It is expected to be available in 2014.

FOR MORE INFORMATION

National Osteoporosis Foundation, 1232 22nd Street, N.W., Washington, D.C. 20037-1292; 202-223-0344; www.nof.org.

New York State Osteoporosis Prevention and Education Program; toll-free 1-888-70-REHAB ext. 4772; Web site: www.nysopep.org. Calcium calculators/ worksheets on-line: www.nysopep.org/pdfs/Prevention_EstimateYourCalcium Intake.pdf.

NIH Osteoporosis and Related Bone Diseases National Resource Center, 2 AMS Circle, Bethesda, Md. 20892-3676; 202-223-0344 or toll-free 1-800-624-BONE; www.osteo.org or www.bones.nih.gov.

BEYOND MEDICATIONS: OTHER TREATMENTS

Alternative and Complementary Therapies

As exciting as new technological and biological advances are, many people see them as only part of their treatment options. There is an ever-growing interest in nonconventional medical treatments. Historically, the medical profession has viewed with considerable skepticism treatments that have not been subjected to scientific testing. Non-Western therapies have been denounced by many scientists as quackery. Despite this skepticism, people have sought *alternative treatments* when traditional medicine offered incomplete relief for chronic conditions such as rheumatoid arthritis (RA). In time, many people began to accept these therapies as *complementary* to conventional medical care rather than rejecting them as replacements for or alternatives to scientifically proven treatments.

Because patients have increasingly turned to complementary therapies, physicians have had to recognize the implications of patients' using both conventional and complementary treatment options. In an effort to be helpful, many medical professionals have attempted to give informed advice to their patients, even in the absence of sound scientific research on most nonconventional treatments. Many hospitals and medical centers have acknowledged the lack of evidence in this area and have developed exploratory programs focused on *integrative medicine.* This new area of medicine is attractive to individuals who want to thoughtfully combine mainstream medicine with complementary therapies. The National Institutes of Health developed the Center for Addiction and Alternative Medicine Research to support rigorous scientific evaluation of complementary and alternative medicine. This NIH program focuses on determining the safety and effectiveness of nonconventional therapeutic approaches.

At this time, many complementary treatments are *still* unproven; hence, you are literally trying them at your own risk. Prospective treatments can range from unproven but potentially useful therapies to potentially harmful therapies, and they may be relatively inexpensive or very expensive. Even if a treatment is inexpensive and carries no risk of physical harm, there is the hidden cost of wasting time on unproven remedies: a person recently diagnosed with RA may miss the opportunity to receive proven and effective treatment during the valuable window of opportunity that occurs early in the course of RA. It is during this window of opportunity that conventional treatments are most effective in preventing structural damage from RA. Another concern is that there is very little quality control in the dietary supplement industry which produces most herbal and alternative medicine preparations, and this creates the potential for many problems. *Always discuss with your doctor all therapies that you are contemplating, so that he or she can steer you away from those treatments with potential health risks.*

If complementary medicine is of interest to you, you will need to become engaged in gathering information and exploring your choices. Your physician may be willing to give you some guidance in choosing practitioners of a given treatment type, *if* he or she has had good experiences with complementary therapists. Always be honest with your doctor about treatments that you are considering. The best way to reduce your risk with unproven treatments or remedies is to *give your doctor the full story,* so he or she can follow you thoughtfully, with complete information. We cannot endorse or recommend any complementary therapies, but we will give you some guidelines to consider when making these decisions. You will also note that many treatments just make sense and are already well on their way into mainstream medicine.

This chapter will focus on some common therapies and disciplines. It is by no means an exhaustive list or assessment. Many of the approaches discussed below involve the use of dietary supplements; these will be discussed more fully in the next chapter. Since this is such an expansive area of interest, we will only be able to scratch the surface of treatment options.

AROMATHERAPY

We all know how certain aromas can help us to recall pleasant memories. Clearly, different scents can elicit different feelings and emotions. The fragrance industry has long understood how scent enhances attitude—"invigorating" morning shower soaps, "sensual" perfumes, "relaxing" bath salts, "power" cologne. Different scents affect smell receptors in your nose, which communicate with parts of your brain, creating different sensations and other effects. In recent years, researchers have discovered that some forms of aromatherapy may have healing properties. Ancient cultures recognized this thousands of years ago, when essential oils were used routinely in Greek, Roman, and Egyptian baths.

Aromatherapy most often uses essential oils (fragrant, highly volatile liquids produced by aromatic plants). They can be absorbed through the skin by way of massage, baths, compresses, facials, lotions, or ointments. Topical applications of several botanical oils are approved in Europe for relieving symptoms of RA. Some of these include camphor, eucalyptus, fir needle, pine needle, and rosemary. A study of arthritis patients in Korea (Kim et al., 2005) found that aromatherapy reduced pain and symptoms of depression. They used the following essential oils: lavender, marjoram, eucalyptus, rosemary, and peppermint. Many people find relief by applying essential oils in a warm compress wrapped around a painful joint. Another approach to aromatherapy uses a vaporizer, diffuser, or steam inhaler, so the person can inhale the aroma. A therapist can present you with different scents to determine which make you feel best. Also, there are many boutiques and spas where you can test essential oils on your own. Whether it is the relaxing scent of lavender or the familiar scent of vanilla that soothes you, you can have fun experimenting. Some essential oils commonly suggested for arthritis are rosemary, lavender, juniper, eucalyptus, cypress, pine, fir, and ginger. Remember that relaxing the mind and body helps to alleviate discomfort. Combining your favorite scent with a warm, soothing bath and calming music can help erase even the worst day.

Do not take any of these oils internally. Essential oils should be diluted in another oil before being applied to the skin. People with eczema or sensitive skin should test a small area first to see if the oils are irritating to them. Keep the oils away from your eyes. People with asthma should discuss inhalation methods with their physician *before* trying them.

AYURVEDA

Ayurveda has been a traditional medical system in India for more than three thousand years. It is a comprehensive system that is still widely practiced in India. Its focus is on mental, spiritual, and physical balance. It approaches illness through lifestyle modifications and a wide range of natural therapies. According to Ayurveda, people, like the universe, are made of five elements and the soul. The five elements in their biological form in the body are known as *doshas.* All functions of the body and mind are dependent on the state of these doshas. Different doshas are associated with different physical and personality characteristics. Customized treatments are based on these body-soul-energy "types." An individualized Ayurvedic program may include selected herbs and supplements, meditation, massage, exercise, oil pulling (see below), and purification regimens that may involve fasting, baths, and purging. In Ayurveda, diet, meditation, and healthy lifestyle practices promote physical and spiritual well-being. Be very cautious about unmonitored fasting or purging. The use of herbs or mixtures of various herbs and other substances is common practice. Some Ayurvedic herb mixtures are an area for concern, because there is no standard of quality control (see next chapter).

Yoga is a practice that stems from ancient Ayurvedic healing. It is often used as part of an Ayurvedic program to bring "union" to the body, mind, and spirit, but it can be performed without embracing the full Ayurvedic principles and practices. Read more about yoga as an exercise in Chapter 9.

Oil Pulling

Oil pulling is an Ayurvedic practice that dates back thousands of years. It involves using oils (historically sesame or sunflower oil) and swishing the oils around the mouth and teeth for 10 to 20 minutes and then expelling the oil. It is important not to swallow because it is believed that the oils draw out toxins, which purifies the body. Modern practitioners of this therapy more frequently use coconut oil. Ancient practitioners claimed that it cured many diseases and slowed aging! As unconventional as this seems, there is often wisdom in ancient practices. It is now apparent that oil pulling is highly effective in killing harmful bacteria in the mouth. Many oils, in particular coconut oil, have antibacterial and antifungal properties. The oils seep into the pockets and crevices around the teeth and draw out harmful bacteria and inflammatory toxins.

Modern researchers have studied the oral health benefits of oil pulling and found a reduction in plaque, gingivitis, and periodontal disease (Amith et al., 2007). Chapter 1 described the very strong link between periodontal disease and RA, and Chapter 5 reviewed research that demonstrated an improvement in RA symptoms with nonsurgical treatment of periodontal disease. This said, to date there have been no valid studies looking at the effect of oil pulling on RA. Certainly, this apparently harmless and age-old practice may be considered as an addition to your oral hygiene regimen. If you do start oil pulling with coconut oil, make sure that you spit the fluid into a container and dispose of it in a garbage can or wastepaper basket. Coconut oil is solid when it cools and can plug up your plumbing!

BODYWORK

Multiple forms and styles of bodywork can be used to relieve pain and tension. Massage is the most common. Massage is defined as the manual manipulation of soft tissues of the body by movements such as rubbing, kneading, rolling, or pressing for therapeutic purposes. Manipulation of the tissues increases blood flow and warmth. Common techniques include Swedish, sport, trigger point, and deep tissue massage; myofascial release; acupressure; and rolfing.

If you are having a severe flare, any bodywork may be too uncomfortable for you. If you are not too sore or swollen, however, and your physician agrees, massage may be an option to relieve symptoms. Most qualified massage therapists know several techniques and can adjust to your specific problems. *Always tell a massage therapist that you have RA* and which joints are involved. If you are not sure what type of massage to ask for, we would recommend Swedish massage, with its gentle stroking and kneading motions. This technique promotes circulation of blood and lymph and muscle relaxation without harsh motions, rigorous stretching or overzealous manipulation, which can hurt tender or vulnerable joints.

Acupressure, like acupuncture, uses acupoint locations on meridians (see "Chinese Medicine" below). Pressure on these points is incorporated into general massage. Japanese acupressure, called *shiatsu*, also focuses on acupoints. Shiatsu is usually practiced on a floor mat and can involve stretching, which may present a problem for those with significant RA.

Deep tissue massage techniques, myofascial release, and rolfing involve deeper massage, which helps many people but may be too aggressive for those with tender joints and muscles. More focused forms of bodywork include reflexology and craniosacral therapy. When you are having any sort of bodywork, *speak up right away if what you are experiencing is painful or uncomfortable in any way.*

ENERGY WORK

The basis of some alternative treatment relies in the notion that our bodies are an elaborate energy system with an intricate array of energy pathways. Many forms of therapy actually rely on the concept of energy movement—unblocking and stimulating energy channels in the body. It is believed that pain and other forms of illness are the result of a disruption in our body's energy pathways. Acupuncture is the best known of this type of therapy. However, many forms of bodywork, such as acupressure and meridian tapping, share the belief that our bodies have energy channels or meridians that can be positively manipulated for improvement in health.

It is postulated that our environment can adversely influence the flow of energy in our bodies. Our air is congested with microwaves, radio frequencies, cell phone signals, television signals, appliance and other electrical background noise, as well as countless other forms of electrical chatter. How this electrical noise affects health is unknown. On a happy note, our own planet, Earth, is still our largest source of energy. It has been proven that different geographical areas have more electrical "energy" than others. Electromagnetic hotspots like Delphi and Stonehenge have been tested and shown to have subtle differences in energy. Religious temples are often built near natural springs or in areas with high quartz levels—both known for electromagnetic energy and healing. Walking around your own home with a sensitive voltmeter will demonstrate variations from room to room!

A new therapy known as "earthing" stems from the observation that we are removed from the good electrical energy of the earth because we no longer have physical contact with the ground—instead, we have rubber soles, buildings, cars, and other things between us and the earth. Proponents suggest that connecting directly with the surface of the earth allows for the transfer of healing electrons from the earth to us. This transfer of energy into our bodies has purported anti-inflammatory benefits. The concept of healthful electromagnetic energies and healing is very exciting and requires more research. Keep an open mind but be wary of commercial aspects and any exaggerated claims.

BREATHING TECHNIQUES, BREATH THERAPY, OR BREATHWORK

It may seem unusual to consider breathing as a form of therapy, but breathing techniques are an important part of many complementary and alternative therapies (for example, massage, yoga, tai chi). Breathwork is closely linked to most forms of relaxation therapy. Many people believe that breathing exercises are so important that even alone they should be considered a form of therapy. During our busy lives, we mostly survive on quick, shallow breaths. Each time we yawn—an automatic, full, deep, diaphragmatic breath—our bodies are trying to tell us that we need something more. Breathing exercises are beneficial in bringing oxygen to tissues, promoting blood flow, and enhancing other physiologic functions, such as digestion.

Breath is the simplest technique that connects the body and mind. Deep breathing techniques have been shown to slow the heart rate, promote relaxation, improve emotional well-being, and enhance vitality. Focused breathing brings you clearly into the moment. Many people find that breathwork, particularly when combined with meditation, provides an opportunity for self-discovery or spiritual awakening. Sounds almost too good to be true, doesn't it?

Breathing techniques include three phases: inhalation, retention, and exhalation. Whenever you are feeling stressed, take a long, deep breath through your nose; make your diaphragm move rather than your chest as you breathe in; hold the air in a few seconds and breathe out slowly through your mouth. You will be surprised how even a few breaths make a difference. As aptly described by Andrew Weil, M.D., author and expert in breathwork, "the simplest and most powerful technique for protecting your health is absolutely free—and literally right under your nose."

CHINESE MEDICINE

Chinese medicine involves ancient principles and practices. The flow of vital life energy, called *Qi* (pronounced *chee*), is central to this discipline. Qi flows in channels called *meridians* that can become blocked, causing your Qi to be out of balance. When Qi is out of balance, illness can occur. Arthritis is believed to be a deficiency of Qi. The goal of Chinese medicine is to balance the yin and yang—opposing forces of nature. Chinese treatments used to balance the flow of Qi include acupuncture, acupressure, tai chi, Qi-gong, and Chinese herbs. Chinese herbs are generally mixtures of various herbs and other substances. The exact amount of active ingredients in a preparation is difficult to determine, due to variations in the quality of herbs. The potential for contaminants in mixtures is also a cause for concern (see "Chinese Herbs" in next chapter). Please refer to Chapter 9 for more on tai chi and Qi-gong.

Acupuncture

Acupuncture has become a very popular treatment in the United States in the past twenty years; it has been practiced in China for over three thousand years. Treatments are still given in traditional Chinese medicine environments, but they have also found their way into conventional treatment arenas such as pain clinics and physicians' offices. More than six thousand physicians (including this book's author) have completed the largest recognized acupuncture training program for medical doctors in the United States. Acupuncture involves inserting extremely thin solid needles at specific points (acupoints) along meridians to balance the flow of Qi and improve health, according to Chinese theory. How acupuncture works is not completely understood. Western researchers propose that acupuncture may stimulate deep sensory nerves that tell the body to release natural painkillers, called endorphins. Recent scientific study has shown that acupuncture decreases the body's production of inflammatory cytokines such as TNF, IL-1, and IL-6 (McDonald et al., 2013) (discussed in Chapters 1 and 14). Although human research reports are mixed, some studies have shown an improvement in pain and morning stiffness after acupuncture (Wang et al., 2008). To date, there has been no scientifically valid study that proves acupuncture can halt the damaging effects of RA. However, it if helps your symptoms and improves your general sense of well-being, it may make a good complement to your medical treatment.

Almost all Western practicing acupuncturists use disposable needles, and you should not accept treatment with reused needles. Definitely make the acupuncturist aware of any artificial joints you have, so he or she can use extra care. Treatments are not as painful as you might expect. You may feel a slight pinch that lasts a few seconds. Generally speaking, it takes at least four treatments before any improvement is seen. If you are fearful of needles, you may want to consider acupressure. *Acupressure* uses similar points but instead of needles uses firm sustained pressure to "open channels." Techniques of acupressure are often incorporated into massage or bodywork.

MUSIC AND SOUND THERAPY

It probably sounds silly to consider music a form of therapy. Intuitively, we all realize that different types of music elicit different feelings and emotions. Music and sound therapy involves the controlled use of sounds in the treatment of disorders. Soothing music can promote relaxation and relieve stress. Familiar environmental sounds, like a running stream, a waterfall, or birds singing, can calm the mind and create a positive mood. Researchers have suggested that soothing sounds can stimulate production of endorphins, the body's natural painkillers. As simple as these notions are, we infrequently take advantage of this simple remedy. So, take some time to listen to your favorite music today.

OTHER MIND-BODY THERAPIES: MINDFULNESS AND OTHERS

Although often considered to be in the realm of complementary medicine, the concept of the importance of the mind-body connection is thousands of years old and is represented in ancient Eastern and Western medical systems and religions. Eastern practices of yoga, tai chi, and Qi-gong rely heavily on mind-body practices. (See Chapter 9 for more on these exercises.) We have witnessed the power of mind-body healing for decades in the medical field, through the *placebo effect.* When people are given a **placebo** ("sugar pill") instead of a real medication in scientific studies, they often get an *objective* improvement in their symptoms. This is likely because they have a powerful belief that they will be better. There is a flip side of this coin: if you have a strong belief that a negative outcome will occur, the chances of its happening are greater. This self-fulfilling prophecy is called the *nocebo effect*—people can literally worry themselves sick. So, clearly, we need to harness the mind's powers for good and avoid hexing ourselves with negative predictions.

In the last several decades, Western societies have incorporated these concepts into mainstream medicine. *Biofeedback,* for example, is commonly used to help people cope with pain, anxiety, and tension. People learn skills that help them identify and respond to changes in their own bodies. In Chapter 7 we addressed some techniques that have been used to decrease stress, anxiety, and tension. You may wish to read that chapter again, to remind yourself of the benefits of meditation, biofeedback, imagery, progressive relaxation, and prayer.

In the 1990s the interest in alternative and complementary healing practices soared in the West. Conventionally trained physicians like Andrew Weil and Deepak Chopra opened the mainstream door for holistic, mind-body medicine. They have attempted to integrate traditional healing practices with recent breakthroughs in medical science. There is considerable scientific evidence demonstrating that how we feel—emotionally, mentally, and spiritually—can have profound effects on our body's physical health.

Many have written on healing as a natural internal power that we all possess. The practices by which we can enlist these inner resources are as variable as each individual who seeks discovery. They all have in common the basic principle of finding and developing your own inner capacity to get to a stronger, better place both mentally and physically.

One area that has been of particular popular interest has been the practice of *mindfulness*, which we touched on in Chapter 7. Rooted in Buddhism, mindfulness-based meditation involves focusing on experiences of that moment without judgment or emotional reaction. Often you cannot change what is occurring in the present moment, but you can change your relationship to that experience. By practicing mindfulness exercises, you develop an open awareness of internal and external events without being caught up in the details, thus reducing stress and its consequences. Incorporating these practices into day-to-day life nurtures awareness, insight, and compassion for yourself and others. Research suggests that mindfulness-based meditation may actually reduce inflammation (Rosenkranz et al., 2012).

Stepping around life's clutter to connect with your own innate intuition and strengths is a journey worth taking. Whether through traditional practices of faith and prayer or through less common spiritual exercise, tapping the power of your inner self will help you master your RA, as well as other challenges that life throws your way. Again, as powerful as these strategies may be, they work best as *an adjunct to* and not *a replacement for* conventional treatment.

NATUROPATHY

Naturopathy is medicine based on "natural remedies." Naturopathic medicine tends to focus on healthy lifestyle, nutrition, and exercise. Naturopathic treatments use herbs, supplements, counseling, massage, spinal manipulation, and diverse other approaches. A naturopathic physician (N.D.) usually undergoes a four-year training program. These practitioners may also specialize in other types of therapy, such as acupuncture or homeopathy. Many people appreciate the naturopathic emphasis on symptom control, exercise, and diet. A well-informed N.D. will encourage you to continue your conventional medications and to ask your rheumatologist about any herbs, supplements, or exercise recommendations. A naturopathic doctor who leads you away from conventional assessment and treatment should be avoided, since valuable treatment time can be lost.

SPA THERAPY, HYDROTHERAPY, AND BALNEOTHERAPY

Spas are one of the oldest forms of therapy for patients with arthritis. The practice of "taking the waters," bathing in and drinking mineral waters, is ancient and widespread. The question is whether the benefit is from the hydrotherapy or from the minerals and other natural ingredients in the natural spas. *Hydrotherapy* involves the therapeutic use of water, steam, or ice. Techniques include baths, compresses, showers, steam rooms, and whirlpools. Hydrotherapy alone has been shown to increase strength, balance, and range of motion of joints.

When hydrotherapy occurs in natural spas, hot springs, or mineral-rich waters, it is called *balneotherapy*. Whether natural spas confer additional benefits to hydrotherapy is not clear. Natural spa waters include many minerals, such as sodium, magnesium, calcium, iron, potassium, arsenic, lithium, manganese, bromine, and iodine. There has been speculation that everything from natural radon to Dead Sea bath salts have special "healing" properties. For example, there have been at least four studies that have shown benefits of Dead Sea salts for people with RA (www.deadsea-health.org). The Dead Sea salts have only 12 percent to 18 percent sodium chloride (NaCl), unlike ocean salt, which has 97 percent NaCl (Ma'or et al., 2006). The rest of the Dead Sea minerals are bromide, calcium, magnesium, and potassium. Trace amounts of these minerals are thought to be absorbed through the skin and into the cells. The importance of minerals is discussed in the nutrition chapter (Chapter 18). People with RA are often deficient in these minerals. It does give one pause for thought as we await further research.

HOMEOPATHY

The theory of homeopathy was developed by a German physician, Samuel Hahneman, in the 1700s. His theory was based on three principles: the "law of similars," the "minimum dose," and "the single remedy." Homeopathic theory holds that if a large amount of a substance causes specific symptoms in a healthy person, smaller amounts of the same substance can treat those same symptoms in someone who is ill. People are given minute amounts of substances that would *cause* illness if given in larger amounts. These highly diluted substances theoretically stimulate the body into a healing mode. Treatments are prescribed based on symptoms and personality rather than on the disease itself. Remedies are made from plants, minerals, and animals.

Very little research has been performed using this type of treatment for RA. There have been a few small trials with conflicting results, more showing benefit than not (Brien et al., 2011). These researchers suggest that the homeopathic practitioner's approach to complete exploration of each person's emotional, spiritual, and physical well-being may play a role in the improvement. There is no doubt that personal empowerment has tremendous potential in improving health outcomes. Professionals who practice homeopathy include naturopathic physicians (N.D.s), doctors of medicine (M.D.s), dentists, chiropractors, and acupuncturists.

GUIDELINES FOR EVALUATING UNPROVEN TREATMENTS

Educate yourself using trusted resources.

When considering alternative forms of therapy, avoid these:

- Treatments that offer *miracles* and *cures*. If it sounds too good to be true, it usually is.

- Treatments for which testimonials (patients' stories) are the only proof of the therapy's effectiveness.

- "Secret" treatments, ones which you are urged not to discuss with other people.

When choosing a practitioner:

- Personal references are always best. Start by asking your doctor, support group, or local Arthritis Foundation.

- The state or national credentialing organization for a particular discipline will sometimes provide referrals.

- Ask for credentials, certifications, or license information.

- Find out where the therapist trained.
- Find out how long the therapist has been in practice and where.
- Find out how much experience the therapist has had with RA patients.
- Do not pay in advance for a series of treatments; pay as you go.
- Make sure the therapist is willing to work with your conventional doctor.
- Speak with your regular doctor before you begin any form of treatment.

Be skeptical of practitioners who:
- Have a "conspiracy theory" for mainstream medicine and pharmaceutical companies; particularly avoid those who ask you to stop your medications.
- Sell high-priced supplements, particularly if the ingredients are not listed.
- Recommend computer-scored "nutrient deficiency tests" as a basis for selling you vitamins and supplements.
- Offer pseudoscientific diagnostic tests that cannot be obtained from your regular doctor.
- Engage in multiple-level marketing, that is, ask you to be a salesperson for them.
- Have moved several times in a short span of years.

FOR MORE INFORMATION

The Arthritis Foundation offers the following brochure free by e-mail or postal mail: "Complementary Therapies." To order from the Arthritis Foundation Store, call 1-800-283-7800 or go to www.afstore.org.

For further information on complementary and alternative medicine for practitioners and the public, contact NIH National Center for Complementary and Alternative Medicine (NCCAM), P.O. Box 8218, Silver Spring, Md. 20907-8218; toll-free 1-888-644-6226, 1-866-464-3615 (TTY). The NCCAM Clearinghouse is an NIH-funded information service for the public, to enhance understanding of complementary and alternative medicine. Its Web site is http://nccam.nih.gov.

Nutrition: Diets, Nutrients, and Nutritional Supplements

NUTRITION AND RA

The idea that a person can completely control rheumatoid arthritis (RA) by dietary means is very compelling to most people. It certainly would be exciting if we could achieve a complete remission through dietary manipulation and "natural" means. Unfortunately, at this time there is no diet *proven* to halt the progression of RA—but that doesn't mean that dietary manipulations have no potential benefits in the management of RA. Modern conventional medicine has not had a strong presence in the efforts to find dietary measures to diminish the symptoms of RA or other chronic conditions. The medical community's efforts have largely been focused on the pharmacologic approach to illness. It didn't start that way. Even Hippocrates, the ancient Greek physician who is considered the father of Western medicine, relied heavily on "the healing power of nature" (or *vis medicatrix naturae* in Latin). In about 400 BC, he declared, "Let food be thy medicine and medicine be thy food."

We are grateful that in recent decades dedicated individuals have pursued a dietary approach to wellness with scientific precision as well as passion. These holistic experts have seen benefits in their dietary practices and have been able to freely disseminate their ideas with the advent of the Internet. Broad public interest in nutrition has prompted the attention of Western researchers as well as mainstream clinicians. Unfortunately, dietary research is very challenging to perform because of the many variables that impinge on any study, including environmental differences, cultural differences, lifestyle factors, and ongoing medical management. Also, funding by industry is limited, because there are no products to patent, and that is the usual motivation for funding such research. Despite this, there are many sources that promote certain foods as *functional foods*. These are foods that are thought to contain biologically active components that enhance health and presumably reduce illness. Some research suggests *avoidance* of specific foods as an approach to controlling RA. In some instances, there is scientific evidence suggesting benefit for a given approach, but often there is just conjecture.

This chapter starts with a discussion of the critical importance of weight management in RA then looks at specific foods and food groups and what we know about them *as they relate to RA*. We will focus on three basic premises and investigate them:

1. Some foods and food patterns are likely unhealthy for *all* people, including, for our purposes, people with RA; avoiding these foods is recommended.

2. Some foods and food groups may aggravate arthritis in *specific* individuals with specific food sensitivities; a trial of elimination may be worth considering, with your doctor's consent.

3. Some foods may be beneficial in reducing the symptoms of RA by virtue of their own healthful constituents; incorporating these foods into your diet is advisable.

We will look at some special diets that may influence RA and make some common sense recommendations that will be appropriate for *most* individuals with RA. Finally, we will look at how the most popular dietary supplements, which include vitamins and minerals, herbs, and other supplements, relate to RA.

Please remember that *only* the disease-modifying antirheumatic drugs (**DMARDs**) and **biologics** have been *proven* to halt the progression of rheumatoid arthritis. First and foremost, the inflammation of RA must be controlled, to prevent damage to the joints. Controlling RA inflammation nearly always involves the use of medications. If changing dietary habits proves highly effective, your doctor can always reduce your medications at a later time when your condition is better.

The following information is provided to help you make sense of the tremendous amount of data and persuasion you will be exposed to by commercial interests, Internet searches, and well-meaning friends. Some of this practical dietary information is well proven and can be safely incorporated into your daily meal planning, while some is less well studied and is offered with the suggestion that you "stay tuned." You will notice that there will be conflicting information and claims. There are many schools of thought regarding what constitutes a healthful diet in general. The same is true of dietary recommendations for people with RA. Any supplementation or significant dietary change should be discussed thoroughly with your physician. Until we have more scientific information on dietary manipulation and its effects on RA, we suggest that you follow a healthy, balanced diet that promotes a healthy weight.

THE IMPORTANCE OF WEIGHT MANAGEMENT IN RA

A person's diet must be both well balanced and nutritious to maintain energy stores and to keep muscles functioning well enough to protect the joints. Ideally, the number of calories you consume each day will maintain your healthy body weight. In some people with very active RA, weight loss may be a problem. More commonly, however, weight gain is the problem. There are several reasons for this. Taking medications that increase appetite (for example, corticosteroids) can result in weight gain. In addition, many people with RA have muscle loss, which decreases the body's metabolic rate; the body doesn't burn as many calories, so it stores them instead. Arthritis often limits physical activity, also resulting in decreased calorie use.

Lastly, when inflammation is brought under control, the body needs fewer calories. Studies have shown that when rheumatoid inflammation is very active, the body burns 12 percent more calories than when inflammation is under control (Roubenoff et al., 1994). Feeding inflammation requires considerable energy, and so, when less energy is required, caloric needs drop. Therefore, it is very common for people to gain weight as their arthritis improves. Many people often wrongly blame their medications for weight gain when it is really just a function of getting better and needing fewer calories. The weight gain is actually a good sign for these people. However, to then maintain a healthy weight, the person needs either to reduce caloric intake or expend more energy in the form of physical activity. Also exercise will help you to regain muscle that has been lost and this will increase your metabolic rate. (Strengthening exercises are best for building muscle mass; a safe approach to exercising with RA is described in Chapters 9 and 10.)

Although achieving and maintaining a healthy weight is particularly challenging in people with RA, it couldn't be more important. There are now considerable data that suggest that obesity increases the risk of developing RA. Some researchers believe that the "obesity epidemic" has contributed to the recent rise in the incidence of RA (Crowson et al., 2013). Further research indicates that being overweight also increases the severity of RA and makes it harder to get inflammation under control. This may be because some inflammatory cytokines are actually stored inside fat cells. Consequently, these cytokines are called *adipokines* because they are produced by adipose (fat) tissue. So, the more of these cells that you have, the more inflammatory cytokines you produce. Our bodies have two forms of fat, called white adipose tissue and brown adipose tissue. Excessive accumulation of white adipose tissue in the midsection, or "belly fat," appears to produce the most inflammatory adipokines. It's a relief to know that stored abdominal fat is usually the first to be lost.

So how do you know how many calories to eat to maintain or to lose weight? There are numerous free calorie calculators available on the Internet (put "calorie calculator" into your search browser). You will fill in your age, current weight, goal weight, height, gender, and activity level. This will give you a good place to start. A dietician or nutritionist will also be able to give you that information. If you are gaining weight, you'll need to cut back calories. Replacing high-fat and sugar rich foods with fiber rich foods will increase your sense of fullness while decreasing calories. Fiber also slows the absorption of sugar and limits insulin surges that contribute to weight gain (more on that process below).

Next, we will discuss the different food groups individually and review the existing research results, both positive and negative, as they relate to RA. Remember, the story of nutrition and RA is a work in progress, and you will need to remain open to new ideas and research as this story evolves.

SPECIFIC FOOD GROUPS AND RA

Fats and Oils

Over the past twenty years, our society has been obsessed with eliminating fat from our diets in an effort to manage weight and reduce heart disease. Simply replacing fat calories with carbohydrate calories has been detrimental in our fight against obesity. Also, we have learned that inflammation may well be the major culprit in heart disease, and we are beginning to understand that high carbohydrate intake may have an effect on our intestinal bacteria and on inflammation. In addition to this, healthful fats are necessary in our diet. Fats supply nutrients called essential fatty acids and are important for absorption of fat-soluble vitamins A, D, E, and K. So, we are beginning to reassess our previous assumptions that all fats are bad for us. There are three major classes of fats: saturated fats, monounsaturated fats, and polyunsaturated fats. Polyunsaturated fats are composed of fatty acids that can be further classified as either omega-3 fatty acids or omega-6 fatty acids. Because our bodies do not have the necessary enzymes to create these fatty acids, they are referred to as *essential fatty acids*.

Saturated fats are found in animal fat, dairy products, and some vegetable oils, such as coconut and palm oil. It has been taught that these fats can be harmful if consumed in excess, because they can increase cholesterol and the risk of heart disease. However, it appears that all saturated fats are not created equal! Coconut oil, for instance, may actually have health *benefits*. Studies have shown a low incidence of heart disease in countries that have coconut oil as their primary fat. Researchers in India (Sircar and Kansra, 1998) have even shown that there has been an increase in heart disease as people replaced coconut oil with other vegetable oils. Coconut oil is made up of a unique group of fat molecules called *medium-chain fatty acids*. There is growing evidence that these molecules may have antibacterial, antifungal, and antiviral capacity. This oil may have immune system–enhancing elements, making it a very good choice for people with RA. (Also read about "oil pulling" in Chapter 17.) In addition, coconut oil may be the best oil for high-heat cooking, since this fat does not change molecular structure at high temperatures.

Since the 1950s there has been a strong push to replace saturated fats with more "heart friendly" polyunsaturated fats. The wisdom of that directive has been widely questioned, as you will read below. However, polyunsaturated fatty acids (PUFAs) are essential for human health. PUFAs are composed of two families of essential fatty acids: omega-3 and omega-6. Our bodies are incapable of making these essential nutrients, so we must include both in our diets. Omega-3 fatty acids have known health benefits. They are present in certain fish and certain plant seeds. Two omega-3 fatty acids, eicosapentaenoic acid (EPA) and docosahexaenoic acid (DHA), both found in fish oil, have been studied closely; numerous studies show that consuming them decreases joint swelling and pain and morning stiffness (Miles and Calder, 2012). EPA and DHA have also been shown to reduce heart disease by decreasing inflammation, blood clot formation, triglycerides, blood pressure, and the build up of atherosclerosis. Before the 1940s, we ingested more omega-3 fatty acids in the form of cod liver oil, which was commonly used to supplement vitamin D and vitamin A. You will read below about supplements and other sources of omega-3 oil. Today's Western diets are very deficient in all omega-3 fatty acids.

Most vegetable oils have high amounts of omega-6 fatty acids. If consumed in amounts *exceeding* the intake of omega-3 fatty acids, they actually fuel inflammation. This is the major problem with the Western cultural shift to polyunsaturated fats. These oils are taken in overabundance in the American diet. There is considerable research on the *omega-6:omega-3 ratio* and its effect on health. Oils generally contain a mix of saturated, monounsaturated, and polyunsaturated fatty acids. Oils that have mostly omega-6 fatty acids include corn oil, sunflower oil, and safflower oil, all commonly used in fried and processed foods. In some Western diets, the dietary ratio of omega-6 to omega-3 can exceed 20:1. Dietary historians suggest that our Stone Age ancestors had a ratio closer to 1:1. (Read more in the section on ancestral diets, below.) Research has shown that lowering the omega-6:omega-3 ratio can have benefits for several chronic diseases (Simopoulos, 2008). For instance, a dietary intake ratio of 2–3:1 had effects of suppressing inflammation in RA.

In addition to the omega-6:omega-3 ratio, PUFAs present another problem. They are very unstable when subjected to heat and even light. These fat molecules become oxidized and damaged. The body cannot utilize these transformed fats. When ingested in large amounts, these damaged fats become incorporated into our cell membranes making them more fragile and prone to injury. So cooking with these oils is not the best choice.

Foods high in *trans fatty acids* tend to raise LDL ("bad") cholesterol and lower HDL ("good" cholesterol). Trans fat can only be found in unsaturated fats. These foods include those high in partially hydrogenated vegetable oils, like shortenings. Partial hydrogenation (a chemical change) was executed on these oils to increase shelf life. Mandatory food labeling of trans fat content, made law in 2003, forced the oil industry to address this health concern. Commercially fried fast foods, processed snack foods, and some bakery goods use these fats in high amounts. Further regulations are likely forthcoming. Until then, these foods should be avoided.

Monounsaturated fats are considered for the most part to be "good" fats. Foods with mostly monounsaturated fatty acids (MUFAs) include nuts, avocado, and olive oil. Using these oils in place of the omega-6-rich vegetable oils helps to maintain a more healthful omega-6:omega-3 ratio. This is one of the fundamental elements of the Mediterranean diets that we will discuss later. These oils appear best for sautéeing and low-heat cooking. At *very* high heat, these fats can be damaged, but not to the degree of polyunsaturated fats. Saturated fats, such as coconut oil, are best for high temperature cooking since they are the most stable.

Consuming a diet high in omega-3 fatty acids will reduce inflammation. The best way to get the value of fish oils is to increase the amount of oily fish in your diet. Types of oily fish include sardines, salmon, mackerel, herring, swordfish, snapper, anchovy, fresh tuna, and lake trout. In food preparation, using oils that promote a more healthful balance of omega-3 compared to omega-6 fatty acids, such as coconut oil and olive oil, will further reduce inflammation. Trying to improve the omega-3 over omega-6 balance appears to be a worthy endeavor.

Researchers disagree on the role of fat in RA. As mentioned above, many believe that the type of fat intake and the other food groups eaten are the most important factors that contribute to inflammation. Some researchers, however, suggest that low-fat diets may ease the symptoms of RA (Lucas et al., 1981). One study recommended reducing dietary fat content to 10 percent and adopting a vegan diet (McDougall et al., 2002; more below). It should be noted that the very low fat diets studied were also vegetarian for the most part. Although there are differences in professional opinion, all agree that reducing reliance on fried and processed foods and reducing trans fats is very important for general health and for RA.

While we wait for more definitive answers about the influence of fat intake on RA, there are good sense recommendations that we can make. Check all ingredient labels for the type and grams of fat contained. Choose omega-3-rich fish. Choose lean meats (skinless poultry, bison). Consider low-fat toppings, such as salsa, lemon juice, and herbs. Use low-fat cooking methods. Choose sliced turkey or chicken breast over high-fat luncheon meats.

Sugar

Sugars occur naturally in nutrient-rich foods such as milk, fruits, and some vegetables. Added sugar, however, is a large source of "empty" (not nutritional) calories for many Americans. Added sugar is often present in the bread and cereal group and is used in the processing of fruits canned in syrups. Soft drinks have enormous sugar content. Adding sugar to low-fat or no-fat foods is a common practice of the food industry, to improve the taste of these foods. For proof of this practice, compare the labels of skim milk to whole milk. Foods that are high in sugar (or high in carbohydrates that break down rapidly into sugar) are called *high-glycemic foods*. The *glycemic index (GI)* is a measure of how quickly your blood sugar increases after eating a specific food. A maximum GI would be a rating of 100. There are several resources that can tell you which foods raise glucose (sugar) levels the most (see end of chapter for more information). The following are a few examples:

High GI, >70: white rice, white bread, corn flakes, and watermelon

Medium GI, 56–69: spaghetti, plain bagel, raisins, and brown rice

Low GI <55: meat, fish, nuts, most vegetables, and legumes

It is now clear that high-glycemic foods not only contribute to obesity but also contribute to inflammation. We spoke above about how obesity can cause inflammation because white fat tissue produces cytokines called adipokines that cause inflammatory changes as well as cardiovascular disease. High sugar intake promotes obesity by causing surges of insulin, which directs our bodies to store fat. When glucose (sugar) levels rise in the blood, our bodies make insulin in an effort to bring the blood levels of glucose down. Insulin acts like a key to open the fat cell for storage of that extra energy as fat. If there is no glucose available, there is no insulin, and fat cannot be stored. This is why low carbohydrate/high fat diets are successful for fat loss, even though they are high in calories. *Fat storage requires insulin.* Insulin surges also make us crave more carbohydrates, and it becomes a vicious cycle. Chronically eating high glycemic meals causes levels of insulin to soar. At times, this can cause a *reactive hypoglycemia*, which is actually *low* blood sugar. In order to protect itself, the brain provokes a stress response to produce glucose. It also produces adrenalin and other stress hormones that increase inflammation.

High-glycemic diets cause inflammation by another mechanism: feeding unhealthy bacteria. Sugars and processed carbohydrates are very dense in carbohydrate concentration; they are said to have a high *carbohydrate density* (Spreadbury, 2012). They are easy to digest, and when they are digested, they flood the bowel with a high concentration of glucose. Unfortunately, these high levels of sugar feed the inflammatory bacteria in the bowel. These unhealthy bacteria then compete with and may prevail over the healthy bowel bacteria. As described in Chapter 1, the imbalance in bowel bacteria can lead to inflammation.

It appears that unhealthy bacteria in our mouths also have a sweet tooth (pardon the pun). There is evidence that when sugars, flours, and other refined carbohydrates are introduced into the diets of indigenous people unaccustomed to them, the people's dental health declines and periodontal disease escalates. Periodontal disease is caused by the growth of these pathologic (bad) bacteria, particularly *Porphyromonas gingivalis*. You will remember from Chapter 1 the growing evidence that periodontal disease and its associated bacteria have been linked to the development of RA. Unfortunately, when we ingest these carbohydrates, we are feeding more than just our own bodies!

Avoidance of sugars and refined carbohydrates does not mean that you can't enjoy sweet foods. Whole fruits are not as dense in carbohydrates as refined sugar because they have fibrous cell walls throughout the intact fruit. This limits the release of sugar into the bowel. The natural fiber also slows the absorption of the sugar, which improves blood glucose levels and prevents the surges of insulin that promote the storage of fat and subsequent weight gain. In fruit juices, however, these fibrous cell walls have been broken down in processing and become *carbohydrate dense.* This is why most fruits have a medium glycemic index but fruit juice has a high GI.

People often inquire about the safety of artificial sweeteners. There is a growing concern that these substances may harbor risks that we do not fully comprehend. We suggest sticking with whole fruit as the treat of choice. However, there are two sweeteners that do not raise blood sugar and are found in nature. Natural Stevia, a South American herb, was approved in the United States as a food supplement in 2008. Less readily available is the powder of a fruit called Luo Han Guo. This fruit (actually in the gourd family) originally comes from the mountains of China, where it has been taken for centuries as a medicinal herb.

Bread, Cereals, Rice, and Pasta

There is no doubt that carbohydrates are an excellent source of energy. They can also be an excellent source of fiber, particularly if they are made with *whole grain*. Whole-grain products are made from the entire kernel of a grain, which is in fact a mature seed. A kernel of corn, wheat, rice, or other grain consists of three seed parts: bran, germ, and endoderm. In the nutrition world, "whole grain" actually means that the food product must contain all three parts of the grain: the bran (the hard protective layer of the grain), the germ (the embryo of the seed), and the endoderm (the starchy nutrition for the seed) in the proportions that exist in nature. The food product can be whole, split, cracked, or ground. Different grains have different nutrients, so eating a variety of whole grains will provide a range of nutrients. These nutrients include protein, fiber, iron, magnesium, phosphorus, zinc, copper, manganese, selenium, and B vitamins.

Refined grains have been milled (ground into flour) so that only the starchy endosperm remains. Refining grains results in a significant reduction in nutrients. Some refined grains are *enriched*, meaning that some of the vitamins and minerals are added back. Fiber, however, cannot be added back. Refined carbohydrates have a high glycemic index and in the body act more like sugar, with all the implications of sugar as it relates to obesity and inflammation. Whole grain foods *still* raise blood glucose and surge insulin levels, although not as significantly as refined grains do.

Knowing if a food product is truly "whole grain" is more challenging than one would think, due to the creativity of the marketing industry. Buzzwords like "multigrain," "100% wheat," and "contains whole grain" can be deceiving. Read the ingredient list on the food label. The whole grain should be the first ingredient listed. Examples of whole grains include: whole wheat, whole oats, oatmeal, whole-grain corn, popcorn, brown rice, wild rice, quinoa, whole-grain barley, buckwheat, bulgur, and whole rye. The Harvard School of Public Health recommends a helpful calculation. They suggest using a *carb-to-fiber ratio* of 10:1. The product should contain one gram of fiber for every 10 grams of total carbohydrate on the food label. That is about the same ratio as an unprocessed grain. For example, if a food label reveals that the food has 25 grams of total carbohydrate, divide that number by 10. The fiber content should be at least 2.5 mg. If it contains less than that, it either isn't whole grain or has additional sugar or artificial sweeteners added.

Whole grains are considered to be a very important source of fiber. High-fiber carbohydrates are made of two forms of fiber: soluble and insoluble. Soluble fiber dissolves in water while insoluble fiber does not. Soluble fiber can help lower cholesterol by binding to fats in your food and reducing fat absorption. It also regulates blood sugar by limiting the absorption of sugar. Some examples of soluble fiber–containing foods are oats, some fruits and vegetables, beans, and barley. Insoluble fiber promotes proper bowel function by adding bulk to the stool. In the large bowel, fiber assists fermentation, thus promoting the growth of beneficial bacteria. Sources of insoluble fiber include whole wheat, bran, and some vegetables. Most people do not consume enough fiber. The National Fiber Council recommends 32 grams of fiber per day. The average American consumes less than half of that.

Despite the beneficial elements of whole grains, there are some people who cannot tolerate specific components of grains. There are numerous potential causes of this intolerance. The most commonly recognized intolerance is a reaction to *gluten*. Glutens are proteins found in many grains, including wheat, rye, barley, and some other grains. There are several forms of *gluten intolerance*. The most severe of these is *celiac disease*. People with celiac disease, like people with RA, appear to have a genetic predisposition to the condition. Two genes, HLA-DQ2 and HLA-DQ8, appear to put people at risk; but, as with RA, not everyone with celiac disease has these genes. People with the at-risk genetic footprint react against a gluten protein called *gliadin*. An enzyme in the digestive tract called *tissue transglutaminase* breaks down gliadin, modifying it. The immune system, led by T cells, reacts against the protein and also against the small bowel, causing damage. Bloating, diarrhea, and malnutrition can result. The definitive way to diagnose celiac disease is by small bowel biopsy. Celiac disease occurs in about 1 percent of the population.

Celiac disease may be only the tip of the iceberg. Gluten intolerance *without* celiac disease appears to be much more common; the exact prevalence is unknown. People who are sensitive to gluten can experience a broad range of symptoms that you might not recognize as food related. Some of these are fatigue, headache, mental fogginess, and joint pain. Can you be tested to see if this is an issue for you? Yes and no. Yes, there are blood tests. Some blood tests are geared to look for evidence of damage to the gut: *anti-transglutaminase antibodies* and *endomysial antibodies*. These are likely to be present if you have true celiac disease, with its resultant damage to the GI tract. Small bowel biopsy by endoscopy is the only definitive diagnostic test, because some people with known celiac disease have normal blood tests. Then, there are tests that look for an immune reactivity against the gluten protein gliadin: *anti-gliadin antibody IgG* and *anti-gliadin antibody IgM*. Most people with celiac disease have these antibodies but some do not. These tests can also be positive in people who have gluten sensitivity without celiac disease (gut involvement). The above-mentioned tests are all readily available. The problem is that some people have these antibodies without any symptoms that *they are aware of*, and the significance of this is unclear.

Also, many people without gliadin antibodies have known and proven intolerance to grains. This is easier to explain. They may be reacting against another protein in the grain that is not the gluten protein, gliadin. One such protein that is getting more attention recently is *wheat germ agglutinin* (WGA), which is not in the gluten family but in the *lectin* family. (You will read more about lectins under legumes.) There are commercial tests available to look for reactivity against other grain proteins, including the lectin, WGA. However, this testing is not widely available or may not be covered by some insurers at the time of this writing. This, however, is an area of growing interest in the medical field, so things should change.

To summarize, it is possible to have:

- biopsy-proven celiac disease with the *presence* of gluten antibodies

- biopsy-proven celiac disease with the *absence* of gluten antibodies

- the presence of gluten antibodies *without* biopsy-proven celiac disease but *with* gluten intolerance symptoms

- the absence of gluten antibodies *with* grain intolerance symptoms due to intolerance to other grain proteins that are not gluten

- the presence of gluten antibodies *without* any known symptoms

If this weren't confusing enough, there are also individuals who have a *true allergy* to some grain proteins, most notably in wheat. Their symptoms are more allergic in nature, as would be expected. The can include itchy rash, hives, itchy eyes, nasal congestion, and asthma. Testing for true allergy and not sensitivity or intolerance involves more traditional allergy testing. Grain allergies can be identified by specific blood tests or skin tests administered by an allergist.

And lastly, as we mentioned under the above section on sugar, high-glycemic foods (including refined grains) can cause inflammation for several reasons that have nothing to do with gluten or grain protein intolerance or allergy.

Because many individuals' arthritis symptoms are aggravated by grains, people with RA may wonder if an attempt at eliminating grains from their diet for a short period is reasonable. There are many experts who believe that grains or their constituents may provoke inflammation. Some physicians recommend a trial of a grain-free/gluten-free or grain-free/sugar-free diet to find out if it helps an individual patient with inflammatory conditions. (More below under special diets.) This would be something you should discuss with your doctor. When attempting restrictive diets such as gluten-free, grain-free, or low-glycemic diets, people often unwittingly reduce their intake of beneficial nutrients, like fiber. It is important to try to get at least 32 grams of fiber per day in your meals. If trying a restricted diet, you will need to consider other sources of fiber. In addition to whole grain, fiber can be found in vegetables, fruits, and legumes, as well as in the form of supplements such as psyllium. Some non-grain high-fiber foods to consider in these situations are cauliflower, green beans, flax seed, and peas.

Fermented Foods

We have already looked at the importance of colonizing the gastrointestinal tract with good bacteria. Good intestinal bacteria assist in the digestion of food and the synthesis and absorption of important vitamins and other nutrients. There is also compelling evidence that healthy bowel bacteria support a healthy immune system. Many ancient cultures added fermented foods, like raw yogurt, fermented milk, kefir, and miso, to their diets to promote good health. Unfortunately, today's highly processed commercial forms of yogurt often contain added sugar or sugar substitutes. Also, stringent pasteurization processes in the United States can reduce the number of beneficial bacteria in yogurt. As a matter of fact, yogurts in the United States are not even required to contain live cultures! Consider trying kefir, a form of fermented milk inoculated with kefir grains. If you are creative, you can make homemade cultured milk, rice milk, and coconut milk using kefir cultures from your local health food store. Try adding more fermented foods like sauerkraut, miso, kimchi, and sour pickles to your diet to support a healthy bacterial balance in your intestines.

Vegetables

All experts and nutritionists agree on the value of vegetables for general health and for inflammatory conditions. Vegetables provide **antioxidants,** such as vitamins A, C, and E, carotenes, and flavonoids. Antioxidants have been shown to reduce some of the damage that can be caused by inflammation. Vegetables are also rich in B vitamins, vitamin K, and minerals, such as potassium, phosphorus, iron, magnesium, calcium, zinc, selenium, copper, and manganese. Vegetables, particularly when eaten raw, are also important sources of fiber, enzymes, and the probiotic bacteria that help support a healthy balance of bowel bacteria. Raw organic cabbage is particularly high in probiotics. Cooking vegetables deactivates some enzymes and reduces the antioxidant levels, so eating a good share of your vegetables raw makes good sense.

Different vegetables supply different amounts and types of nutrients. Dark green leafy vegetables, orange vegetables (carrots, pumpkin), and tomatoes pack plenty of vitamin A. Broccoli, peppers, tomatoes, cabbage, potatoes, and leafy greens are good sources of vitamin C. Vitamin E is found in dark leafy vegetables. Okra, peas, and yellow corn provide B vitamins. Dark green leafy vegetables, broccoli, and asparagus are ready sources of folic acid. White and sweet potatoes are excellent sources of potassium. Vegetables with the deepest, brightest colors usually are the most nutritious, and choosing foods with different colors will also give you a variety of food pigments. Pigments contain phytochemicals, which can act as antioxidants. Capers, dill, red onion, and kale are rich in the flavonoid quercetin. Kale, turnip greens, dandelion, spinach, and swiss chard provide the carotenoid lutein. Lycopene is a carotenoid found in red tomatoes. Carrots, winter squash, tomatoes, green beans, and cilantro have high levels of alpha-carotene. Beta-carotene can be found in butternut squash, carrots, orange bell peppers, and pumpkins. The list of beneficial nutrients is exhaustive and increasing. Consuming a variety of antioxidants is beneficial.

Because vegetables (and fruits) are a prime source of potassium, this is a good place to discuss the *sodium:potassium ratio* and its significance. It has been estimated that in the Paleolithic era, people consumed 11,000 mg of potassium and 700 mg of sodium daily (Eaton et al., 1985). Today, the average American consumes over 3000 mg of sodium and about 2600 mg of potassium. The dominance of sodium over potassium in our diets has been linked to heart disease. A study by the Centers for Disease Control found that consumption of food with a sodium:potassium ratio of <1 was protective against heart disease (Yang et al., 2011). For example, consuming 1000 mg of sodium and 1200 mg of potassium would equate to a ratio less than one, since you are eating less sodium than potassium. It has been hypothesized that this reduction in heart disease risk may be due to decreased inflammation. Although there have been no formal trials specifically looking at manipulating the sodium:potassium ratio in regard to RA, there was a small study that looked at potassium supplementation in a group of people with RA with low potassium levels. In this small study, supplementation with potassium resulted in a significant reduction in pain in the potassium treated group (Rastmanesh, 2008). Although there has been at least one study that looked at potassium intake and its possible effects on RA, we do not suggest taking extra potassium to treat RA, because this can be dangerous in some people. Rather, we suggest having a diet rich in vegetables and fruits and limited in sodium-rich processed foods; this will support a healthy ratio. Later, we will discuss ancestral-type diets. Because these diets favor potassium-rich fruits and vegetables, the potassium intake in such diets can exceed 9000 mg. Sodium intake drops to about 726 mg per day with the removal of processed foods, which also supports a healthy ratio (Cordain, 2002a). Always discuss your diet with your doctor, particularly if you have other health issues, such as heart, liver, or kidney ailments.

Fruits

Like vegetables, fruits are important sources of vitamins, minerals, and antioxidants. Fruits, particularly unpeeled and raw, are an excellent source of fiber. Orange-colored fruits (mango, cantaloupe, apricots, peaches) are high in vitamin A and other antioxidant carotenoids. Citrus fruits, kiwi, strawberries, and cantaloupe are loaded with vitamin C. Fruits, with their many colorful varieties, are rich in pigments and vary in types of antioxidants. Here is a short list of some fruits and their predominant pigment: blueberry, black raspberry, concord grape (anthocyanin); red grape skin (resveratrol); citrus (hesperidin); red apple, red grapes (quercetin). As with vegetables, deeply pigmented fruits appear to have a particularly high antioxidant capacity. Consider a wide mix of berries, cherries, grapes, plums, apples, peaches, guava, mango, citrus, pomegranate, and other colorful fruits. Dried fruits maintain most of the nutrient value of fresh fruit and remain an excellent source of fiber. Watch out for the added sugar; also with so much water removed from dried fruits, a serving will naturally contain much more sugar than a serving of the whole fruit.

Plan a diet with various colors of fruits in order to get a broad range of pigments and antioxidants. Choose fresh, whole fruits. Canned fruits are often laden with extra sugar. Fruit juices usually go through a pasteurization process that can destroy some vitamins and minerals. With the fiber removed, the food value of juice is decreased and the effect on blood sugar and insulin is increased. Also, additional sugar is frequently added to fruit juices. Even whole fruit increases blood sugar to some degree. Different fruits raise blood sugar by different degrees, though. Trying to choose most of your fruits from the low-glycemic category will help manage your sugar levels and help with weight control. Fruits with GI scores of less than 55 are digested slowly and produce a more gradual increase in sugar. They will not spike insulin levels *as much* as high-GI fruits. Although there is a range in each fruit category, examples of some fruit types that fall below 55 are apples, pears, oranges, peaches, cherries, grapes, and strawberries. Some high-GI fruits (GI greater than 70) are watermelon, dates, and canned fruits.

Meat, Poultry, Fish, and Eggs

This group of foods provides needed proteins, B vitamins, iron, and zinc. As we discussed above, choosing fish as a dietary mainstay is particularly recommended for people with RA, given the known benefit of omega-3 oils in decreasing inflammation. Furthermore, a Swedish study (DiGiuseppe et al., 2013) revealed that long-term intake of a diet rich in salmon and other fatty fish resulted in a 50 percent reduction in risk of developing RA. Poultry with the skin removed makes a convenient choice for weekly meal planning. Although red meat is an excellent source of protein and iron, a British study reported that people who had the *highest* consumption of red meat were two times more likely to develop RA (Pattison et al., 2004a). Limiting red meat appears to make sense for this and other health reasons. Of course, choose leaner cuts of beef, pork, and veal and trim away all visible fat. When you do eat red meat, consider eating organic, grass-fed, pasture-raised beef, which is leaner and has other possible advantages over grain-fed beef. Buying free-range poultry and eggs also improves food quality. Broil or roast meats rather than frying them.

Legumes

Legumes and nuts constitute the other major source of protein for humans. Well known legumes include kidney beans, pinto beans, and lentils. Legumes commonly thought of as other food types include peanuts (not really a nut), peas and green beans (not really vegetables), and soy (not really a grain). Legumes are among the best non-animal proteins and are critical in many vegetarian diets. They are also high in fiber, phytonutrients, folate, iron, zinc, calcium, and magnesium.

Some people can have difficulties digesting legumes. Legumes are gluten free but often contain *lectins*. Lectins, proteins that are found in many food groups, can be detrimental to health for some sensitive individuals. But not all lectins are harmful nor are they always present in high enough levels to be harmful. The levels of potentially troubling lectins appear to be highest in grains, legumes, and dairy. Lectins are very sticky molecules that can bind to human tissues, including the intestinal lining. It is thought that lectins can damage the intestinal wall and lead to "leaky gut" syndrome, which can lead to inflammation. ("Leaky gut" is discussed in Chapter 1.) Why doesn't everyone have problems then? Some people may react more due to their genetics. Others may react because their bowel has been previously injured by some other cause, leaving the lining unguarded. People who have a healthy balance of gut bacteria to begin with appear to have a protective barrier to prevent lectins from sticking. These beneficial bacteria produce *mucin* and *secretory IgA*. Mucin binds to lectins preventing them from sticking to the intestinal wall. Secretory IgA also binds to lectins, preventing them from wreaking havoc with the bowel lining. This is another example of the importance of healthy balance of bowel bacteria.

Legumes also contain *phytates*, compounds that can bind to dietary minerals and slow their absorption. A legume's phytate and lectin levels can be reduced to some extent by prolonged soaking, slow cooking, sprouting, and fermenting. Keeping a food journal will help you determine if legumes are creating any problems for you.

Nuts and Seeds

Nuts, including almonds, Brazil nuts, hazel nuts, macadamia nuts, pecans, pine nuts, pistachios, and macadamia nuts, are an excellent source of protein, fiber, and other nutrients. Nuts vary in the types of nutrients they contain. Walnuts are high in alpha-linolenic acid (ALA), an omega-3 acid that we will discuss below. Almonds are excellent sources of vitamin E, potassium, magnesium, and other antioxidants. Cashews contain oleic acid, the same fat that is in olive oil, as well as vitamin K, magnesium, and iron. Macadamias are rich in thiamine and manganese. Pistachios are packed with the antioxidants lutein and zeaxanthine. Hazelnuts provide vitamins A, C, and E. Pecans are sources of vitamin A, beta-carotene, and numerous minerals. Brazil nuts are an excellent source of selenium, an important antioxidant.

As with other foods, varying the nuts in your diet will broaden the range of nutrients you receive. Dry roasted nuts have no added fat; oil roasted nuts are higher in fat calories. Honey roasted nuts have sugar added, which should be avoided. Blanched nuts have the skins removed, taking away some of the benefits. Raw, unroasted nuts have the most benefits, because they have been unaltered by heat or chemicals. Raw almonds are difficult to find due to pasteurization mandates in the United States that became effective in 2007. Although nutritious, nuts must be eaten in moderation, because they are very high in omega-6 fatty acids. As we discussed above, omega-6 fatty acids are essential for our health but have to be balanced with omega-3 fatty acids to prevent inflammation. Increasing your intake of omega-3 oils and not overindulging in sources of omega-6 oils will help keep the *omega-6:omega-3 ratio* down so you can enjoy these nutritious foods. Some people with RA find that some nuts aggravate their RA.

Seeds are also superb sources of fiber, protein, and nutrients. Some seeds are high in the omega-3 acid ALA; these include flax seeds, chia seeds, and hemp seeds. Pumpkin seeds (also known as pepitas) are rich in carotenoid antioxidants. Sunflower seeds are packed with vitamin E, B vitamins including folate, and the minerals selenium and copper. Sesame seeds are high in calcium, magnesium, iron, and phosphorus. Seeds high in ALA have a more healthful omega-6:omega-3 ratio than most nuts (not more than walnuts). Other seeds have ratios similar to nuts and so need to be eaten in moderation.

Milk, Yogurt, and Cheese

Milk products provide protein, vitamins, and minerals, particularly calcium. Adequate calcium intake is important with RA, because of the risk of **osteoporosis.** Cheese is a particularly rich source of vitamin K2, which protects your heart, brain, and bones.

Some people with RA cannot tolerate milk or milk products. They may have an intolerance to milk proteins, such as *casein* and *whey,* or they may have difficulties with the milk sugar, lactose, which means they have *lactose intolerance,* an insufficiency of the enzymes needed to break down lactose. Several small studies have shown that dairy products can worsen RA symptoms in some people (Cordain, 2000). If you are one of these people and you enjoy butter you might try making *ghee,* a form of clarified butter. This process removes some of the offending milk proteins. Instructions for making ghee are given on many Internet sites. There may be miniscule amounts of lactose that remain but this should not be an issue except for people with severe lactose intolerance. There are also commercial butter oils available from which the lactose and casein have been removed. If you have true milk allergies, it is, of course, best to avoid all milk products.

SPECIAL DIETS

The promise of dietary "cures" for rheumatoid arthritis is alluring, and books and Web sites touting such cures abound. Although there is much written on this subject, scientific studies on the impact of special diets have been scant, often poorly designed, and inconclusive. This is fortunately slowly changing. However, one need not read long before finding that the supposedly curative dietary strategies conflict with each other. However, within each strategy, there may be elements that will prove helpful for *some* individuals. Researchers are beginning to look closely at diet and its relationship to arthritis. Patients and physicians will be eager to hear the results. Here are some commonly discussed special diets for RA.

Elimination Diets

Elimination diets or exclusion diets are based on the premise that *some* individuals have sensitivity to specific foods and that eating those foods can cause symptoms that may include aggravation of rheumatoid arthritis. The diet strategy in these situations is to *avoid* the offending food. We have touched on many of the suggested culprits above, including dairy, wheat and other grain constituents, corn, oats, legumes (including soy and peanuts), beef, pork, and eggs. Also sometimes incriminated are foods that contain solanine: tomatoes, white potatoes, peppers, eggplant, and other vegetables in the "nightshade family."

Most food intolerances are not a result of allergies in the usual sense of the word. More commonly, they are reactions of the immune system to specific foods. Historically, research studies have looked for antibodies against different foods in the *blood* of people with RA to look for evidence of an "immune reaction." These studies have not been useful. New studies have made us look at the research protocols differently. As mentioned numerous times in this book, an immune reaction in the gastrointestinal tract can be a major trigger for inflammation in the body. Researchers in Oslo, Norway, decided to look there for answers (Hvatum et al., 2006). They had people with known RA consume various foods, including gliadin (gluten protein), oats, cow's milk, soy, pork, codfish, and eggs. Then they took samples of the fluid from the jejunum (part of the small intestine) and looked for antibodies. They found that the intestinal fluid from patients with RA contained higher levels of antibodies to these offending food proteins than did that taken from people who did not have RA. Testing of blood samples at the same time did not reveal the same increase in antibodies. How these antibodies worsen RA is unclear. It may be that the gut antibodies form immune complexes that circulate to the blood and joints and contribute to inflammation. This is another example of how the gastrointestinal part of the immune system may play a prominent role in some patients with RA.

Elimination diets are based on the notion that the aggravating foods can be identified by systematically eliminating suspect foods. Elimination diets can begin with a complete diet with subsequent exclusion of one food or food group at a time while observing symptoms. A more rigorous approach involves *starting* with a very limited diet, such as a pure vegan diet, or even fasting. Rarely, these diets can begin with medically monitored *elemental diets*, which are liquid diets composed of amino acids, fats, sugars, vitamins, and minerals. Culprits are then determined by systematically *adding back* common offending foods, one at a time, for example: nightshades (tomato, potato, eggplant), gluten containing foods (wheat, barley, rye, malt), legumes (beans, soy, peanuts), corn, dairy, eggs, pork, and citrus. Highly restrictive diets clearly need to be guided by a licensed professional.

As you will read in the next sections, studies have shown that exclusion-type diets have been useful in identifying triggers for arthritis symptoms in some people. Some experts in the field suggest that as many as 30 to 40 percent of patients with RA might benefit from an elimination diet followed by food reintroduction to identify culprit foods that they could then continue to exclude (Rayman and Pattison, 2008). This is a much higher percentage of individuals than we have believed historically. If you are going to pursue this type of diet, it is best to work with a health professional knowledgeable about nutrition, to make sure that you are meeting your nutritional requirements while you are limiting foods. Remember, if you remove a group of foods, you need to replace its vital nutrients in other ways. For example, when removing dairy products, add calcium and vitamin D supplements. Elimination diets can be harmful if they are followed for a prolonged time without paying attention to nutritional needs.

Fasting

In several studies, fasting has been shown to reduce the *symptoms* of RA. The benefits appear to be short-lived, however, and symptoms return when a regular diet is resumed. A German review of this topic (Muller et al., 2001) found four studies showing that fasting, followed by a vegetarian diet, was associated with some benefit. Since fasting is not sustainable and may be harmful, it is *not recommended* as an option and clearly should not be attempted without your doctor's permission and supervision. A more exciting angle, however, is that researchers are looking at fasting patients to determine what changes may be responsible for reducing inflammation. One Norwegian study (Fraser et al., 2000) showed that the inflammatory cytokine called IL-6 was reduced in these patients. Fasting is not practical, but finding practical ways to duplicate this effect would be a great breakthrough. As you read in Chapter 14, some *biologic* medications are also focused on reducing IL-6.

Vegetarian Diets

There are several degrees of vegetarian diets. Many people choose not to follow a strict vegan diet (no dairy, eggs, fish, or meat). Some may eat dairy products (lactovegetarian), eggs (ovovegetarian), or fish (pescovegetarian). Researchers at the University of Kupio in Finland have published several reports on the use of an *uncooked* vegan diet for RA (Hanninen et al., 2000). An uncooked vegan diet consists of vegetables, roots, nuts, germinated seeds, sprouts, cereals, fruits, and berries. This diet is often called a *"living food* diet." It is high in fiber, carotenoids, flavonoids, vitamins C and E, lycopene, and lutein. Some foods included in the research diet were fermented foods. These foods contain living lactobacilli, a beneficial bacterium that decreases inflammation by improving the bacterial balance in the gastrointestinal tract. Patients with rheumatoid arthritis following this diet were reported to have improvement in symptoms, although blood test measures of inflammation did not change. The authors of the study report were not able to demonstrate if the symptomatic relief came from the vegan diet or the addition of fermented foods.

A small study was devised to see if a very-low-fat vegan diet improved RA (McDougall, 2002). No animal products or additional fats or oils were added to food beyond the food's natural content. The diet was composed of cereals, beans, potatoes, rice, fruits, and vegetables. Within the diet, the participants were moved from a total food intake of 49 percent carbohydrate, 32 percent fat, and 17 percent protein to one of 76 percent carbohydrate, 10 percent fat, and 13 percent protein. The study was only four weeks long, but a decrease in stiffness, joint pain, and morning stiffness was reported. No change in laboratory test results was noted.

There are other small studies that show that vegetarian diets can reduce the signs and symptoms of RA. In a small but intensive Norwegian study (Kjeldsen-Kragh, 1999), the researchers designed a staged diet as compared to having one single diet throughout the entire study. This dietary intervention started with a 7- to 10-day fast consisting mainly of teas and vegetable juice. A vegan and gluten-free diet then followed. After 3.5 months, the experimental group added back dairy, alcohol, citrus, and gluten-containing foods, one at a time, as individually tolerated. Hence, the experimental group ended with an individually modified lactovegetarian diet for the last 9 months of the study. The experimental group participants noted improvement in arthritic symptoms compared to people in a control group on a well-balanced diet without restriction. Blood tests that indicate inflammation showed reduced inflammation in the vegetarian group. A review of similar studies suggests that a fast followed by a vegan or lactovegetarian diet can have a long-term benefit on symptoms of RA for up to 45 percent of people (Rayman and Pattison, 2008). Again, this approach is something that would need to be guided by a physician.

With vegetarian diets, it is not clear if the benefit to people with RA comes from eliminating animal-derived products or from increasing fruits and vegetables. Some researchers favor the elimination hypothesis, believing that meat is a major factor contributing to the inflammation of RA (Grant, 2000). Other reports dispute this theory, including a recent study on nurses in the United Kingdom (Benito-Garcia et al., 2007). This study did not confirm an association of meat, protein, or iron intake with the development of RA. Because plants are rich natural sources of vitamins, minerals, and antioxidants, these nutrients might explain some of the benefit of a vegetarian diet. A third hypothesis relates to the ever-growing body of evidence that an imbalance of intestinal bacteria increases inflammation and may even act as a potential trigger for the development of RA. Vegetarian diets help this balance. In the Finnish study mentioned above, researchers showed evidence that vegetarian diets with fermented foods increased beneficial gut bacteria. In the Norwegian study, the vegetarians had less evidence of antibodies against the bacterium *Proteus mirabilis,* which is a known pathologic (bad) gut bacterium. This again supports the hypothesis that the improvement in RA activity may be related to positive effects of the vegan diet on the balance of gut bacteria.

Since eliminating animal products can seriously decrease protein intake, you should work with a nutritionist or dietitian if you wish to do this. Professional nutritionists can help you plan meals that meet your daily requirements, particularly of amino acids, B vitamins, iron, and calcium. Remember that good muscle health is critical to properly functioning joints. Your muscles require essential amino acids, the building blocks of protein and muscle, and meat is a major source of amino acids.

Gluten-Free Diet

Glutens are a mixture of proteins that are found in many grains, including wheat, rye, and barley. Above, we discussed the implications of gluten intolerance and celiac disease. Recent studies have even shown that people with celiac disease and people with rheumatoid arthritis share some predisposing genes for each condition (Zhernakova et al., 2011). Despite the common link, there have been no studies to date that have looked at eliminating *only* gluten to see if that one dietary manipulation would help RA. However, in a Swedish study (Hafstrom et al., 2001), researchers compared a gluten-free vegan diet with a well-balanced normal diet in a one-year trial. Results showed an improvement in symptoms as well as an improvement in inflammation blood tests. The study also showed that levels of antibodies against gliadin (a gluten protein) and beta-lactoglobulin (a milk protein) decreased in the group of patients with RA who had a good response to a gluten-free vegetarian diet. Since this study was both vegetarian *and* gluten-free, the benefits could have been from either intervention or a combination of both interventions. However, the decrease in gliadin antibodies in the people who responded to the diet suggests that *some* people with RA may derive benefit from a gluten-free diet. It should be pointed out that in this study there was no difference in the participants' x-rays at year's end. Hence, despite improvements in symptoms and laboratory tests, joint erosions were not halted by diet alone during this one-year study.

Mediterranean Diet

The traditional Mediterranean diet involves a high intake of olive oil, fruits, vegetables, nuts, seeds, legumes, and whole grain cereals; a moderate intake of fish and poultry; a low intake of dairy products, processed meats, and sweets; and wine in moderation with meals (Willett et al., 1995). A recent article in the prestigious *New England Journal of Medicine* has brought considerable attention to this diet by the lay public, media, and the medical community (Estruch et al., 2013). It reported on a very large study in Spain that showed that the Mediterranean diet supplemented with either extra-virgin olive oil or a mix of nuts (walnuts, almonds, hazelnuts) reduced the incidence of major cardiovascular events (heart attacks and strokes) by 30 percent compared to a low-fat diet. This echoes what we have said earlier about the type of fat being more important than the amount of fat when it comes to health risks. We also know that inflammation and cardiovascular disease go hand in hand.

So, is the Mediterranean diet beneficial for people with RA? A 1999 Harvard study looked at the benefits of the Mediterranean diet in Greek residents. They found that those who consumed more olive oil and more vegetables were less likely to develop RA (Linos et al., 1999). The results of a later Swedish study (Skoldstam et al., 2003) indicated that RA patients who changed to a Mediterranean diet had a decrease in painful, swollen joints, an increase in physical function, and improved vitality. In Glasgow, researchers looked at the results of an educational program for people with RA that focused on cooking and eating a Mediterranean-type diet. When compared to people who were given a generally accepted healthy diet, the women on the Mediterranean diet reported less pain and morning stiffness (McKellar et al., 2007).

As you will recognize after reading the sections above, the Mediterranean diet is high in omega-3 fatty acids and monounsaturated fat and has minimal saturated fats. This creates a favorable omega-6:omega-3 ratio, likely playing a role in reducing inflammation. The diet is also rich in olive oil. Extra-virgin olive oil contains a compound called *oleocanthal* that has natural anti-inflammatory effects similar to ibuprofen (Beauchamp et al., 2005). The diet is also rich in dietary fiber, having a favorable effect on bowel bacteria. Vegetable-enriched diets are also a source of antioxidants, which, as we know, limit the damage of inflammation.

Ancestral Diets

"Ancestral diets" reflect the food patterns of our hunter-gatherer ancestors, who lived before the agricultural revolution. Hunting and fishing provided the predominant source of protein and fat. Wild plant foods such as berries and root vegetables were the sources of carbohydrate. Diets were composed of unprocessed animal and plant foods, with no grains, flour, sugar, or refined fats. This diet was high in protein, fiber, and potassium and much lower in sodium and carbohydrates. Our bodies genetically adapted and evolved to thrive on this diet over the millennia. With the advent of agriculture, the consumption of sugar and grain-based foods increased markedly as did the development of obesity and chronic diseases. The premise is that our genetic blueprint, evolved for a hunter-gatherer existence, has not changed significantly, though most people's eating habits have changed dramatically.

There are several modern-day diets that attempt to recreate this style of eating. Walter Voegtlin, with *The Stone Age Diet* (1975), was among the first to introduce a contemporary version of this diet as a means to improve health. Gaining more consumer interest, the Paleolithic diet, or the Paleo Diet, has been popularized by Loran Cordain (Cordain, 2002b). Contemporary recommendations vary, but in general, ancestral diets consist of fish, eggs, grass-fed beef, poultry, vegetables, mushrooms, root tubers, nuts, and fruit, and they exclude grains, dairy, legumes, and refined or processed foods.

There are many explanations as to why the composition of this diet may have benefits in RA. Most of these have been discussed in detail above in other sections: increasing the content of omega-3 fatty acids in the diet, improving the omega-6:omega-3 ratio, reducing the consumption of carbohydrate-dense foods, reducing gluten consumption, reducing some lectin consumption, increasing fiber, improving the potassium:sodium ratio, and increasing dietary nutrients such as vitamins, minerals, and antioxidants. Despite these rationales for the benefits of this diet in people with RA, there have been no formal studies yet. As an aside, in the few years prior to this writing, I have recommended an 8- to 12-week trial of this diet to several patients with RA who have expressed an interest in dietary efforts to help manage inflammation. It is a challenging diet to follow and requires considerable planning. However, from those who have been able to follow the diet, the feedback has been very favorable. This observation is no substitute for sound research and does not imply that the author recommends treating RA with diet alone.

RECOMMENDATIONS

As you can see by the above information, dietary recommendations for RA are quite varied, and confusing. And sources of information often conflict with each other! Don't be frustrated by this, though, because it means that researchers are interested in this very important aspect of treating RA. There have been dramatic insights into diet and RA and much more knowledge is needed. Be ready to learn and respond to this new research as it becomes available. For now, the following general recommendations seem to make sense for most people with RA.

- Eat a variety of green and colorful vegetables to optimize nutrients, particularly antioxidants.
- Eat vegetables rich in potassium, such as spinach and beet greens.
- Incorporate raw foods into your diet as much possible.
- Eat foods as they are found in nature; for instance, choose chicken breast over a hot dog.
- Eat whole foods that are naturally fiber rich whenever possible.
- Choose whole fruit for treats and vary the selection to broaden nutrients, particularly antioxidants.

- Eat organic produce when it is financially possible for you to do so.
- Eat locally grown produce as it is available.
- Eat pasture-raised beef, poultry, and eggs as available and affordable.
- Eat fish one to three times per week if possible.
- Eat more omega-3 fats than omega-6 fats.
- Eat fermented foods as a source of probiotics.
- Avoid or minimize processed food.
- Avoid or minimize refined sugar.
- Minimize high-glycemic food as much as possible.
- Avoid artificial sweeteners.
- Choose a diet moderate in salt and sodium.
- For high-temperature cooking use coconut oil, butter, ghee, or palm oil.
- For low-heat cooking use olive oil, avocado oil, or macadamia oil.
- Do not cook with safflower, sunflower, corn oil, canola oil, soybean oil, or shortening.
- Balance the food you eat with physical activity.
- Maintain or strive for a healthy weight.
- Keep a food journal to see if certain foods aggravate your RA.
- Discuss restricted diets with your doctor before trying any.
- If you drink alcoholic beverages, do so in moderation.
- Drink at least five eight-ounce glasses of water per day.
- Read food labels.

A WORD ON NUTRITIONAL SUPPLEMENTS

Scientists are becoming increasingly interested in using food supplements as adjuncts to standard medication, and consumer interest in food supplements has exploded in the past few decades. This interest was supported in Congress by the passage of the Dietary Supplement Health and Education Act of 1994 (DSHEA). This law removed regulatory barriers that were said to be "limiting or slowing the flow of safe products and accurate information to consumers." As you have seen when reading magazines or watching television, this has allowed the supplement industry considerable leeway in making vague claims about effectiveness. The theory was that "consumers should be empowered to make choices about preventive health care programs based on data from scientific studies of health benefits related to particular dietary supplements." The Food and Drug Administration (FDA) regulates safety, manufacturing, and labeling, while the Federal Trade Commission (FTC) has jurisdiction over advertising claims for food supplements, under its consumer protection function.

A very important part of the DSHEA, however, has not been fully implemented. This is the section on strict manufacturing requirements, commonly called good manufacturing practices (GMPs). The law allows the FDA to require that dietary supplements meet GMPs for potency, cleanliness, and stability. Unfortunately, at the time of this writing, the criteria are not being measured or monitored by anyone except the manufacturer. Amounts of active ingredients can still vary considerably between brands. There is little monitoring of additives, dyes, or contaminants. The FDA does not have to review or approve supplement ingredients or products before they are marketed. Currently, it is only *after* injury or harm to consumers has been proved that the FDA can use its authority and resources to remove a supplement from the market.

Many physicians are reluctant to consider or even discuss any form of food supplementation, because of lack of quality control regulations, the scarcity of research studies, the potential for harm, and the possibility of drug interactions. Many physicians will listen and try to help if it is within their capacity, if you are interested in trying supplements. Drug-supplement interaction data are becoming more available to interested physicians, but information is far from complete. If your doctor is not interested and you have a strong wish to pursue this avenue, you may need to negotiate with your doctor. *Above all, do not take a supplement and hide the fact from your doctor.* It may be dangerous for your health and will certainly be harmful to a trusting doctor-patient relationship. You may never receive your doctor's endorsement of a supplement, but he or she needs to be informed that you are taking it, to be on guard for negative effects and to be knowledgeable about your health.

Despite lack of scientific evidence, America has spoken. Food supplements constitute a multibillion-dollar business, if for no other reason than because they offer hope to many with chronic conditions. Fortunately, some supplements do hold promise for relief of arthritis symptoms, but we must overcome the quality control problems and get confirmatory evidence of effectiveness and safety. As a consequence of these circumstances, the number of funded studies for research on food supplements has increased markedly in the past years.

Guidelines for Evaluating Nutritional Supplements

Until science catches up to demand and regulation of supplements improves, patients are taking supplements at their own risk. There are some general principles that will help you lessen, but not remove, these risks. Here are some basic strategies to follow when making decisions about supplements.

When purchasing supplements:

- Consider only products from large companies, pharmacies, or reputable health food stores.
- Be cautious with Internet, mail order, magazine, or "infomercial" purchases unless the brands are well known.
- Look for ingredients with the U.S.P. notation, which indicates that the manufacturer has followed standards established by the U.S. Pharmacopoeia; adherence to these high standards is voluntary.

Make certain that the label of the supplement contains:

- Serving size
- Name and amount of active ingredient
- Name and place of manufacturer, packer, or distributor
- Directions for use

Avoid products offering or claiming:

- "Secret" ingredients
- A "cure," "breakthrough," or "new discovery"
- Only personal testimonials (patient stories) to show effectiveness
- A "quick fix" for chronic problems
- "Cure-alls" or claims to improve a wide range of unrelated problems
- To be "scientifically proven" but providing no references
- No side effects (even placebos have side effects)
- To "detoxify" or "purify"
- Wisdom of the ages as proof of safety: "time tested," "ancient remedies"

Always discuss with your physician any product you are considering using. Review with your doctor or pharmacist any potential drug interactions between the product you are considering taking and medications you are already taking. Go on-line and research interactions for yourself as well.

As with any medicine, try only one new supplement at a time, to accurately determine benefit or side effects. Keep a record of the brand, the dose, and the time when you take it. *Never* take a greater amount than the label recommends. You *can* overdose on supplements.

VITAMINS AND MINERALS

Vitamins and minerals are critical to health. As much as possible, the recommended daily nutrients should be consumed through diet rather than via supplements. When a busy lifestyle makes it difficult to eat a well-rounded diet, we often recommend that patients take a high-quality, high-potency daily multivitamin with minerals that includes extra B vitamins and antioxidants. Low-quality vitamins may contain the right amounts of nutrients, but the nutrients may not be adequately absorbable, especially minerals, which are difficult to absorb in their original form. High-quality daily vitamin and mineral supplements often contain "chelated" minerals, which are more easily absorbed by the body. If you take more than one supplement, be certain to add up the individual vitamins and minerals from each supplement to avoid exceeding daily maximum amounts. This is particularly important with fat-soluble vitamins, which can accumulate in the body and cause toxicity. Don't forget to count the nutrients contained in drinks and shakes that are fortified with extra vitamins and minerals.

Many vitamins and minerals have been scrutinized to determine whether they could help in the treatment of rheumatoid arthritis. Reported vitamin and mineral deficiencies in people with RA have included deficiencies in vitamins A, C, D, B5, B6, B12, E, and folic acid (B9), and in calcium, magnesium, zinc, and selenium. There is a growing scientific rationale for the use of dietary supplements as *adjuncts* in the treatment of inflammatory disorders like RA (Darlington, 2001). However, *no vitamin or mineral supplement has been proven to reduce the risk of structural damage that can be caused by rheumatoid arthritis.*

Vitamins

Vitamin A

Vitamin A is a fat-soluble vitamin with antioxidant properties. Its plant-derived precursor is beta-carotene. Because vitamin A is required for normal immune system function, there is some interest in its role as a supplement for people with RA. A Johns Hopkins study showed that patients with low blood levels of beta-carotene and retinol, as well as vitamin E, were more likely to develop RA (Comstock et al., 1997). The results of this study make us question if increased antioxidant intake can have a protective role against the development of RA. This concept was tested in the Nurses' Health Study (Costenbader, 2010). In this 24-year study, increased antioxidant use (including vitamins A and E) did not appear to protect against RA in this group of women. There have also been no studies demonstrating benefit of vitamin A supplementation for people who already have RA. Vitamin A is toxic in high doses. Beta-carotene overdose is less common. It is best to get this vitamin from your diet. Foods high in vitamin A include fortified milk, leafy vegetables, sweet potatoes, carrots, and apricots.

B Vitamins and Folate

Water-soluble B vitamins include thiamin (B1), riboflavin (B2), niacin (B3), pantothenic acid (B5), pyridoxine (B6), cyanocobalamin (B12), and folate (B9). A 1960s study showed people with RA to be deficient in B5 (Barton-Wright et al., 1963). Another small study showed some reduction in symptoms of RA after supplementation with B5 (General Practitioner Research Group, 1980). Good food sources for vitamin B5 are soybeans, lentils, eggs, grains, and meat.

Low levels of vitamin B6 have been noted in people with RA, particularly those with significant inflammation (Roubenoff et al., 1994). Some researchers have suggested that vitamin B6 is utilized in greater amounts when inflammation is present. One study revealed that women with RA had lower B6 levels and higher homocysteine levels (Woolf, 2008). Low B6 and high homocysteine levels have been be linked to heart disease. This may be one of the contributors to the increased risk of cardiovascular disease that has been seen in people with RA. Researchers in Taiwan have found that supplementing vitamin B6 resulted in decreased inflammation as measured by level of the pro-inflammatory cytokines IL-6 and TNF (Huang et al., 2010). Foods rich in B6 include garlic, turnips, and fish.

Vitamin B12 is important for the development of new red blood cells. Anemia can be a problem in people with RA, so getting adequate amounts of B12 is crucial, particularly when taking the medication methotrexate. Leafy green vegetables, legumes, peanuts, sunflower seeds, whole grains, meat, fish, and dairy products all contain B12. Again, I recommend taking a multivitamin with extra B vitamins.

Like vitamin B12, folate (folic acid) is important for red blood cell development. It also helps lower homocysteine, high levels of which are linked to heart disease. Folate is not stored in the body, so it is important to get it in foods or supplementation regularly. Treatment with methotrexate is known to interfere with folic acid metabolism. This is why it is currently recommended to prescribe folic acid supplementation (1 mg or 1000 mcg per day) while taking methotrexate. A diet rich in folic acid is recommended. Most multivitamins include folic acid. Daily recommendations are 200 micrograms per day, but higher doses are needed for people who are taking methotrexate. Foods high in folic acid include leafy green vegetables, legumes, broccoli, and dried beans.

Vitamin C
Vitamin C (ascorbic acid, ascorbate) is a water-soluble antioxidant. As such, it may have benefits for inflammation. Vitamin C is also important for tissue repair and formation of collagen, the main protein in joint tissue and bone. A British study found that people with lowest dietary intake of vitamin C increased their risk of developing RA more than threefold (Pattison et al., 2004b). It is also believed that while performing its antioxidant duties ascorbate gets depleted from the body, which would explain at least in part why people with established RA can have low levels of vitamin C in their blood (Situnayake, 1991). But does that mean that vitamin C supplementation will help RA? There is too little research to say. However, a recent report from the Riordan Clinic in Witchita, Kansas, revealed that high-dose intravenous vitamin C improved inflammation (decreased CRP) in patients with RA (Mikirova et al., 2012). Until more information is available, keep your eyes open for new research and enjoy a diet high in vitamin C–rich foods. Citrus fruits (oranges, grapefruit, strawberries) and most vegetables (broccoli, red peppers, green peppers) are high in vitamin C.

Vitamin D
Vitamin D is likely the most important vitamin to consider for people with RA. It is fat-soluble and may be acquired by diet, though most vitamin D is derived from exposure of the skin to ultraviolet B (UVB) light from the sun. Vitamin

D has long been known for the important role it plays in calcium absorption by the body. It clearly also is important for the prevention and treatment of osteoporosis, which can occur in RA (see Chapter 16 for more on preventing and treating osteoporosis). But research has shown that its importance goes far beyond calcium absorption and preserving bone health. Of all the nutrients studied in the past decade, none has gotten more attention than vitamin D. There have been hundreds of reports documenting newly recognized benefits of this critical vitamin. Given the enormity of these reports, this discussion will be limited to its influence on RA.

Vitamin D appears to have a critical role in the proper functioning of our immune system. In retrospect, we have had evidence of this for some time. Historically, before the advent of antibiotics, we sent people with tuberculosis to "take in the air." It was likely the exposure to sunlight, rather than outside air, that improved the immune system in these people. And many great-grandmothers will recall that a teaspoon of cod liver oil, a rich source of vitamin D, kept their children well through the winter months in years gone by.

More recently, there has been evidence that links vitamin D deficiency to several autoimmune diseases, including multiple sclerosis, diabetes mellitus, systemic lupus erythematosus, inflammatory bowel disease, and rheumatoid arthritis. Some early research suggested that vitamin D might have a protective role in RA (Deluca and Cantoma, 2001). A small, uncontrolled study in Yugoslavia revealed that treatment with high-dose vitamin D resulted in an improvement in disease activity (Vojinovic et al., 1999). RA is more prevalent in northern latitudes, which have less sun exposure and a higher incidence of vitamin D deficiency (Vieira et al., 2010).

Several reports confirm that vitamin D deficiency is common in people with RA. Others hypothesize that this deficiency may represent a risk factor for RA development and worsening of the disease once present (Gatenby et al., 2013). Some researchers suggest that the degree of rheumatoid activity parallels the deficiency (Kostoglou-Athanassiou et al., 2012). Vitamin D deficiency has also been found to be a cause of widespread muscle pain that improves with supplementation. Vitamin D supports muscle health, which is important for joint protection and for balance. There have not been *controlled* studies to determine if vitamin D *alone* improves the symptoms or outcome of RA. These trials would be ethically challenging to perform given that other medical interventions would have to be postponed. However, there is enough information available for us to know that vitamin D supplementation has a beneficial effect on autoimmunity. Vitamin D appears to have a very important role in *immune tolerance*, which is what allows our immune systems to decipher between potential invaders and our own tissues.

As you read in Chapter 16, the recommended dose of vitamin D in adults is 600–800 IU per day. There is considerable controversy among experts in this area. After reviewing all opinions, I use the following protocol: Test blood levels of 25-hydroxy-vitamin D (25-OH-Vitamin D). Adjust the vitamin D supplementation to achieve a minimum level of 32 nanograms/milliliter (ng/ml). Try to attain a level between 40–60 ng/ml for best results. In my experience, the average amount of vitamin D supplementation required to achieve these goals is 2000 IU per day. You should not take this amount of vitamin D supplementation without the advice of your doctor and monitoring of blood levels.

Foods high in vitamin D include fortified milk and cold-water fish, such as salmon, sardines, mackerel, herring, anchovy, and lake trout.

Vitamin E
Vitamin E is a major antioxidant, possibly the most important one. It is crucial for maintaining a normal immune system. A small study showed low levels of vitamin E in inflamed rheumatoid joints (Fairburn et al., 1992), and other research indicated low amounts of vitamin E in the blood (Kajanachumpol et al., 2000). Several studies have suggested that people with RA may not be consuming enough vitamin E, but does taking vitamin E supplements prevent RA? A large study, called the Women's Health Study, found that vitamin E supplementation did not reduce the risk of developing RA (Karlson et al., 2008). Vitamin E supplementation has been reported to have some benefit for symptoms of RA in several small studies, but others did not confirm this (Canter et al., 2007). Because of mixed results, some experts recommend a trial of vitamin E (up to 400 mg per day) for up to three months to see if there is a decrease in pain (Rayman and Pattison, 2008).

Care should be exercised not to exceed the maximum dose of vitamin E. High doses can interfere with natural blood clotting and can interfere with the blood thinner Coumadin (warfarin). Review all supplements with your doctor. Foods naturally high in vitamin E include whole grains, nuts, seeds, poultry, and fish.

Minerals

Calcium
Adequate calcium intake is critical to prevention of the bone loss associated with RA. (See Chapter 16 for details on calcium supplementation.)

Copper

Reports suggest that some people with RA are deficient in copper (DiSilvestro et al., 1992), but there is *no* definitive evidence that oral supplementation with copper can help treat or slow RA. Many people advocate wearing copper bracelets for arthritis. One study suggests that trace amounts of copper dissolve in the body sweat and are absorbed by a process called "dermal assimilation" (Walker and Keats, 1976). Wearing copper is a benign treatment that we have no objection to. Foods high in copper include dried beans, shellfish, nuts, seeds, whole grains, vegetables, and chocolate. Supplementation of daily diet beyond a multivitamin with minerals is not recommended.

Selenium

Selenium is an essential trace mineral that has important antioxidant functions. Studies have indicated a low level of selenium in some people with severe RA (Tarp, 1995). Finnish studies suggest that low selenium and low vitamin E levels may be a risk factor for *developing* RA (Knekt et al., 2000). Studies also suggest that selenium levels decrease as a response to inflammation (Rayman and Callaghan, 2006). Although studies disagree on the therapeutic value of selenium supplementation for people who have RA, at least three studies have demonstrated measurable improvements (Rayman and Pattison, 2008). We need further study to determine if there is any benefit to selenium supplementation. For now, until we have more evidence about using selenium for RA symptoms, it is best simply to add selenium rich foods to your diet or make certain that your multivitamin contains selenium. Brazil nuts contain 68–91 mcg per nut according to the Office of Dietary Supplements (see end of chapter for more about ODS). The recommended daily allowance (RDA) for adults is 55 mcg per day so keep your intake of these nuts below three per week to avoid excessive selenium. Food sources of selenium include Brazil nuts, liver and other organ meats, fish, shellfish, and lentils.

Zinc

Zinc levels have been shown to be low in some people with RA. This trace element is necessary for some antioxidant activity. Studies designed to determine the effectiveness of zinc supplementation in treating RA have been contradictory (Rayman and Callaghan, 2006). Given the importance of this mineral in overall human health, we recommend aiming for at least the RDA for this nutrient. Vegetarians need to be extra conscientious about getting this nutrient. Grain and legumes, which are the best non-animal source of zinc, also contain *phytates* that can bind to zinc and limit its absorption (see about legumes above). Also, zinc intake can suppress copper absorption, so if you take additional zinc, make certain that you are taking adequate copper as well. Foods high in zinc include seafood, red meats, organ meats, egg yolk, whole grains, and legumes. If you take a multivitamin, it seems prudent to take one that includes zinc.

HERBS AND PLANT-BASED MEDICINE

Herbs and medicinal plants were a cornerstone in ancient systems of medicine for hundreds of years. Many standard pharmaceutical medications are biological compounds that have been derived from plants. Their manufacture and standardization are carefully monitored and they must meet strict regulations. Unlike pharmaceutical drugs, medicinal herbal preparations and phytonutrients are not necessarily produced with careful attention to standardization and quality control. Many people believe that herbs and other botanical supplements cannot be harmful because they are "natural." But, just as medicinal herbs can have good effects, they can also have bad effects. For all intents and purposes, herbs are medicines that do not have to pass the rigorous guidelines established by the Food and Drug Administration for effectiveness or safety.

With the current flurry of interest in herbal medicine, many companies are manufacturing these products. Some are legitimate, high-quality manufacturers, but others use processing techniques that include additives or use parts of the plant that are not proven to be therapeutic. There is little or no oversight regarding how an herb is planted, cultivated, fertilized, chemically treated, harvested, or preserved. Cases of contamination have particularly been a problem with Chinese and Ayurvedic herbs, requiring the removal of tainted products from the market. Contaminants, additives, and improper packaging, handling, or storage will remain a concern until the FDA gains regulatory oversight of this industry and good manufacturing procedures can be enforced.

We are all optimistic about the prospect of safer natural remedies. Although there are exciting new studies about herbs and health, we suggest that you *use extreme caution when using herbal treatments*. In addition to the above quality and standardization issues, there are two other particular concerns. First, very little is known about drug-herb interactions with rheumatoid medications. Second, treatment for RA usually requires several different types of medications, and adding to that complexity may confuse the picture considerably if a side effect does occur. If you do consider herbal remedies, do your research. Scrutinize the manufacturer's credentials. Use companies with reputations for high-quality products. With little-known companies, look for quality certifications from third parties, such as Good Manufacturing Practices (GMP), the International Organization for Standardization (ISO), or Safe Quality Food (SQF). Also, companies that require certified organic ingredients tend to have more stringent processing standards. But above all, please keep your doctors informed. With the growing interest in medicinal herbs and plants, more research on herb-drug interactions is inevitable.

The herbs discussed in this section are commonly advertised for the treatment of RA. At this time, there is very little research to support their use in treating RA.

Boswellia

Boswellia (*Boswellia serrata*) is an herb that has been used for centuries in Ayurvedic medicine (traditional medicine from India). Modern research shows that it has potent anti-inflammatory characteristics. Research in animal models of inflammation shows that Boswellia may work by reducing the number of neutrophils that infiltrate the **synovium** in arthritis (Nanjundaiah et al., 2013). (Chapter 1 describes how the neutrophil, a white blood cell, is involved in joint inflammation.) Despite this research, published reports on the use of this phytonutrient in RA reveal conflicting results (Etzel, 1996; Sander et al., 1998). Given the inconsistent research regarding this herb, its use in treatment of RA cannot be endorsed at this time.

Bromelain

Bromelain is an extract of the pineapple plant. Studies reveal that this plant enzyme has anti-inflammatory effects. It is commonly used in Europe to reduce swelling after injury. It is also available in the United States. Its benefit in RA has not been proven. One small study (Cohen et al., 1964) suggested that bromelain might help reduce swelling and impaired joint mobility. Several small studies have shown some improvement in patients with osteoarthritis. There is very little evidence at this time that this herb will make a meaningful difference in RA. Bromelain can also thin the blood and therefore may have the potential for a *drug interaction* with Coumadin (warfarin), heparin, and possibly with aspirin and NSAIDs. There is also a possibility of interaction with tetracycline antibiotics. Clearly, if you are taking minocycline for RA you should *avoid* this herb.

Cat's Claw

Cat's claw (*Uncaria tomentosa*) is made from the bark of a Peruvian vine; its use in South America dates back hundreds of years. Although it is frequently used to treat RA, studies of its effectiveness are scant. One very small study did show a modest benefit for tenderness in the joints when added to either sulfasalazine or hydroxychloroquine (Mur et al., 2002). Cat's claw has the potential for *drug interactions* with blood thinners such as Coumadin (warfarin) and heparin.

Chinese Herbs

The list of ancient Chinese herbs is lengthy. Many combinations are used. Unlike "Western herbs," Chinese herbs are often difficult for the layperson and even physicians to understand. In the United States, there are concerns about the lack of standardization and quality control. Chinese herbal preparations tainted with aristocholic acid, a possible kidney carcinogen, have been discovered. The result was an FDA-ordered recall and an increase in our concern about purity. If you are determined try these preparations, please purchase the herbs from a certified practitioner or an acupuncturist who is experienced and certified and who has a longstanding commitment to your community. Committed professionals would be more likely to use high-quality herbs from a reputable source and to help you determine if there are potential negative interactions with other medicines you are taking. Always inform your physician of these treatments.

Curcumin

Curcumin, an extract of the spice turmeric, has also been used for many years in Ayurvedic medicine. In the 1970s and 1980s Indian researchers confirmed its mild anti-inflammatory effects. This herb is widely used in India for RA. In the past decade, this phytochemical has been confirmed to have significant anti-inflammatory, antioxidant, and anti-cancer activities. There are numerous human studies under way looking at its potential benefit in a wide range of inflammatory diseases and cancer. There have been studies that show it may be effective in periodontal disease (Guimaraes et al., 2011). We know that periodontal bacteria have been linked to the development of RA (see Chapter 1). A recent Indian study compared curcumin to the NSAID diclofenac in patients with RA (Chandran and Goel, 2012). Curcumin was found to be superior to diclofenac for the reduction of pain and swelling. Although this is a very exciting finding, the study was a small one. Also, this phytochemical has not been widely studied for herb-drug interactions. Curcumin can theoretically have drug interactions with blood-thinning drugs like aspirin, NSAIDS, heparin, warfarin, and others. Because curcumin can cause gallbladder contraction, its use should be approved by your physician, particularly if you have gallbladder problems.

Devil's Claw

Devil's claw (*Harpagophytum procumbens*) comes from the root of an African plant. It is used in Europe as an anti-inflammatory treatment for rheumatoid arthritis. Although this herb is commonly used, there is no direct proof of its benefit for RA. It may cause a *drug interaction* with the blood thinners like Coumadin (warfarin) and Plavix (clopidogrel); it may also lower blood sugar.

Feverfew

This herb has been used for many years to treat headaches and arthritis. It has potent anti-inflammatory effects because of one of its components, parthenolide. Despite this, one small study showed no benefit to its use in treating RA (Heptinstall et al., 1989). A potential *drug interaction*: use of feverfew with NSAIDs might increase NSAID side effects such as stomach and kidney problems.

Ginger

Ginger is a common spice used in tea, soda, and food and has long been employed medicinally. In at least Ayurvedic and Chinese herbal traditions it has been used for inflammation. In animal models of inflammation, ginger extract has been shown to reduce levels of cytokines IL-1, IL-2, IL-6, and TNF (Nanjundaiah et al., 2013) (see Chapter 14 about these cytokines). Ginger's benefit for RA has not been definitively proven. In large amounts, it may irritate the stomach, and it may interact adversely with blood thinners.

Yucca

Yucca has been used for many years by Native Americans for arthritis. Although there have been no large studies in RA patients, researchers are interested in this medicinal plant. A recent review suggests that yucca has anti-inflammatory, antioxidant, and anti-protozoa (type of bowel microbe) activity (Cheeke et al., 2006). Based on these findings, further studies are warranted. For now, there is no documented evidence of its effectiveness in RA.

OTHER SUPPLEMENTS

Antioxidants

Above we have discussed vitamins and minerals that have antioxidant activity, most notably vitamin A, vitamin C, vitamin E, selenium, and zinc. What exactly does antioxidant mean? An antioxidant inhibits the oxidation of other molecules. During the inflammatory response, a chemical reaction called oxidation occurs and immune cells produce "free radicals." These toxic byproducts wreak havoc on the immune system and create damage to organs and tissues. Antioxidants act like a clean-up team to get rid of these toxic byproducts. There are many other antioxidants that are under investigation for treatment of inflammation as well as a host of conditions that are thought to be a consequence of inflammation. The research is very exciting but really is just in its infancy and beyond the scope of this text to cover. As you read in the food sections above, many and varied antioxidants can be obtained by consuming a healthful diet rich in whole foods, in particular, fruits and vegetables.

Glucosamine Sulfate and Chondroitin Sulfate

Glucosamine and chondroitin are substances that occur naturally in the body, manufactured versions of which have become part of mainstream medicine. The combination of glucosamine and chondroitin is frequently used for treatment of osteoarthritis. Formal studies have been mixed in demonstrating symptom relief and long-term benefit for patients with *osteo*-arthritis (degenerative arthritis). Theoretically, the effectiveness of these supplements lies in their benefit to cartilage that has been broken down by the forces of wear and tear. Unfortunately, these supplements have not been shown to help with the symptoms or progress of rheumatoid arthritis. This is almost certainly because the damage from RA comes from inflammation and not from wear and tear. These two supplements do not directly affect inflammation in a meaningful way.

Fish Oil and Essential Fatty Acids: EPA, DHA, ALA, and GLA

We read above about the importance of fish oils and the omega-3 fatty acids DHA and EPA in our diets. The best way to get adequate amounts of these substances is to have a diet rich in foods containing these oils. However, your doctor or other health care practitioner may recommend additional supplementation.

Fish oil supplementation for RA has been more rigorously studied than any other natural remedy. Several studies have determined that fish oil supplementation can reduce the pain and swelling of RA. The most influential of the published studies have been led by Dr. Joel Kremer at the Albany (New York) Medical Center. The omega-3 fatty acids in fish oil are thought to be responsible for its anti-inflammatory effects. The two most important of these are the long-chained fatty acids EPA (eicosapentaenoic acid) and DHA (docosahexaenoic acid). Supplements of these substances have been shown to reduce both the number of swollen joints and morning stiffness (Kremer, 2000). There have been numerous reviews and studies of this topic since (Rayman and Callaghan, 2006). Research has shown noted improvements in the following: painful, swollen and tender joints, morning stiffness, NSAID use, and evidence of inflammation by laboratory analysis.

Not all fish oils are equal. Cod liver oil, for example, is very high in vitamin A and vitamin D as well as omega-3 fatty acids. These fat-soluble vitamins can build up in your body and cause toxic effects; therefore, you should keep track of the content of fat-soluble vitamins in all supplements you take. Other possible complications include bloating and gas. Fish oil also has blood-thinning characteristics. This may present the potential for a *drug interaction* when combined with an anticoagulant medication (prescription blood thinner) such as Coumadin (warfarin) or heparin. In people at risk for bleeding, combining fish oil with aspirin or NSAIDs may not be advisable. Always ask your doctor.

Other sources of DHA and EPA include krill and squid oil. An alternative for vegetarians can be derived from several strains of algae that produce DHA. Recently, it has been discovered that there is a strain of algae that also produces EPA. Algae produced DHA and EPA (algal "fish" oil) is now commercially available (Ovega-3). To achieve an anti-inflammatory effect, most sources recommend between 3 to 4 grams of EPA and DHA in food or supplementation with the advice to minimize omega-6 oils in the diet. Achieving a daily minimum of 3 grams of EPA and DHA would require around six to seven servings per week of a fish like salmon (Rayman and Pattison, 2008). Eating this much salmon or similar fish is not practical and may not be safe, considering the possibility of toxic contaminants like PCBs, dioxins, and mercury (Rayman and Callaghan, 2006). Even if anti-inflammatory doses are not possible or tolerated, lower doses have been found to reduce the risk of heart disease, which can be an issue in people with RA.

Another omega-3 fatty acid that has gotten attention is alpha-linolenic acid (ALA). Although our bodies cannot make EPA and DHA for the most part, we have a *limited* ability to make them if our diet is rich in the short-chained fatty acid, ALA. Flaxseed oil is the richest food source, but ALA is also found in walnut, canola, and soybean oil. But can we convert ALA into enough EPA and DHA to have significant anti-inflammatory and cardiovascular benefits? There has been very little research using ALA in the treatment of rheumatoid arthritis. A small study in Finland (Nordstrom et al., 1995) compared flaxseed (high in ALA) to safflower seed (high in linoleic acid, an omega-6 fatty acid). After three months, there was no difference in arthritis symptoms or the blood levels of DHA and EPA between the two groups. Although a small trial, the results suggest that sticking with the proven omega-3 fatty acids, DHA and EPA remains prudent when they are being used to treat inflammation.

Contrary to this previous information, there are certain omega-6 fatty acid derivatives that may help inflammation. Gamma-linolenic acid (GLA) is an essential fatty acid found in evening primrose oil, borage oil, and black currant oil. There is some evidence that GLA may help RA symptoms (Zurier et al., 1996). Be careful about GLA supplements; they can have *drug interactions* with blood thinners.

Probiotics, Prebiotics, and Fiber Supplements

We have reviewed how disruption of the bacterial balance in the gut may be a trigger for RA and how a diet with plenty of fiber-rich foods (vegetables, nuts, seeds, fermented foods) can help promote a healthy balance. If you cannot get the 32 grams of fiber recommended, a fiber supplement may be in order. Natural psyllium supplements without additives such as sugar or synthetic ingredients will help meet this requirement if you cannot meet it by diet, though diet is the preferred approach.

Probiotic supplements are also available which can help replace the healthful bacteria in the bowel. There are hundreds of good bacteria in our intestines. Probiotics contain a variety of live organisms that potentially confer health benefits. But does probiotic supplementation help RA? A Finnish study tested the probiotic *Lactobacillus rhamnosus* GG (Hatakka et al., 2003). There were some subjective improvements in a sense of well-being but no changes in laboratory test results. A Canadian study looked at *Lactobacillus reuteri* RC-14 and *Lactobacillus rhamnosus* GR-1 in people with RA (Pineda et al., 2011). The patients on the probiotic appeared to function better, but there were no other changes in symptoms or blood tests. In the United States, researchers looked at the effects of *Bacillus coagulans*. This study reported an improvement in pain and a decrease in inflammation tests. Hence, probiotics might offer some potential benefits for RA. Probiotic supplements vary considerably as to which bacterial strains they contain and in what potency. If you are considering probiotic supplementation, ask your doctor for recommendations regarding specific brands. There are also supplements called *prebiotics*, which consist of nondigestible ingredients that provide nutrients for beneficial microbes. A diet high in fruit and vegetable fiber from a variety of sources will almost always suffice, though. Chicory root, Jerusalem artichokes, raw garlic, onions, asparagus, and bananas are particularly good prebiotic sources.

Recommendations regarding Specific Supplements

- Follow the recommendations for evaluating supplements given above.

- Review all supplements with your doctor.

- Try to get most nutrient needs from food.

- Nutrient needs that cannot be met by diet alone should be discussed with your doctor; particularly of worth in RA are vitamin D and fish oil.

FOR MORE INFORMATION

The Arthritis Foundation offers *Nutrition and Your Arthritis* and the *Arthritis Today Supplement and Vitamin Guide.* They can be ordered in printed form or can be sent free by e-mail from the Arthritis Foundation Web site: www.arthritis.org/.

The University of Sydney offers the official Web site for the glycemic index and international GI database. The Web site is updated frequently and is offered free to the public. Visit www.glycemicindex.com for more information.

Nutrition.gov is a collaborative, multi-sponsor site that provides food and nutrition information from across the federal government. It provides multiple links and resources in the area of nutrition, weight management, dietary supplements, and other food related topics. Web site: http://www.nutrition.gov.

The Office of Dietary Supplements (ODS) of the National Institutes of Health provides fact sheets that give a current overview of data on individual vitamins, minerals, and other dietary supplements. It provides other publications (such as *Dietary Supplements: What You Need to Know)* and the PubMed Dietary Supplement Subset. PubMed is a service of the National Library of Medicine and contains publication information and brief summaries of articles from scientific and medical journals. The ODS Web site address is: http://ods.od.nih.gov; the PubMed Dietary Supplement Subset Web site address is: ods.od.nih.gov /Research/PubMed_Dietary_Supplement_Subset.aspx.

The U.S. Department of Agriculture offers *The Food and Nutrition Information Center* (FNIC), whose mission is to collect and disseminate information about food and human nutrition. FNIC continues to add services and resources in the area of nutrition, food safety, dietary supplements, and other related topics. FNIC Web site: http://fnic.nal.usda.gov.

MedlinePlus is the National Institutes of Health's Web site for health care consumers. From this site, you can browse information on dietary supplements and herbal remedies. Visit: http://www.nlm.nih.gov/medlineplus/druginfo /herb_All.html.

19

Surgery for Rheumatoid Arthritis

Sometimes, despite timely medical therapy, rheumatoid arthritis (RA) continues to cause inflammation and joint damage. When other therapies haven't been successful, surgery may be necessary. Surgical techniques are constantly being improved, providing new alternatives to help people with RA.

Surgery is recommended for a variety of reasons, the most common of which is to control severe pain caused by inflammation or damaged joints. Surgery may also be advised to repair ruptured ligaments or tendons or to remove inflamed synovial tissue that has not responded adequately to other therapy and which threatens to cause joint damage. Surgery may be recommended as the best treatment to retain or restore function in a specific joint.

Some surgical procedures are intended to provide temporary relief and to prevent damage over the long term. Others are corrective measures aimed at improving the function of joints that have already been damaged.

SURGEONS SPECIALIZING IN THE TREATMENT OF RA

Your primary care doctor or **rheumatologist** may recommend that you have a consultation with a surgeon to determine whether a surgical procedure will help you. The specific problems you are having and which joints are involved will to some extent determine the type of surgeon you see. The expertise of the surgeons practicing in your geographical area will also influence your choice.

Surgeons who specialize in performing surgery on bones and joints are called **orthopedic surgeons.** These professionals perform surgical procedures on the large joints—shoulders, elbows, hips, and knees. Many also have expertise in surgeries on the smaller joints of the hands and feet. Some orthopedic surgeons are experts in specific types of surgery, such as joint reconstruction or arthroscopic surgery.

Hand surgeons are generally highly specialized; most of them have training in either orthopedic surgery or **plastic surgery.** Often they will have obtained specialized training in surgery of the upper extremities. If they have had this formal fellowship training, they can be certified as hand subspecialists.

Podiatrists (doctors of podiatric medicine) are specialists in the medical and surgical treatment of foot ailments. Many podiatrists perform surgery on the feet of people with RA. This is an area of expertise which they share with some orthopedic surgeons.

TYPES OF SURGERY

Some of the basic types of joint surgeries are discussed below. For an animated view of these surgeries, visit the Arthritis Foundation's on-line site Surgery Center, which presents surgery animations and provides other timely information (www.arthritis.org/conditions-treatments/surgery-center).

Arthroscopic Surgery

By inserting a pencil-sized scope called an **arthroscope** through a small incision in the skin, a surgeon or rheumatologist is able to look inside a joint without putting the patient through major surgery. Being able to see the inside joint structures helps the surgeon determine what conditions are creating problems. While the surgeon is examining the inside of the joint, he or she can take a biopsy of tissue within the joint to confirm a diagnosis or perform simple corrective procedures, such as removing damaged **cartilage.**

More extensive surgical procedures such as **ligament** and **tendon** repairs can also be performed through an arthroscope. Arthroscopic synovectomy (see below) is another common procedure.

Synovectomy

Synovectomy is the name of the procedure that is intended to halt the effects of destructive **synovitis** by removing this inflammatory tissue. The affected **synovium** (joint lining) is removed surgically to prevent it from damaging cartilage and other joint structures. Although very effective in reducing joint pain and swelling, synovectomy should not be viewed as providing a permanent cure, because the synovium can grow back, and complete removal of all synovial tissue is not possible.

Synovectomy can be performed through an arthroscope. This approach has an advantage over open surgical synovectomy in that it avoids cutting and opening the joint capsule. For this reason, recovery from arthroscopic synovectomy is generally quite rapid.

Although it is more invasive, an open surgical synovectomy also has certain advantages. It provides the surgeon a better view of, and improved access into, the total joint, thereby facilitating thorough removal of the inflamed synovial tissue.

Synovectomies are frequently performed in the wrist, elbows, and knees. This surgery is often combined with tendon repair or reconstruction or with bone resection (see below).

Tendon Reconstruction or Transfer

RA can damage or even rupture surrounding tendons and ligaments. If the tendon is ruptured, it can be reconstructed by connecting a separate but intact tendon to the ruptured one. This procedure is known as *tendon transfer*. Rupture is most common in the tendons that travel along the top of the hands down to the fingers.

Joint Fusion

Joint fusion, or *arthrodesis*, is a surgical procedure that permits bone to be connected to bone across a joint. This procedure is performed only on painful and unstable joints, most commonly in the wrists, feet, ankles, and thumbs. It very effectively decreases pain and improves stability, but it permanently inhibits motion in the fused joint. For this reason, joint fusion is rarely performed on the shoulder or hip.

With longstanding RA involving the neck, the vertebrae can become unstable because of ligament and bone loss caused by the synovitis. In severe cases, an operation to fuse the vertebrae may be required to increase stability.

Osteotomy and Bone Resection

Osteotomy is a procedure that involves cutting and repositioning bone to improve joint alignment and to compensate for deformity. This procedure is performed less frequently than it once was, because improved joint replacement procedures provide more effective treatment.

Sometimes a section of bone is removed (*resected*) from the bone end nearest the joint. This form of bone resection is a simple procedure and is performed on joints in the shoulders, elbows, wrists, and feet to improve the joint's range of motion and to relieve pain.

Joint Replacement

New techniques of joint replacement, or *arthroplasty*, have dramatically improved the outlook for people with RA. In arthroplasty, a severely damaged joint is reconstructed. This may involve only resurfacing the damaged ends of bones on either side of the joint and realignment of the joint, or it may involve replacing the entire damaged joint with an artificial one.

In the past, total joint replacement was performed only in older, inactive individuals who had less chance of wearing out their new joints. However, current trends in surgery reflect the opinion that preserving function is mandatory for good health, and therefore the use of artificial joints in younger, more active individuals has increased. Total joint replacement is frequently performed in the knees, hips, and shoulders, with excellent results. Replacements for the elbows, wrists, and ankles are available, but the outcome is not as predictable. New designs are continually becoming available, however, and will likely provide better and more consistent results.

Artificial joints can be attached to the bone by two different methods. In the first, surgeons insert the stem of the replacement joint into a hole drilled into the bone; the hole is filled with a special cementing material. This method is less painful and facilitates rehabilitation with faster healing, but the cement may crack and the joint may loosen in time, particularly in very active individuals.

Surgeons can also utilize cementless joint replacements, the second method of attaching the artificial joint to the bone. In this method, the replacement stem, which has small pores in it, is inserted snugly into a perfectly matched hole in the bone. The patient's own bone slowly grows into the pores to provide stability. If successful, this method of replacement has the benefits of increased strength and durability, with (theoretically) a decreased need for additional replacement surgery in the future. The procedure's disadvantages include a prolonged rehabilitation and potential problems with delayed healing, as well as bone growth inadequate to support and stabilize the replacement. This bone growth inadequacy may be more likely to occur in individuals with RA whose bones have already been weakened by arthritis and some medications.

Joint replacements do not last forever, which is why many doctors favor postponing replacement until it becomes absolutely necessary. The newer techniques and materials have increased the life of a replacement joint to 15 years or more, under good conditions. Efforts to prolong the life of the replacement with joint protection measures such as weight management are very important. If the replacement breaks down, *revision arthroplasty* is often very successful.

PREPARING FOR AND RECOVERING FROM SURGERY

Before Surgery

Be certain that your *surgeon* is aware of *all* of the medications you are taking, particularly nonsteroidal anti-inflammatory drugs (**NSAIDs**), **immunosuppressants, corticosteroids,** and **biologics.** Remember to include over-the-counter medications, such as ibuprofen and aspirin, and all herbal preparations. To reduce the risk of excessive bleeding, NSAIDs are generally discontinued before surgery. Because surgery can lead to higher than normal risk for infection, medications that can inhibit or suppress the immune system are generally stopped for a short time before and after surgery. This would include medications such as methotrexate, leflunamide, any of the biologics, and Xeljanz. Make sure that you discuss your medications with *both* your prescribing physician and your surgeon when you are making plans for surgery.

If you are scheduled to have general anesthesia, tell your surgeon about any history of neck or jaw discomfort. Some surgeons request that a neck x-ray be taken in individuals who have had RA a long time. These precautions are often taken before general anesthesia is administered.

Before you undergo any joint replacement surgery, make certain that your orthopedic surgeon is aware of *any* infections you have, including skin breakdown and bladder infections. It is possible for infection to spread to the new joint by way of the bloodstream, so your surgeon will want to treat the infection if possible before proceeding. A common problem that people neglect to mention to their surgeon is severe dental caries (cavities) or tooth decay. Whether or not you have tooth decay, scrupulous dental hygiene is essential after a joint replacement, to avoid spreading bacteria into the new joint.

Ask your physician well in advance of the surgery whether it is possible for you to reserve your own blood in case you need blood during the procedure. Receiving your own blood is called an *autologous transfusion* and is the safest kind of blood transfusion. The medication *erythropoietin* can be administered to people with **anemia** to stimulate the production of red blood cells; this should make it possible for someone with anemia to put blood aside in advance in case it is needed during surgery.

Before having surgery, do some home planning. Think about preparing meals ahead and freezing them. Arrange for help with everyday tasks in advance so you will be prepared after surgery. Rearrange furniture and equipment so you can get to what you need easily and safely. Too many people only consider these issues after the surgery is performed. *Plan ahead.*

During Your Recovery

You can increase the extent and speed of your recovery by actively participating in rehabilitation both before and after surgery, so the best advice is to follow the instructions of your **physical** and **occupational therapists** closely. When you are able to exercise after surgery, be certain to discuss with your orthopedic surgeon any exercise program involving the joint that has been operated on. Speak with your doctors about restarting any medications that were temporarily discontinued. Before restarting medications that can suppress the immune system, make certain that a member of your orthopedic team has evaluated your surgical wounds for signs of infection.

FOR MORE INFORMATION

The Arthritis Foundation publishes "Surgery and Arthritis: What You Need to Know," a free pamphlet. Go to www.afstore.org or call 1-800-283-7800 to order a copy. Also visit www.arthritis.org/conditions-treatments/surgery-center, to reach the AF's Surgery Center, which has very useful and specific surgical information.

PRACTICAL MATTERS

20

Disability Benefits, Insurance, and Other Financial Matters

There's no getting around the fact that rheumatoid arthritis (RA) can sometimes interfere with a person's ability to work. Stiffness, pain, decreased mobility, and fatigue may present problems for someone whose employment involves an eight-hour or longer workday. Thanks to the advent of new treatments, most people will not need special accommodations. However, if necessary, employers are expected to make reasonable accommodations to help an employee keep working, under the *Americans with Disabilities Act* (*ADA*). People with RA often find it helpful to talk with their employers about arranging for increased flexibility in work hours and creating an arthritis-friendly workplace. These modifications can help a person with RA avoid interference with work because of minor flare-ups. Another possibility is a job-sharing program, in which two people each work half-time to fulfill the duties of one full-time job.

We stress the fact that persons with RA are *differently abled*, rather than disabled, and that, with creative planning, flexibility, and understanding, a person with RA often can remain fully engaged in his or her job. This is what many people would prefer to do, but sometimes, despite a person's best creative efforts, it is not possible to continue being employed as before. This is particularly true for people with a physically demanding job that requires repeated use of inflamed joints.

A person with RA who is having problems at work would be well advised to discuss the situation with his or her doctor and a social worker. If the best decision seems to be to make a change, the person might consider pursuing another form of employment, making arrangements with his or her employer to change jobs within the same company (or to change the description and duties of the present job), or applying for disability benefits. This decision, of course, is highly personal. The choice you make depends on your work experience, education, age, financial responsibilities, degree of arthritis involvement, and the advice of your health care team.

DISABILITY BENEFITS

Should your doctor suggest that you stop working, you may be eligible for disability benefits. These benefits vary greatly depending on the coverage offered by your employer and the availability of benefits for which you may be eligible. The definition of *disability* varies considerably among benefit providers, too. The following kinds of disability benefits may be available to you.

Commercial and Employment Disability Programs

Some companies offer short-term or long-term disability insurance as part of a benefits package. If disability insurance is an *optional* benefit in which you have chosen to participate, premium payments may be deducted from your paycheck. Disability benefits are often available for military or civil service employees.

Some people purchase individual disability policies from private insurance companies. Before signing up for disability insurance, read the insurance contract carefully to determine how long you need to be disabled before benefits begin and how *disability* is defined. Some policies are quite restrictive in these regards and may not be worth the investment.

With any private disability policy that you purchase, through work or privately, consider paying the premium with after-tax dollars. In this way, if you need the benefits in the future they will not be taxed.

State Disability Policies

Some states have disability insurance programs. People enrolled in these programs contribute a portion of the premium by way of a payroll deduction. Benefits are generally paid in proportion to the amount contributed to the fund. Your doctor will be familiar with your state's disability benefits and can tell you how to join the program.

Social Security Disability Benefits

You may be eligible for federal benefit programs if you are disabled by your arthritis. The definition of *disability* is based on your present and projected inability to perform *any* kind of work. You may be considered disabled by Social Security standards if:

- your arthritis prevents you from being gainfully employed and
- your condition is expected to last for at least one year or to result in death.

Social Security officers will review your history, medical records, and personal physician's reports to determine whether you are disabled under Social Security criteria. A physical examination by a consulting physician may be requested by the agency if additional information about your current physical condition is needed. The reviewers will determine whether your arthritis matches disability standards set forth by an objective *listing of impairments*.

According to Social Security regulations, to qualify as having disabling RA, a person must show proof of persistent joint pain, swelling, or tenderness in multiple joints. Signs of joint inflammation (swelling and tenderness) must have been present for at least three months despite therapy and must have resulted in decreased function of those joints. It must be expected that the arthritis will remain a physical impairment for longer than twelve months. The results of such RA laboratory tests as **ESR** (erythrocyte sedimentation rate), **rheumatoid factor, anti-CCP** (anti-citrullinated peptide), and biopsy (see Chapter 3) should also be abnormal. Other factors taken into consideration include pain, fatigue, ability to perform basic work-related activities, age, education, past work experience, and transferable skills. The process of determining eligibility for benefits may take several months to complete. It is a good idea to keep in touch with the Social Security office during this time, to monitor the progress being made on your case.

The Social Security Administration offers two disability programs, the Social Security Disability Insurance (SSDI) program and the Supplemental Security Income (SSI) program. Rules regarding eligibility for the two differ. SSDI benefits are based on work history, while SSI is based on financial need. Neither of these programs is designed to cover short-term or partial disability, as some private policies do.

Social Security Disability Insurance (SSDI). These Social Security benefits are funded through FICA taxes paid by both employees and employers. You may be eligible if you meet the disability standards described above. You and certain members of your family may qualify for SSDI if, in addition:

- you have sufficient work credits (determined by your length of employment, how recently you have worked, and the age at which you became disabled) or

- you are not engaged in substantial gainful activity (SGA) (in 2014, SGA was defined as not having earnings of more than $1,070 per month on average).

Benefits usually begin after six full months of disability. The amount of your monthly disability benefit is based upon your lifetime average earnings covered by Social Security. You can obtain an estimate of your disability benefit from a Social Security office. Ask for a Social Security statement that displays your earning record and provides an estimate of your disability benefit. Payments are larger for people with dependents. Benefits may be adjusted if you are eligible for other federal disability benefits or for state, civil service, or military disability benefits. After twenty-four months of receiving SSDI, an individual qualifies for Medicare insurance.

Supplemental Security Income (SSI). This program is funded through general revenue funds. Again, to receive SSI benefits, you must be qualified as disabled according to the Social Security standards mentioned above. Unlike for SSDI, to be eligible for SSI you do not have to have a work history; instead, you must prove financial need, sufficient limitation of income and resources.

In determining financial need, the Social Security office will take into consideration the income and assets of your spouse, if you are married. Not all income and resources are included in determining eligibility, however; a portion of your monthly income, the value of food stamps, and most home energy assistance funds are not counted as income. Your personal home as well as burial plots (and money saved for burial costs) also do not count as resources. Automobiles and life insurance policies are generally not counted unless their value exceeds the limits set forth by SSI regulations.

If you think you will need SSI, you should apply at any Social Security office as soon as you become disabled. Before going to the office, be sure to call the national toll-free number for the agency. Social Security staff will answer many of your questions, tell you what records and documents to have ready, and direct you to the nearest Social Security office. You can speed up the application process by having all requested documents in hand when you make application. The office will send your completed application to the Disability Determination Services (DDS) in your state. The DDS will review your medical history and available records. Occasionally, a further medical consultation is requested. Decisions regarding your claim will be sent to your home. If you are denied benefits, information on the appeal process will also be sent.

Benefits will begin immediately after your application has been approved. The length of time required to qualify varies considerably, depending on the nature of your disability, your needs, and the accessibility and complexity of your medical and financial information. The benefit amount varies from state to state. Medicaid benefits may or may not begin immediately upon SSI approval. Medicaid eligibility also varies from state to state (your local Social Security office will be able to provide you with information about benefits in your state).

Vocational Rehabilitation Benefits

Vocational Rehabilitation (VR) agencies are present in every state because of the Rehabilitation Act of 1973. To be eligible for VR benefits, your disability *must directly interfere with your ability to work.* VR services can include counseling, job training, educational opportunities, rehabilitation and assistive technology, financial assistance, job placement, and on-the-job assistance. VR programs are run by state agencies and each state has different services and eligibility requirements.

If you are receiving Social Security benefits as a result of your disability, you may be automatically referred to VR. If you are not receiving SSDI or SSI, you may still qualify for VR in some states in which VR finances are available. The resources of each state differ markedly, because the funds available reflect contributions allocated to the program by the state legislatures. Please look under "For More Information" at the end of the chapter for the Job Accommodation Network (JAN), which provides a list of state vocational rehabilitation agencies.

Return to work programs. The *Ticket to Work and Work Incentives Act of 1999* substantially expanded opportunities for people receiving Social Security benefits to return to work on a trial basis. These work incentives and Ticket to Work programs allow trial work periods while the person continues to receive cash benefits and Medicare coverage. This act has removed some difficult obstacles for the many people who wish to try to return to work. With the new treatments for RA, this has been a very valuable change in Social Security rules. The rules differ between SSDI and SSI, so contact the Social Security office for details. (See end of chapter for contact information.)

HEALTH INSURANCE

Private Health Insurance

If you are working and your employer provides health insurance benefits, you may not have the option of selecting a specific form of insurance or a specific insurance carrier. (*Note:* If you are insured through a group plan at work and then lose your job or begin to consider another job, *do not* drop your health insurance. More information on this is given below.)

If you do have a choice when it comes to health insurance, we recommend that you examine carefully several types of policies and look into several insurance carriers before making a decision. Choosing wisely is important, especially because it is sometimes difficult to make changes in insurance coverage if your health deteriorates in any way. Fortunately, the Affordable Care Act of 2010 has made it easier for many people who have pre-existing medical conditions to purchase health insurance coverage. It is not possible to measure the act's impact this early in its history, but the hope is that many people in need of care will be able to see physicians and other health care providers more easily and at less cost.

Selecting the best form of health insurance involves choosing among many variables. This is a challenging process, since health insurance options have become very complex. Get a pencil and pad or computer and compare options, side-by-side. Asking the following key questions may help you choose wisely.

- Is there a deductible? (And can you afford to pay that deductible each year? Read more about high deductible plans below.)

- Are there large co-payments? (If so, do lower premiums offset that expense?)

- What percentage of expenses are you responsible for after the deductible has been met? (Would you prefer to pay higher premiums in exchange for paying a lower percentage of a covered expense?)

- Is there an annual "cap" on the amount you have to pay for *all* medical expenses, also called an "out-of-pocket maximum"? (For your protection, there should be.)

- Is there a prescription policy? (We recommend that you enroll in an insurance plan that pays most of the cost of prescription drugs, because arthritis medications can be extremely costly. The cost of biologics can easily exceed $20,000 per year at the time of this writing. Make sure that there is *not* a cap on prescription coverage by the insurance company; make sure that there *is* a cap on your prescription contribution; make sure that you do not choose a "generic only" drug plan.)

- If the plan is an HMO (health maintenance organization), PPO (preferred provider organization), or other restricted physician panel plan, is your choice of physicians too limited? Is there a rheumatologist and an orthopedic surgeon experienced in joint surgery on the *preferred provider* staff? (If the services of these specialists aren't provided, can you get the insurance carrier to agree to pay for the services of such specialists if needed?)

- Are you permitted to use only specific hospitals and specific physical therapy services? (If so, find out—by asking your present doctor, if necessary—whether the permitted service providers have a good reputation for treatment of RA.)

- Do the primary care doctors in the plan readily refer their patients for specialty consultation? (They ought to.)

- Does your policy cover physical therapy, occupational therapy, and the services of a podiatrist? (If not, you'll probably want to choose a different policy.)

- Will your policy cover *durable medical equipment* (DME) such as splints, braces, orthotics, walking aids? (If there is an additional premium for this coverage, you'll have to decide whether you would prefer to pay the cost of these aids out of pocket as necessary or whether it is better for you to pay the additional premium on a regular basis. Unfortunately, a DME option is not available in many plans today.)

- Is there a *pre-existing illness* clause that may limit payment for costs related to your RA? (As of 2014, most health insurance plans cannot refuse to cover you or charge you more just because you have a pre-existing condition. However, there are a few exceptions, so check to be sure your RA expenses are covered.)

With the rising costs of medical insurance, many employers have changed to high deductible health plans (HDHPs). These policies have lower premiums but have deductibles from $1,250 to over $5,000. Meeting these deductibles out-of-pocket can be very challenging. The U.S. government has made provisions for the creation of a tax-favored savings account called a health savings account (HSA). To qualify for an HSA, your annual deductible has to be over $1,250 for an individual or $2,500 for a family (as of 2014). You can contribute to this savings account, often pretax, from your payroll. You can use the money to pay for *covered* medical expenses until you have met your deductible. Any money that you do not use will roll over into the next year. (Do not confuse an HSA with a flexible spending account [FSA], which cannot roll over into the next year but also covers eligible medical expenses and is removed from payroll before taxation. See below.) For many people, high deductible plans are cost effective. However, meeting the high deductible with after-tax money takes away a lot of the cost advantage. For example, if you are in the 30 percent tax bracket, a $1,500 deductible would cost you over $2,140 in earned income! So, look into HSAs if you are considering these plans. In your planning, always assume that you will have to pay the whole deductible.

COBRA

It is critical that you examine your insurance options if your employment status is about to change. Be very careful: you may experience a time lapse before finding another insurance carrier to cover you. A federal law, COBRA (Consolidated Omnibus Budget Reconciliation Act) requires that, in most cases, employees be allowed to convert their group insurance into an individual policy that will be guaranteed at the group premium rate for a given time period. However, before you discontinue your coverage under your former employer's group plan—or allow your former employer to discontinue your coverage—be sure to review your new policy and be certain that it has gone into effect. You will have to pay the premium for this new insurance, of course.

While you are covered under COBRA, explore other options: can you obtain coverage under your spouse's policy, for example, or can you get group insurance through a new job or a professional society? What are the current options in the HealthCare.gov Health Insurance Marketplace? Take every possible precaution to prevent a lapse in coverage. Our experience tells us that insurance carriers are often most reluctant to provide comprehensive coverage to people with chronic medical problems. This is why we emphasize the importance of holding on to one health insurance policy until another one has gone into effect.

Government Health Insurance

Medicare. People may qualify for this federally funded health insurance program if they are over age 65 *or* if they have received Social Security Disability

Insurance for more than twenty-four months. Medicare insurance options have become very complex over the past decade.

There are two parts of traditional Medicare: Part A and Part B. Part A covers in-patient hospital care and is financed through FICA taxes. Part B covers a percentage of doctors' fees, x-rays, and diagnostic tests. This portion of Medicare is financed through monthly premiums paid by the individual.

Traditional Medicare insurance provides limited coverage. It does not pay for medications, for example. In addition, many physicians will not "accept assignment" (the amount that Medicare agrees a given service should cost) as full payment because this reimbursement is significantly less than the average fee charged by physicians. Medicare also requires the insured person to pay a significant deductible as well as an additional 20 percent of *approved* assignments. Consequently, it is wise to purchase a private supplemental health insurance policy which will help pay the costs that Medicare does not cover. Many of the private insurers also offer a Medicare Part D prescription policy that can be purchased with the Medicare supplement plan.

Over the past decade, the number of people who choose traditional Medicare with a supplemental insurance has decreased. Many private insurance plans offer a growing list of insurance plan options for Medicare patients, including HMOs, PPOs, and Medicare Advantage Plans. The important thing to understand is that when you sign up for these products, you are *no longer* under the rules of the traditional Medicare plan. Each plan has a *separate* set of rules, costs, and restrictions by which you must abide. There is no easy way to simplify the process of choice. Use the same key questions that we listed above under private insurance. Compare your options side-by-side, looking at your individual needs. See the end of the chapter for helpful resources.

Medicaid. This health insurance is jointly funded by the federal and state governments and is available to individuals with low income. Disabled persons with low income may also be eligible. In most states, most individuals who qualify for SSI will automatically qualify for Medicaid. Other eligibility qualifications vary extensively among states, and these qualification criteria are constantly changing in response to the constantly escalating costs of health care. Many private insurance companies offer insurance plan options for Medicaid patients. This situation varies considerably by community. Your doctor may be able to help you in making this decision.

Because the fees paid to physicians from traditional Medicaid are extremely low, many physicians in private practice are unable to accept this form of health insurance. Federally funded clinics, hospitals, and university centers, however, will usually accept Medicaid insurance, especially if you reside in their region.

VETERANS ADMINISTRATION BENEFITS

The Veterans Administration (VA) offers both health care and disability help to veterans who qualify. Although service-connected disabilities are covered by the VA, rheumatoid arthritis generally does not qualify as a service-connected disability, and so eligibility for treatment of RA would depend on other criteria, such as your income and ability to pay. The benefit specialist at the local VA center can assist you by outlining the options available to you. If you are a veteran, find out what benefits you are eligible to receive.

INCOME TAXES

Having RA can be quite expensive, especially with the advent of the biologic medications. For tax purposes, the question is whether your expenses in any one year are high enough to be tax deductible. Generally, medical and dental expenses are only deductible when they reach extremely high levels—currently, more than 10 percent of your adjusted gross income. If you spend a large amount of money for health care, however, you may be able to get some assistance in the form of a tax break. The tax code defines eligible itemized deductions for medical expenses as amounts paid for the "diagnosis, cure, mitigation, treatment, or prevention of disease, and for treatments affecting any part or function of the body." Qualifying expenses may include capital expenditures for special equipment or for home improvements if their main purpose is medical care: building ramps; widening doors; changing counter heights or fixtures; installing railings, handrails, or grab bars; modifying hardware; and so on. Generally a doctor's order will suffice to qualify for a deduction of reasonable costs. Other deductible expenses are car modifications, chiropractic and dental care, medications, eyeglasses, trained animals for assistance, hearing aids, home care, health insurance premiums, *qualified* long-term care contracts, stop-smoking programs, and *physician-directed* weight loss programs.

Tax laws change continually, so you (and your accountant) will need to keep abreast of them. Currently, you can refer to the following Internal Revenue

Service publications for information: 502 ("Medical and Dental Expenses"), 524 ("Credit for the Elderly or the Disabled"), and 907 ("Tax Information for Persons with Handicaps or Disabilities"). To order these publications, call 1-800-TAX-FORM or get them on line at www.irs.gov/forms-&-pubs.

If your health care expenses are high but not high enough to be deductible on your income taxes, there may be other options. Many employers offer a "cafeteria/flexible benefits" program or flexible spending account (FSA) (under section 125 of the Internal Revenue Code) which allows you to use *pretax* dollars to pay for eligible health costs. In this way, you do not pay income taxes on income that you spend on health care. Find out whether such a program is available where you or your spouse works. If not, you may be able to promote some interest in the program in the personnel or human resources department.

Whatever your insurance or tax situation, save all of your receipts for any expenses that relate to your RA, including home modifications or special expenses that are a result of your arthritic condition.

FINANCIAL HELP FOR RA TREATMENT

Treatment for RA can be very costly. Many of the makers of RA medications offer financial assistance programs. Some of these resources and company-sponsored programs are listed at the end of Chapter 14. Most high-cost RA drug makers offer co-pay assistance for RA patients who do not have Medicare. Unfortunately, because of Medicare rules, pharmaceutical companies cannot *directly* offer any financial assistance to Medicare patients. Many companies have sponsored independent foundations, which can bypass federal rulings because the foundations are not owned or controlled by the pharmaceutical company. However, due to the great demand for help, funds are limited. Listed at the end of Chapter 14 are several other resources to consider if you are having difficulty covering the cost of your medications.

FOR MORE INFORMATION

The Job Accommodation Network (JAN) is a service provided by the U.S. Department of Labor's Office of Disability Employment Policy (ODEP). JAN is the leading source of free guidance on accommodating people with disabilities in the workplace. A list of state Vocational Rehabilitation agencies can be found at www.askjan.org/cgi-win/typequery.exe?902. Telephone 1-800-526-7234 or 1-877-781-9403 (TTY), or visit the Web site www.askjan.org.

For numerous publications and other information about Social Security benefits, contact your local Social Security office or write or call the national office: Social Security Administration, Office of Public Inquiries, 6401 Security Blvd., Baltimore, Md. 21235-6401; toll-free 1-800-772-1213, TTY 1-800-325-0778; Web site www.socialsecurity.gov.

Call the above number for the following Social Security publications: "Disability Benefits," "Your Ticket to Work," "Working While Disabled: How We Can Help," and "A Summary Guide to Employment Support for Individuals with Disabilities under the Social Security Disability Insurance and Supplemental Security Income Programs."

To contact the Social Security "Work Site" for specific information and help regarding work, disability, work incentive programs, and vocational rehabilitation, call toll-free 1-866-968-7842, TTY 1-866-833-2967, or check the following Web sites: www.socialsecurity.gov/disability; www.socialsecurity.gov/work; www.choosework.net.

Contact your local chapter or the national office of the Arthritis Foundation for copies of the free pamphlet "Arthritis and the Workplace."

HealthCare.gov is the official Web site of the Health Insurance Marketplace. This is a federal government site that helps you find, compare, and buy health insurance. Visit www.HealthCare.gov or call 1-800-318-2596 or 1-855-889-4325 (TTY).

About income taxes, IRS forms, and publications, write to: Internal Revenue Service, Technical Publications Branch, W:CAR:MP:FP:P, 1111 Constitution Ave., N.W., Washington, D.C. 20224; or call 1-800-TAX-FORM (1-800-829-3676). The Web site is www.irs.gov.

The Medicare Rights Center is a national, nonprofit consumer service organization that helps people with Medicare understand their rights and benefits. National Helpline: 1-800-333-4114. For general information: www.medicarerights.org. For Medicare benefit questions: www.medicareinteractive.org.

Other Issues

SURFING THE NET: EMPOWERMENT OR DECEPTION?

We have arrived conclusively in the information era. The Internet has allowed us to get up-to-date information. It has given both patients and physicians access to resources that were not available in preceding decades. Universities, professional associations, legitimate advocacy groups, national public service programs, and not-for-profit organizations like the Arthritis Foundation provide valuable information on-line to people with RA. The abundance of resources is very exciting and has been long awaited by people looking for cutting-edge information. At the same time, the Internet is available to profiteers, pseudo-experts, and unqualified practitioners who prey on the pain and suffering of others. Many promoters pose as legitimate organizations or foundations in an effort to deceive people, making false promises in exchange for their victims' hard-earned money. You should avoid these sites and fight the understandable urge to try their products.

The Internet sites we list in this book present balanced information. Some of these sites are sponsored by the pharmaceutical industry; they promote products, but they also give great insight into RA. They are certainly worth investigating. However, keep in mind that they may reveal a bias toward the medication being marketed. We would also like to give you a few guidelines for choosing Internet sites as you surf the Web.

Consider sites that:

- represent organizations known to be legitimate, such as the Arthritis Foundation (remember that most legitimate "institutes," "foundations," and "associations" do *not* promote products)
- are associated with universities or medical centers
- are federally sponsored, such as those from the NIH, USDA, or FDA
- are recommended by legitimate authorities

Avoid sites that:

- are selling a specific therapy
- use "official" sounding but unfamiliar names (check out "Questionable Organizations: An Overview" at www.quackwatch.com
- do not list references for their "science" or "research"
- do not give an address (Post Office boxes do not count)
- do not give a telephone number to call if you want to ask questions
- accuse the medical profession and pharmaceutical companies of conspiracy

CLINICAL RESEARCH

What Is Clinical Research?

Exciting and promising new medications for the treatment of RA are around the corner. In the United States, all new therapies must go through stringent testing and receive approval from the Food and Drug Administration (FDA) before they are made available to the public. Testing ensures that new treatments are both safe and effective. Clinical trials of new treatments are conducted by physicians in medical offices, hospitals, teaching universities, and research centers under the direction of a pharmaceutical company and the FDA.

How Do Clinical Studies Operate?

Clinical trials are generally conducted in three phases:

Phase I
The first step in a clinical trial program for a new product candidate is a Phase I clinical trial. Phase I trials are designed to screen a substance for safety and to find the maximum safe dose.

Phase II
Phase II studies are undertaken to establish dosing and duration of treatment. Therapeutic effectiveness and safety are also evaluated.

Phase III

The final phase in a clinical study is designed to confirm effectiveness in larger patient populations and to continue monitoring for rare but significant side effects. Phase III trials are conducted in large groups of patients and generally compare the new product to another treatment.

Should I Participate in a Clinical Trial?

Participation in a clinical trial is completely voluntary. Before joining a study, a volunteer will receive an *informed consent* form, which should provide detailed information about the treatment, the potential side effects, the kind and number of visits that will be required, and any procedures that may be done. The physician and staff conducting the study should review with you any questions you have. They will also discuss treatment options that are *not* part of the research study, so you can understand the range of options available to you. Study participants have the right to *withdraw their consent at any time* during the study. The decision to participate in a clinical study is a very personal one. Volunteers are needed to bring these exciting new therapies to the public, and many people enjoy contributing to the research effort and having the opportunity to be the first to try a new therapy. In addition, these studies also may give you access to very expensive medications like the biologics without any out-of-pocket expenses. On the other hand, many people prefer to wait until a therapy is fully tested. As always, your physician will help guide you in these decisions. Never let anyone pressure you into joining a study that you are not comfortable with.

TRAVEL TIPS

Sometimes people with RA give up vacation trips and other activities involving travel because they are afraid that they'll encounter insurmountable obstacles or barriers when they're away from home. Traveling is a wonderful pastime, though, and one you need not deny yourself. With careful planning, people with RA can travel almost wherever they choose.

Medical Tips for Travelers

Always discuss your vacation plans with your doctor. Ask him or her to recommend physicians where you are going who will consult with you and treat any unexpected problems that arise.

Take along one or two weeks' worth of medication *beyond* what you expect to need, as well as extra clearly written prescriptions from your doctor, in case your trip is prolonged unexpectedly.

Keep your medication separate from your luggage; that way, if your luggage is misplaced or stolen, you will still have your medication. It's best to keep your medication with you.

Carry a description of your medical problems and a list of your medications on your person. This information will be very useful if, in an emergency, you are unable to speak. Wearing a Medic Alert bracelet or necklace designating your medication allergies and other important medical information is a good idea. (For more information about acquiring a bracelet write: Medic Alert Foundation, 2323 Colorado Ave., Turlock, Calif. 95382; or call 1-888-633-4298 or visit www.medicalert.org.)

If you have syringes or needles, carry a note from your physician explaining why you need them. A physician's note for needles or syringes may be required for security reasons during flights and may be required on other forms of transportation or when you are driving across national boundaries. Best to be prepared. The author provides her patients with a note asking that biologics not go through the x-ray equipment. Tests on the safety and potency of biologics exposed to these x-rays have not been performed to date. Let airline agents and screening personnel know *in advance* about any artificial joints or metal shoe inserts that may trigger detectors.

If you are planning to travel out of the country, find out what your health insurance will cover in terms of medical care in other countries. Additional, temporary coverage is sometimes available. Always purchase trip insurance for large, expensive trips, in case you have a serious flare-up and are unable to travel as scheduled.

Driving Tips

Stop the car frequently, and get out and stretch. This will help you avoid stiffness and soreness.

Rental cars often have such features as tiltable steering wheels, cruise control, and power steering. Rental cars with wide-angled rearview and sideview mirrors (helpful if you have arthritis in your neck), adjustable headrests, and auto aids such as padded steering wheels and right- and left-hand controls are also sometimes available. A call to the car rental company in advance could facilitate access to these features.

In cold weather, have someone else warm up the car before you get into it.

Lever aids that can be put on door and ignition keys help those who find it difficult to turn a key because of arthritis in the fingers.

Grab handles can be attached to the ridge of the roof to help you get in and out of the car.

Keep medications in the glove compartment rather than in the trunk, so they will be more protected from extreme changes in temperature.

Pack snacks and a beverage so you can take your medications on schedule. Set your cell phone alarm or carry a small folding travel alarm clock to remind you to take your medication. When you are away from your normal routine and distracted by new things, it can be easy to forget a dose.

Neck, back, and seat cushions in various styles and materials are available to support painful areas. Special seat-belt cushioning can be added to decrease shoulder discomfort.

When Traveling by Air

Notify the airline in advance of any special needs you have. Airline personnel can help you with your luggage and assist you in boarding and getting off the airplane. Airlines can often accommodate special diets.

Try to travel during light air traffic hours and the least busy weeks of the year. It's best to avoid crowds.

Never be embarrassed to ask for assistance. Do not hesitate to use the "pre-board" option.

If possible, find a flight that will deliver you to your destination without stopping in another city on the way, *especially if the flight involves changing planes*. If it isn't possible to book a nonstop flight, allow for adequate time between flights. Arrangements can be made to have a wheelchair or cart transport you and your luggage to the next departure area.

Request a bulkhead seat (the first row of seats in a section) or an exit-row seat for more room. During flight, do simple range-of-motion exercises, particularly with your hips, knees, and feet, and when you are getting close to your destination.

Carry as little luggage as possible onto the airplane. Heavy luggage should be sent through normal airline luggage processes. Consider buying rolling carry-on hand bags, with long extendable handles, to minimize the stress on your hands and wrists.

If you are wheelchairbound, use the restroom before boarding the plane. Restrooms on board are often not easily accessible for someone in a wheelchair.

When planning a hotel or motel stop, call in advance to find out whether their facilities will meet your needs. If the facilities will make it difficult for you to maneuver or if they will force you to exert energy that you would rather save to use elsewhere, then you'll probably want to find someplace else to stay. Ask these questions:

- How close is the parking lot to my room?
- Where are the elevators in relationship to my room?
- Is it possible to book a room that has a bathroom with tub and toilet grab bars?
- (If you are in a wheelchair) Are there ramps, and are the doors to the room and bathroom wide enough to accommodate a wheelchair?

PREGNANCY AND CHILDBIRTH

Deciding whether or not to have children is a momentous decision for anyone. It is natural to have concerns about the health of a potential child, and most people think about this before or during pregnancy. Women of childbearing age who have RA will have specific questions about how their illness might affect their body and their unborn child.

Can I Become Pregnant?

Fertility is generally not affected by RA. During severe flare-ups, however, fertility may be temporarily lower in some individuals. But you should not count on this as a method of birth control, since it is not a failproof method.

How Will Pregnancy Affect My RA?

More than 75 percent of women see improvement in their RA during pregnancy. After delivery, most of them find that their arthritis returns to its pre-pregnancy level.

How Will My RA Affect My Unborn Child?

The health of the fetus and newborn infant does not appear to be affected adversely by RA, although this question has not been studied adequately for us to state unequivocally that this is so.

We do know that certain arthritis medications can compromise your baby's health. If you are considering getting pregnant or if you are sexually active and are not using birth control, you *must* discuss your medications with your primary care physician and obstetrician. *This is important for men as well as women.* There are several arthritis medications that need to be discontinued months or weeks before conception takes place or the child might be affected. Chapters 12 and 13 provide general recommendations about drugs, pregnancy, and breastfeeding, but your own doctor can best advise you on this subject.

Can I Breastfeed My Infant?

In most circumstances, breastfeeding is an option, although there is some evidence that breastfeeding can increase the risk of postpartum flare in RA (Barrett, 2000). If a flare-up occurs, medications may be necessary to calm it. Medications, routine or for a flare-up, can be excreted in the breast milk, and breastfeeding is not recommended for women taking some RA medications. Please discuss breastfeeding with your doctor.

Will My Child Have RA?

After reading the discussion earlier in this book about the role of genes in the development of RA, you may be wondering whether this is a condition that will be passed on to your children. Remember, though, that genes tell only part of the story. We do not know exactly what triggers the development of RA. It is true that a person who has a close family member with RA or another autoimmune condition has a higher likelihood of developing RA than the general population. We do not feel that the small increased risk of passing on RA should influence a person's decision about childbearing. The vast majority of children born to a parent with RA do not develop the condition. You also have read in Chapter 1 about **epigenetics**—how environmental factors can trigger genetic changes that increase the risk of developing RA. Teaching your child healthy lifestyles by example will likely further reduce the risk that he or she will develop RA in the future.

Will I Be Able to Care for My Baby?

This is perhaps the most difficult question. Caring for a baby requires a great deal of energy and stamina on the part of the caregiver. Performing frequent diaper changes and carrying around an extra 10 to 20 pounds can put a serious strain on tender joints. Feedings at two o'clock in the morning tire out even the healthiest parents. And, as we have discussed, joint stress, fatigue, and exhaustion can make arthritis and its symptoms worse.

You and your partner need to discuss these issues honestly with each other. You both need to be committed to creating and carrying out a plan that will allow the person with RA to get adequate rest. Putting aside extra funds for child care assistance is an excellent idea. Using disposable diapers will help, so that you don't have to manipulate diaper pins and wring out soiled diapers. You may want to invest in a carrier for holding the infant and get advice from an **occupational therapist** about how you can carry the baby while putting the least amount of stress on your joints. Plan ahead, and make certain that your plans include the toddler years.

IMMUNIZATION FOR THE PERSON WITH RA

Should I Get a Yearly Flu Shot?

Many physicians recommend yearly influenza, or "flu," vaccinations for people with RA. This is because RA is a chronic illness and because many people with RA take medications (**immunosuppressants, biologics,** and **corticosteroids**) that can impair the body's ability to ward off an infection like the flu. The flu vaccination is generally safe and effective.

Are There Other Vaccinations That I May Need to Get?

It is recommended that people with RA receive a vaccination against a form of pneumonia called *pneumococcal pneumonia*. This vaccination is called Pneumovax. You may want to discuss this vaccine with your doctor. If you do receive it, keep a written record of it in a safe place, so you can remember when and where you received it should you be asked about it in the future.

All other vaccines should be reviewed with your rheumatologist. "Live" vaccines should not be given with some medications (see Chapters 13 and 14). It is often worthwhile to get vaccinations updated *before* starting medications that can affect your immune system. This is not always possible, though.

FOR MORE INFORMATION

A nonprofit corporation that combats health care fraud has a Web site: www .quackwatch.com.

The Food and Drug Administration has a Web site that provides information on how to spot health fraud: www.fda.gov/forconsumers/protectyourself/health fraud/default.htm.

The Society for Accessible Travel and Hospitality (SATH) is a nonprofit organization dedicated to raising awareness of and removing obstacles for travelers with disabilities. Resources, travel trips, and access information can be found at www.sath.org.

Reliable information on resources for the disabled traveler, including airlines, trains, buses, cruise lines, driving, and travel agents can be found at www.moss resourcenet.org.

Closing Thoughts

In closing, here are ten thoughts and principles that deserve special emphasis. For each person, life is a series of choices. I hope that the choices recommended in this book will nurture you and lead you to greater strength and a better place as you live with RA.

Choose hopefulness. Physicians and scientists have never been in a better position to understand RA and learn new ways of controlling this condition. The current discoveries and future possibilities are incredibly promising.

Choose knowledge. Learn as much as you can about RA. Find trusted advocates like the Arthritis Foundation and become an expert on your condition. This will empower you. This is the first step to self-efficacy—the ability to take control of your condition, both physically and mentally. Self-direction regarding your RA will flow into other aspects of your life in a positive way.

Choose healthy habits. Get a good night's sleep. Limit alcohol. Do not smoke and avoid others who do. Give your body the fresh, clean air it deserves. Balance your activities. There is considerable evidence that a healthy lifestyle reduces the symptoms of RA.

Choose fitness and good nutrition. Nutrition has been discussed in detail in this book. Make informed food choices. You have only one body. Listen to it. Respect it. Treat it as you would any prized possession.

Choose spirit. Feed your spirit as you would your body. Tap into your inner resources. Be open to self-discovery. Live in the present moment. Keep your heart open. Explore disciplines that help you open your spiritual self, such as mindfulness, yoga, tai chi, and religion, all practices that have stood the test of time.

Choose positivity. We have limited reserves of physical and emotional energy. Give yours to appreciation, understanding, compassion, and love. This will give you more energy. Use your energy to learn new things or to exercise or to plan a lovely meal. Don't waste an ounce on disappointment, resentment, guilt, or anger. These will empty the well and keep it dry. (Seek professional help if you are having trouble coping with anxiety or depression.)

Choose beauty. Surround yourself with things of beauty. Listen to great music. Take a walk in nature. Listen to the rain. Put on your favorite fragrance.

Choose joy. Resolve to bring joy and fun to your life. Like all things, even this takes a choice. Make this one, because you deserve it.

Choose communication. Choose to understand and to be understood. Make your needs known. Make sure you know what your loved ones need from you. You may be surprised to learn that the reality is different from what you expected and, possibly, easier to fulfill. Studies show that people with supportive relationships experience less pain.

Choose to simplify. We waste valuable resources on the unnecessary. Simplicity takes some discipline, because many things are competing for our time and attention. It is worth the energy to thoughtfully decide what is important and clear up the clutter in one's life. Only then can you make clear choices about your next step.

Glossary

abduction: Movement of a part of the body away from the midline of the body.

ACPA (anti-citrullinated protein antibodies): Autoantibodies that are detected in the blood of RA patients. (Also see **anti-CCP.**)

adduction: Movement of a part of the body toward the midline of the body.

anemia: Low red blood cell count, which can sometimes result in fatigue and a sense of weakness.

antibodies: Proteins that are formed by the body as a defense against foreign substances (antigens), such as bacteria or viruses; also called immunoglobulins.

anti-CCP (anti-cyclic citrullinated peptide antibodies): Autoantibodies that are detected in the blood of RA patients. (Also see **ACPA.**)

antigen: Substance or material that is detected by the body as foreign.

antioxidant: A vitamin, mineral, or other organic substance that helps prevent damaging effects of substances called free radicals that can cause harm in the body.

arthrocentesis: Procedure to remove joint fluid with a needle; also called joint aspiration.

arthroscope: Instrument used to view the inside of a joint by inserting a small scope through the skin.

articulation: Another name for a joint.

atrophy: Decrease in size.

autoantibodies: Antibodies that, although created by the body, cause the body to react against itself.

autoimmunity: When the body inappropriately makes antibodies or has immune reactions against its own tissues.

biofeedback: Technique by which a person uses his or her own physiologic responses to achieve some control over bodily responses not normally considered consciously controllable.

biologics or biologic response modifier (BRM): Type of medication that is directed at very specific parts of the immune system; made from biogenetically engineered proteins, these medication are given by intravenous or subcutaneous administration.

biomarker: A laboratory test that can be objectively measured and reflects some biologic indicator, such as the risk of getting a condition, the prognosis of the condition, or whether the condition will respond to a specific treatment.

biosimilars: Drugs in the biologics family that are similar although not identical to branded biologic medications.

bone density test: Noninvasive diagnostic test that determines mineral density of the bone and can diagnose osteoporosis.

bursa: Slippery sac that lies between tendons, muscles, and bones, promoting easy movement without friction.

bursitis: Inflammation of the bursa.

capsule: Fibrous sac surrounding the cavity of a joint.

cartilage: Tissue that covers the bone on each side of a joint.

cell: Smallest living component of an organism.

chondrocytes: Cartilage cell.

chronic: Lasting months or years; used to describe condition or illness.

collagen: Structural protein important in the framework of cartilage and bone.

collagenase: Enzyme that breaks down collagen and thus cartilage and bone.

combination therapy: Use of two or more DMARDs at the same time.

complete blood count (CBC): Count of the different kinds of cells (such as red blood cells, white blood cells, and platelets) in a blood sample of a designated size.

connective tissue disease: Condition involving inflammation of the connective tissue (such as joints, skin, muscle). These disorders usually involve autoimmunity. RA is a connective tissue disease.

corticosteroid: Strong anti-inflammatory medication; also called steroid or cortisone.

COX-2 (cyclo-oxygenase-2) inhibitors: New class of NSAID that causes less stomach side effects.

CRP (C reactive protein): A protein found in blood, the levels of which rise in response to inflammation present somewhere in the body.

cytokine: Chemical messenger produced by cells to govern the activity of other cells.

dermatologist: Physician who specializes in care of and treatment of disorders of the skin.

dietitian: Trained specialist who provides information about proper nutrition, special diets, and weight-loss programs.

differential diagnosis: List of potential conditions when a patient presents with a given set of symptoms that can be present in more than one disease.

DMARD (disease-modifying antirheumatic drug): Medication used in the attempt to induce a remission of rheumatoid arthritis.

effusion: Excessive accumulation of fluid.

enzyme: Protein that can cause changes in other substances within the body.

epigenetics: The study of how individual genes can be activated or suppressed by environmental factors.

episcleritis: Inflammation of the outer covering of the eye.

erosion: Deterioration, such as a small hole in cartilage and bone caused by inflammation of the joint lining (synovitis).

erythrocyte: Red blood cell.

ESR (erythrocyte sedimentation rate or "sed rate"): Blood test that reveals the presence of inflammation in the body.

extension: Straightening out of a joint.

extra-articular: Symptom occurring outside the joint.

Felty's syndrome: Complication of rheumatoid arthritis consisting of an enlarged spleen and a low white blood cell count.

flexion: Bending of a joint.

gastritis: Inflammation of the stomach lining.

gelling: Feeling of stiffness upon arising in the morning or after remaining in the same position for a long time.

gluten: The major protein in wheat and some other whole grains.

hematocrit and **hemoglobin:** Measurements of red blood cells.

hyaluronic acid: The major lubricating substance in synovial (joint) fluid.

hypertrophy: Increase in size.

imagery, visualization: Use of images or the imagining of images, such as to promote relaxation or healing.

immune system, immunity: The body's system for defense against foreign substances or what the body perceives as foreign substances.

immunosuppressant: A medication that suppresses the immune system and may thereby reduce symptoms of arthritis.

inflammation: Complex bodily reaction characterized by heat, swelling, redness, and pain.

inflammatory arthritis: Arthritis caused by inflammation in the joints.

interleukin-1 (IL-1): Cytokine known to cause inflammation and damage.

interleukin-6 (IL-6): Cytokine known to cause inflammation and damage.

intravenous: Administered by needle into a vein, usually in the arm.

joint effusion: Excessive fluid in the joint.

kinase inhibitor: New oral form of DMARD that has similar effectiveness to the biologics.

latex fixation: Test used to detect rheumatoid factor.

leukopenia: Low number of white blood cells.

leukotriene: Substance, produced by the body, that is an extremely potent producer of inflammation.

ligament: Cordlike structure that attaches bone to bone across joints, giving them stability.

lymphocyte: Type of white blood cell involved in inflammation and infection fighting.

macrophage: Type of white blood cell that can engulf and destroy foreign substances.

malaise: Vague feeling of illness.

meditation: Discipline in which one directs or focuses the mind.

monoclonal antibody therapy: Using "man-made" antibodies that are designed to bind to specific cytokines, receptors, cells, and other targets in an effort to treat disease.

neuropathy: Nerve problem leading to numbness or weakness.

neutrophil: White blood cell involved in inflammation and infection fighting; also called polymorphonuclear cell.

nodule: Small, painless lump, such as those that can occur over a bony prominence or a tendon.

NSAID (nonsteroidal anti-inflammatory drug): Medication that is used to decrease pain and inflammation.

nurse: Trained health care provider who is knowledgeable about patient care and medical science. There are several kinds of nurses and nurse assistants: registered nurses (RNs), licensed practical nurses (LPNs), nurse's aides, and nursing technicians.

nutritionist: See **dietitian.**

occupational therapist: Person who teaches people how to perform their daily tasks in a fashion that accommodates their physical limitations. The occupational therapist may introduce adaptive equipment that allows independent living or make recommendations for changes in the home and workplace to improve functioning there. An occupational therapist is usually the specialist who designs wrist or hand splints and who teaches relaxation techniques and tips for conserving energy.

ophthalmologist: Physician who is an eye specialist (differs from an optometrist, who measures vision, and an optician, who makes eyeglasses).

orthopedic surgeon: Physician who specializes in surgery of the bones and joints.

orthotics: Development and application of splints, braces, or other additional materials to improve function, decrease pain and inflammation, or prevent deformity.

orthotist: Person who fabricates specialized braces and corrective equipment used to improve the functioning of joints and muscles or reduce pain and inflammation.

osteoarthritis: Most common form of arthritis; also called degenerative joint disease.

osteoclasts: Cells that break down bone.

osteoporosis: Condition resulting from loss of bone density; it increases the risk of fracture.

osteotomy: Surgical procedure that involves removing a piece of bone to realign the joint and reduce deformity.

pannus: Inflamed synovial tissue when it moves along the cartilage and bone and breaks down joint tissue.

pedorthist: Practitioner skilled in the design, manufacture, fit, and modification of prescription footwear and related devices for problem feet.

pericardial effusion: Fluid around the heart.

pericarditis: Inflammation of the covering of the heart (pericardium).

periodontal disease: Infection of the gums and tissues that surround and support the teeth.

pharmacist: Person trained in the preparation of medications. The pharmacist can provide information about drug side effects and drug interactions.

physiatrist: Physician who is an expert in the field of exercise and rehabilitation. The physiatrist generally refers people with rheumatoid arthritis to a physical therapist or occupational therapist for a treatment program.

physical therapist: Person trained to assess a patient's physical abilities and organize an exercise program designed to meet that individual's needs. The physical therapist instructs people with arthritis in methods of joint protection as well as in exercise programs designed to maintain joint mobility and muscle strength or to strengthen muscles and improve fitness and endurance without damaging the joints. A physical therapist also helps people to rehabilitate after joint surgery and to develop strategies of pain control, including heat therapy, cold therapy, hydrotherapy (water therapy), ultrasound, and electrotherapy, and instructs people in the proper use of walking aids.

placebo: Mostly used in research studies, a prescribed treatment that has no innate medicinal value but which the patient believes to be a form of therapy. Often referred to as "sugar pills" but not made of sugar.

plasma cell: Type of white blood cell.

plastic surgeon: A surgical specialist who operates on the skin, underlying tendons, muscles, and other soft tissues.

platelet: Blood cells responsible for clotting.

pleural effusion: Fluid around the lungs.

pleurisy: Inflammation of the lining around the lungs, resulting in pain when inhaling.

pneumonitis: Inflammation of the lungs; also called interstitial lung disease.

podiatrist: Person who is trained solely in medical and surgical treatment of the feet. The podiatrist also makes recommendations about customized shoes and fabricates inserts or specialized orthotics to fit inside shoes to accommodate changes that have occurred in the feet.

progressive relaxation: Relaxation program that focuses on successive regions of the body in a stepwise fashion.

prostaglandin: Substance, produced by the body, that produces and modifies inflammation.

psychologist, psychiatrist: Mental health experts who can help people to cope with the challenges posed by having a chronic condition. A psychologist usually has either a master's or a doctorate degree, whereas a psychiatrist has the M.D. degree and can prescribe medications.

remission: Period of time during which there is no evidence of active disease.

rheumatoid factor: Special form of antibody which is found in 80 to 90 percent of people with rheumatoid arthritis.

rheumatoid nodule: See **nodule.**

rheumatologist: A physician who is board certified in internal medicine and who specializes in the treatment of arthritis and other rheumatic diseases. Most rheumatologists are internists who have had special training in arthritis.

rheumatology: Study of arthritis and related problems as well as the study of diseases of autoimmunity.

scleritis: Inflammation of the white part of the eye, called the sclera.

sepsis: Severe infection in which bacteria get into the bloodstream.

social worker: Person educated and trained to provide information about, and help people connect with, resources they need, such as support groups, counseling, and other local agencies and services. A social worker can also help in solving problems related to finances, insurance, disability, job retraining, home care, housing, and legal issues.

splint: Manufactured support used to stabilize and rest a given joint.

subchondral bone: Bone found directly beneath (*sub*) the cartilage (*chondral*) in a joint.

subcutaneous: The tissue just below the skin; a subcutaneous injection is administered with a needle directed just below the skin.

synovial cells: Cells in the joint lining which include synovial fibroblasts.

synovial fluid: Joint fluid.

synovial joint: Joint that is freely movable, has a synovial lining, and is affected in rheumatoid arthritis; also called a diarthrodial joint.

synovitis: Inflammation of the synovium.

synovium: Joint lining; also called synovial membrane or synovial lining.

systemic: Affecting more than one part of the body.

tendinitis: Inflammation of a tendon.

tendon: Structure that attaches muscle to bone; often surrounded by a tendon sheath.

tenosynovitis: Inflammation of the tendon and surrounding joint lining.

tissue: Body component, such as cartilage, muscle, and bone.

titer: A measurement that indicates the quantity of a substance present in blood.

tumor necrosis factor (TNF): Cytokine known to cause inflammation.

ultrasound, musculoskeletal: A special from of diagnostic imaging that uses sound waves to image the joints and surrounding structures.

vasculitis: Inflammation of the blood vessels.

white blood cell: Cell involved in the complex functions of defense against infection and inflammation.

Bibliography

Adler, C. J., et al. 2013. "Sequencing Ancient Calcified Dental Plaque Shows Changes in Oral Microbiota with Dietary Shifts of the Neolithic and Industrial Revolution." *Nature Genetics* 45: 450–55.

Amith, H. V., et al. 2007. "Effect of Oil Pulling on Plaque and Gingivitis." *Journal of Oral Health and Community Dentistry* 1 (1): 12–18.

Barrett, J. 2000. "Breast-feeding and Postpartum Relapse in Women with Rheumatoid and Inflammatory Arthritis." *Arthritis and Rheumatism* 43 (May): 1010–15.

Barton-Wright, E. C., et al. 1963. "The Pantothenic Acid Metabolism of Rheumatoid Arthritis." *Lancet* 2: 862–63.

Bax, M., et al. 2011. "Genetics of Rheumatoid Arthritis: What Have We Learned?" *Immunogenetics* 63: 459–66.

Beauchamp, G. K., et al. 2005. "Phytochemistry: Ibuprofen-like Activity in Extra-virgin Olive Oil." *Nature* 437: 45–46.

Benito-Garcia, E., et al. 2007. "Protein, Iron, and Meat Consumption and the Risk for Rheumatoid Arthritis: A Prospective Cohort Study." *Arthritis Research and Therapy* 9: R16.

Brien, S., et al. 2011. "Homeopathy Has Clinical Benefits in Rheumatoid Arthritis Patients that Are Attributable to the Consultation Process but Not the Homeopathic Remedy: A Randomized Controlled Clinical Trial." *Rheumatology* 50 (6): 1070–82.

Burnett, P. 2012. "Gut Bacteria and Brain Function: The Challenges of a Growing Field." *Proceedings of the National Academy of Science* 109 (4): E175.

Canter, P. H., et al. 2007. "The Antioxidant Vitamins A, C, E, and Selenium in the Treatment of Arthritis: A Systemic Review of Randomized Clinical Trials." *Rheumatology* 46: 1223–33.

Chandran, B., and A. Goel. 2012. "A Randomized, Pilot Study to Assess the Efficacy and Safety of Curcumin in Patients with Active Rheumatoid Arthritis." *Phytotherapy Research* 26 (11): 1719–25.

Cheeke, P. R., et al. 2006. "Anti-inflammatory and Anti-arthritic effects of *Yucca schidigera*: A Review." *Journal of Inflammation (London)* 3 (6).

Cohen, A., et al. 1964. "Bromelain Therapy in Rheumatoid Arthritis." *Pennsylvania Medical Journal* 67: 27–30.

Colebatch, A. N., and C. J. Edwards. 2010. "The Influence of Early Life Factors on the Risk of Developing Rheumatoid Arthritis." *Clinical and Experimental Immunology* 163: 11–16.

Comstock, G. W., et al. 1997. "Serum Concentrations of Alpha-toco-pherol, Beta-carotene, and Retinol Preceding the Diagnosis of Rheumatoid Arthritis and Systemic Lupus Erythematosus." *Annals of the Rheumatic Diseases* 56 (May): 323–25.

Cooney, J. K., et al. 2011. "Review Article: Benefits of Exercise in Rheumatoid Arthritis." *Journal of Aging Research* 2011: 681640.

Cordain, L. 2000. "Review Article: Modulation of Immune Function by Dietary Lectins in Rheumatoid Arthritis." *British Journal of Nutrition* 83: 207–17.

Cordain, L. 2002a. "The Nutritional Characteristics of a Contemporary Diet Based Upon Paleolithic Food Groups." *Journal of the American Nutraceutical Association* 5 (5): 15–24.

Cordain, L. 2002b. *The Paleo Diet: Lose Weight and Get Healthy by Eating the Food You Were Designed to Eat.* New York: Wiley.

Costenbader, K. H., et al. 2006. "Smoking Intensity, Duration, and Cessation, and the Risk of Rheumatoid Arthritis in Women." *American Journal of Medicine* 119: 503–9.

Costenbader, K. H., et al. 2010. "Antioxidant Intake and Risks of Rheumatoid Arthritis and Systemic Lupus Erythematosus in Women."*American Journal of Epidemiology* 172 (2): 205–16.

Crowson, S., et al. 2013. "Contribution of Obesity to the Rise in Incidence of Rheumatoid Arthritis." *Arthritis Care and Research* 65 (January): 71–77.

Cutolo, M. 2000. "Sex Hormone Adjuvant Therapy in Rheumatoid Arthritis." *Rheumatic Disease Clinics of North America* 26 (November): 881–95.

Darlington, L. G. 2001. "Antioxidants and Fatty Acids in the Amelioration of Rheumatoid Arthritis and Related Disorders." *British Journal of Nutrition* 85 (March): 251–69.

Deluca, H. F., and M. L. Cantoma. 2001. "Vitamin D: Its Role and Uses in Immunology." *FASEB Journal* 15 (December): 2579–85.

DiGiuseppe, D., et al. 2013. "Long-term Intake of Dietary Long-chain n-3 Polyunsaturated Fatty Acids and Risk of Rheumatoid Arthritis: A Prospective Cohort of Women." *Annals of Rheumatic Disease.* 2013-203338.

DiSilvestro, R. A., et al. 1992. "Effects of Copper Supplementation on Ceruloplasmin and Copper-Zinc Superoxide Dismutase in Free-living Rheumatoid Arthritis Patients." *Journal of the American College of Nutrition* 11 (April): 177–80.

Eaton, S., et al. 1985. "Paleolithic Nutrition—A Consideration of Its Nature and Current Implications." *New England Journal of Medicine* 312 (5): 283–89.

Enliven Panel. 2000. "RA and Intimacy" (pamphlet).Wyeth-Ayerst Pharmaceuticals and Immunex Corporation.

Estruch, R., et al. 2013. "Primary Prevention of Cardiovascular Disease with a Mediterranean Diet." *New England Journal of Medicine* 368: 1279–90.

Etzel, R. 1996. "Special Extract of *Boswellia serrata* (H15) in the Treatment of Rheumatoid Arthritis." *Phytomedicine* 3: 91–94.

Evans, S., et al. 2013. "Impact of Iyengar Yoga on Quality of Life in Young Women with Rheumatoid Arthritis." *Clinical Journal of Pain* (January 30) (e-publication ahead of print, 7/30/2014).

Fairburn, K., et al. 1992. "Alpha-tocopherol, Lipids and Lipoproteins in Knee-joint Synovial Fluid and Serum from Patients with Inflammatory Joint Disease." *Clinical Science* 83: 657–64.

Fraser, D. A., et al. 2000. "Serum Levels of Interleukin-6 and Dehydroepiandosterone Sulphate in Response to Fasting or a Ketogenic Diet in Rheumatoid Arthritis." *Clinical and Experimental Rheumatology* 18 (May–June): 357–62.

Gatenby, P., et al. 2013. "Vitamin D Deficiency and Risk for Rheumatic Diseases." *Current Opinion in Rheumatology* 25 (2): 184–91.

General Practitioner Research Group. 1980. "Calcium Pantothenate in Arthritic Conditions." *Practitioner* 224 (1340): 208–11.

Grant, W. B. 2000. "The Role of Meat in the Expression of Rheumatoid Arthritis." *British Journal of Nutrition* 84 (November): 589–95.

Gray, R. G., and N. L. Gottlieb. 1985. "Adverse Reactions from Antirheumatic Drugs." *Rheumatoid Arthritis: Etiology, Diagnosis, Management.* Philadelphia: J. B. Lippincott.

Guimaraes, M. R., et al. 2011. "Potent Anti-inflammatory Effects of Systemically-administered Curcumin Modulates Periodontal Disease in Vivo." *Journal of Periodontal Research* 46 (2): 269–79.

Gul'neva, M., and S. M. Noskov. 2011. "Colonic Microbial Biocenosis in Rheumatoid Arthritis" [in Russian]. *Klinicheskaia Meditsina (Mosk)* 89 (4): 45–48.

Gutweniger, S., et al. 1999. "Body Image of Women with Rheumatoid Arthritis." *Clinical and Experimental Rheumatology* 17: 413–17.

Hafstrom, I., et al. 2001. "A Vegan Diet Free of Gluten Improves the Signs and Symptoms of Rheumatoid Arthritis: The Effects on Arthritis Correlate with a Reduction in Antibodies to Food Antigens." *Rheumatology* 40 (October): 1175–79.

Hanninen, O., et al. 2000. "Antioxidants in Vegan Diet and Rheumatic Disorders." *Toxicology* 155 (1–3): 45–53.

Hardin, J. G., and G. L. Longenecker. 1992. *Handbook of Drug Therapy in Rheumatic Disease: Pharmacology and Clinical Aspects.* Boston: Little, Brown.

Harris, E. D., Jr. 1990. "Rheumatoid Arthritis: Pathophysiology and Implications for Therapy." *New England Journal of Medicine* 322 (May 3): 1277–89.

Hatakka, K., et al. 2003. "Effects of Probiotic Therapy on the Activity and Activation of Mild Rheumatoid Arthritis—A Pilot Study." *Scandinavian Journal of Rheumatology* 32 (4): 211–15.

Heptinstall, P. M., et al. 1989. "Feverfew in Rheumatoid Arthritis: A Double-Blind, Placebo-Controlled Study." *Annals of Rheumatic Disease* 48 (7): 547–49.

Huang, S. C., et al. 2010. "Vitamin B6 Supplementation Improves Proinflammatory Responses in Patients with Rheumatoid Arthritis." *European Journal of Clinical Nutrition* 64: 1007–13.

Hvatum, M., et al. 2006. "The Gut-Joint Axis: Cross Reactive Food Antibodies in Rheumatoid Arthritis." *Gut* 55: 1240–47.

Irwin, M. R., et al. 2012. "Sleep Loss Exacerbates Fatigue, Depression, and Pain in Rheumatoid Arthritis." *Sleep* 35 (4): 537–43.

Kajanachumpol, S., et al. 2000. "Levels of Plasma Lipid Peroxide Products and Antioxidant Status in Rheumatoid Arthritis." *Southeast Asian Journal of Tropical Medicine and Public Health* 31 (June): 335–38.

Karlson, E. W., et al. 2008. "Vitamin E in the Primary Prevention of Rheumatoid Arthritis: The Women's Health Study." *Arthritis and Rheumatism* 59 (11): 1589–95.

Kim, M. J., et al. 2005. "The Effects of Aromatherapy on Pain, Depression, and Life Satisfaction of Arthritis Patients" [in Korean]. *Taehan Kanho Hakhoe Chi* 35 (1): 186–94.

Kinlen, L. J. 1985. "Incidence of Cancer in Rheumatoid Arthritis and Other Disorders after Immunosuppressive Treatment." *American Journal of Medicine* 78, suppl. 1A: 44–49.

Kjeldsen-Kragh, J. 1999. "Rheumatoid Arthritis Treated with Vegetarian Diets." *American Journal of Clinical Nutrition* 70 (September): 594s–660s.

Klareskog, L., et al. 2006. "A New Model for an Etiology of Rheumatoid Arthritis: Smoking May Trigger HLA-DR (Shared Epitope)-Restricted Immune Reactions to Autoantigens Modified by Citrullination." *Arthritis and Rheumatism* 54 (1): 38–46.

Knekt, P., et al. 2000. "Serum Selenium, Serum Alpha-tocopherol, and the Risk of Rheumatoid Arthritis." *Epidemiology* 11: 402–5.

Kostoglou-Athanassiou, I., et al. 2012. "Vitamin D and Rheumatoid Arthritis." *Therapeutic Advance in Endocrinology and Metabolism* 3 (6): 181–87.

Kremer, J. M. 2000. "N-3 Fatty Acid Supplements in Rheumatoid Arthritis." *American Journal of Clinical Nutrition* (January): 349s–351s.

Lahiri, M., et al. 2013. "Using Lifestyle Factors to Identify Individuals at Higher Risk of Inflammatory Polyarthritis." *Annals of the Rheumatic Diseases*, 2012-202481.

Lawrence, R. C., et al. 2008. "Estimates of the Prevalence of Arthritis and Other Rheumatic Conditions in the United States: Part II." *Arthritis and Rheumatism* 58 (January): 26–35.

Levinski, W. K., and J. Lansbury. 1951. "An Attempt to Transmit Rheumatoid Arthritis to Humans." *Proceedings of the Society of Experimental Biology and Medicine* 78 (1): 325–26.

Linos, A., et al. 1999. "Dietary Factors in Relation to Rheumatoid Arthritis: A Role for Olive Oil and Cooked Vegetables?" *American Journal of Clinical Nutrition* 70 (December): 1077–82.

Lucas, C. P., et al. 1981. "Dietary Fat Aggravates Active Rheumatoid Arthritis." *Clinical Research* 29: 754A.

MacGregor, A. J., et al. 2000. "Characterizing the Quantitative Genetic Contribution to Rheumatoid Arthritis Using the Data from Twins." *Arthritis and Rheumatism* 43: 30–37.

Maksymowych, W., and A. S. Russell. 1987. "Antimalarials in Rheumatology: Efficacy and Safety." *Seminars in Arthritis and Rheumatism* 18 (February): 206–21.

Mandel, D. R., et al. 2010. "*Bacillus Coagulans*: A Viable Adjunct Therapy for Relieving Symptoms of Rheumatoid Arthritis According to a Randomized, Controlled Study." *Complementary and Alternative Medicine* 10:1.

Ma'or, Z., et al. 2006. "Antimicrobial Properties of Dead Sea Black Mud." *International Journal of Dermatology* 45 (5): 504–11.

Matthews, D. A., et al. 2000. "Effects of Intercessory Prayer on Patients with Rheumatoid Arthritis." *Southern Medical Journal* 93: 1177–86.

McDonald, J. L., et al. 2013. "The Anti-Inflammatory Effects of Acupuncture and Their Relevance to Allergic Rhinitis: A Narrative Review and Proposed Model." *Evidence-Based Complementary and Alternative Medicine*. Accessed at http://dx.doi.org/10.1155/2013/591796.

McDougall, J., et al. 2002. "Effects of a Very Low-fat, Vegan Diet in Subjects with Rheumatoid Arthritis." *Journal of Alternative and Complementary Medicine* 8: 71–75.

McKellar, G., et al. 2007. "A Pilot Study of a Mediterranean-type Diet Intervention in Female Patients with Rheumatoid Arthritis Living in Areas of Social Deprivation in Glasgow." *Annals of Rheumatic Disease* 66: 1239–43.

McNeal, R. L. 1990. "Aquatic Therapy for Patients with Rheumatic Disease." *Rheumatic Disease Clinics of North America* 16 (November): 915–29.

Melzack, R., and P. Wall. 1983. *The Challenge of Pain.* New York: Basic Books.

Mikirova, N., et al. 2012. "Effect of High Dose Intravenous Ascorbic Acid on the Level of Inflammation in Patients with Rheumatoid Arthritis." *Modern Research in Inflammation* 1 (2): 1177–86.

Miles, E. A., and P. C. Calder. 2012. "Influence of Marine N-3 Polyunsaturated Fatty Acids on Immune Function and a Systemic Review of Their Effects on Clinical Outcomes in Rheumatoid Arthritis." *British Journal of Nutrition* 107: Suppl. 2: S171-84.

Minor, M. A., and N. E. Lane. 1996. "Recreational Exercise in Arthritis." *Rheumatic Disease Clinics of North America* 22 (August): 563–77.

Muller, H., et al. 2001. "Fasting Followed by Vegetarian Diet in Patients with Rheumatoid Arthritis." *Scandinavian Journal of Rheumatology* 30: 1–10.

Mur, E., et al. 2002. "Randomized Double-Blind Trial of an Extract from the Pentacyclic Alkaloid-Chemotype of *Uncaria tomentosa* for the Treatment of Rheumatoid Arthritis." *Journal of Rheumatology* 29: 678–81.

Myasoedova, E., et al. 2010. "Is the Incidence of Rheumatoid Arthritis Rising? Results from Olmsted County, Minnesota, 1955–2007." *Arthritis and Rheumatism* 62: 1576–82.

Nanjundaiah, S. M., et al. 2013. "Review Article: Mediators of Inflammation-Induced Bone Damage in Arthritis and Their Control by Herbal Products." *Evidence-Based Complementary and Alternative Medicine.* Accessed at http://dx.doi.org/10.1155/2013/518094.

Nielen, M. M., et al. 2004. "Specific Autoantibodies Precede the Symptoms of Rheumatoid Arthritis: A Study of Serial Measurements of Blood Donors." *Arthritis Rheumatism* 50: 380–86.

Nordstrom, D. C., et al. 1995. "Alpha-linolenic Acid in the Treatment of Rheumatoid Arthritis: A Double-blind, Placebo-controlled and Randomized Study: Flaxseed vs. Safflower Seed. *Rheumatology International* 14 (6): 231–34.

Ortiz, P., et al. 2009. "Periodontal Therapy Reduces the Severity of Active Rheumatoid Arthritis in Patients Treated with or without Tumor Necrosis Factor Inhibitors." *Journal of Periodontology* 80 (4): 535–40.

Pattison, D. J., et al. 2004a. "Dietary Risk Factors for the Development of Inflammatory Polyarthritis: Evidence for a Role of High Level of Red Meat Consumption." *Arthritis and Rheumatism* 50 (12): 3804–12.

Pattison, D. J., et al. 2004b. "Vitamin C and the Risk of Developing Inflammatory Polyarthritis: Prospective Nested Case-control Study." *Annals of Rheumatic Disease* 63: 843–47.

Pineda, M., et al. 2011. "A Randomized, Double-blinded, Placebo-controlled Pilot Study of Probiotics in Active Rheumatoid Arthritis." *Medical Science Monitor* 17 (6): CR 347–54.

Pischon, N., et al. 2008. "Association among Rheumatoid Arthritis, Oral Hygiene, and Periodontitis." *Journal of Periodontology* 79: 979–86.

Rastmanesh, R. 2008. "A Pilot Study of Potassium Supplementation in the Treatment of Hypokalemic Patients with Rheumatoid Arthritis: A Randomized, Double-Blinded, Placebo-Controlled Trial." *Journal of Pain* 9 (8): 722–31.

Rayman, M. P., and A. Callaghan, 2006. *Nutrition and Arthritis*. Oxford: Blackwell Publishing.

Rayman, M. P., and D. J. Pattison. 2008. "Dietary Manipulation in Musculoskeletal Conditions." *Best Practice and Research, Clinical Rheumatology* 22 (3): 535–61.

Rosenkranz, M. A., et al. 2012. "A Comparison of Mindfulness-based Stress Reduction and an Active Control in Modulation of Neurogenic Inflammation." *Brain, Behavior, and Immunology*. Accessed at http://dx.doi.org/10.1016/j .bbi.2012.10.013.

Roubenoff, R., et al. 1994. "Rheumatoid Cachexia: Cytokine-Driven Hypermetabolism Accompanying Reduced Body Cell Mass in Chronic Inflammation." *Journal of Clinical Investigation* 93: 2379–86.

Sander, O., et al. 1998. "Is H15 (Resin Extract of *Boswellia serrata*, 'Insense') a Useful Supplement to Established Drug Therapy of Chronic Polyarthritis? Results of a Double-blind study" [in German]. *Zeitschrift fur Rheumatologie* 57: 11–16.

Savioli, C., et al. 2012. "Persistent Periodontal Disease Hampers Anti-Tumor Necrosis Factor Treatment Response in Rheumatoid Arthritis." *Journal of Clinical Rheumatology* 18 (4): 180–84.

Scammell, H. 1998. *The New Arthritis Breakthrough*. New York: M. Evans.

Scarvell, J., and M. R. Elkins. 2011. "Aerobic Exercise Is Beneficial for People with Rheumatoid Arthritis." *British Journal of Sports Medicine* 45 (12): 1008–9.

Scher, J. U., et al. 2012. "Periodontal Disease and the Oral Microbiota in New-Onset Rheumatoid Arthritis." *Arthritis and Rheumatism* 64 (10): 3083–94.

Silman, A. J., et al. 1996. "Cigarette Smoking Increases the Risk of Rheumatoid Arthritis. Results from a Nationwide Study of Disease-discordant Twins." *Arthritis and Rheumatism* 39: 732–35.

Simopoulos, A. 2008. "The Importance of the Omega-6/Omega-3 Fatty Acid Ratio in Cardiovascular Disease and Other Chronic Diseases." *Experimental Biology and Medicine* 233: 674–88.

Sircar, S., and U. Kansra. 1998. "Choice of Cooking Oils—Myths and Realities." *Journal of the Indian Medical Association* 96 (10): 304.

Situnayake, R. D. 1991. "Chain Breaking Antioxidant Status in Rheumatoid Arthritis: Clinical and Laboratory Correlates." *Annals of Rheumatic Disease* 50 (2): 81–86.

Skoldstam, L., et al. 2003. "An Experimental Study of a Mediterranean Diet Intervention for Patients with Rheumatoid Arthritis." *Annals of Rheumatic Disease* 62: 208–14.

Spreadbury, I. 2012. "Comparison with Ancestral Diets Suggests Dense Acellular Carbohydrates Promote an Inflammatory Microbiota, and May Be the Primary Cause of Leptin Resistance and Obesity." *Diabetes, Metabolic Syndrome and Obesity Targets and Therapy* 5: 175–89.

Stafford, L., et al. 2000. "Androgen Deficiency and Bone Mineral Density in Men with Rheumatoid Arthritis." *Journal of Rheumatology* 27 (December): 2786–90.

Svartz, N. 1948. "The Treatment of Rheumatic Polyarthritis with Acid Azo Compounds." *Rheumatism* 4: 180–85.

Tarp, U. 1995. "Selenium in Rheumatoid Arthritis: A Review." *Analyst* 3: 877–81.

Tilley, B. C., et al. 1995. "Minocycline in Rheumatoid Arthritis: A 48-Week, Double-Blind, Placebo-Controlled Trial." *Annals of Internal Medicine* 122: 81–89.

Uhlig, T., et al. 2010. "Exploring Tai Chi in Rheumatoid Arthritis: A Quantitative and Qualitative Study." *BMC Musculoskeletal Disorders* 11: 43.

Van der Heijden, I. M., et al. 2000. "Presence of Bacterial DNA and Bacterial Peptidoglycans in Joints of Patients with Rheumatoid Arthritis and Other Arthritides." *Arthritis and Rheumatism* 43: 593–98.

Vieira, V. M., et al. 2010. "Association between Residences in U.S. Northern Latitudes and Rheumatoid Arthritis: A Spatial Analysis of the Nurses' Health Study." *Environmental Health Perspectives* 118 (7): 957–61.

Voegtlin, W. L. 1975. *The Stone Age Diet: Based on In-depth Studies of Human Ecology and the Diet of Man.* Vantage Press.

Vojinovic, J., et al. 1999. "Disease Modifying and Immunomodulatory Effects of High Dose 1 Alpha (OH) D3 in Rheumatoid Arthritis Patients." *Clinical and Experimental Rheumatology* 17 (4): 453–56.

Walker, W. R., and D. M. Keats. 1976. "An Investigation of the Therapeutic Value of the Copper Bracelet: Dermal Assimilation of Copper in Arthritic/Rheumatoid Conditions." *Agents Actions* 6: 454–59.

Wang, C., et al. 2008. "Acupuncture for Pain Relief in Patients with Rheumatoid Arthritis." *Arthritis Care and Research* 59 (9): 1249–56.

Willet, W. C., et al. 1995. "Mediterranean Diet Pyramid: A Cultural Model for Healthy Eating." *American Journal of Clinical Nutrition* 61 Suppl.: 1402s–1406s.

Wolfe, F. 2000. "The Effect of Smoking on Clinical, Laboratory, and Radiographic Status in Rheumatoid Arthritis." *Journal of Rheumatology* 27 (March): 630–37.

Wolfe, F., and M. F. Marmor. 2010. "Rates and Predictors of Hydroxychloroquine Retinal Toxicity in Patients with Rheumatoid Arthritis and Systemic Lupus Erythematosus." *Arthritis Care Research* 62 (6): 775–84.

Woolf, K. M. 2008. "Elevated Plasma Homocysteine and Low Vitamin B-6 Status in Nonsupplementing Older Women with RA." *Journal of the American Dietary Association* 108 (3): 443–53.

Yang, Q., et al. 2011. "Sodium and Potassium Intake and Mortality among US Adults: Prospective Data from the Third National Health and Nutrition Examination Survey." *Archives of Internal Medicine* 171 (13): 1183.

Yeoh, N., et al. 2013. "The Role of the Microbiome in Rheumatic Disease." *Current Rheumatology Reports* 15 (3): 314.

Zhernakova, A., et al. 2011. "Meta-analysis of Genome-wide Association Studies in Celiac Disease and Rheumatoid Arthritis." *Plos Genetics* 7 (2): e1002004.

Zurier, R. B., et al. 1996. "Gamma-Linolenic Acid Treatment of Rheumatoid Arthritis: A Randomized, Placebo-controlled Trial." *Arthritis and Rheumatism* 39 (November): 1808–17.

Index